Terpenes and Terpene Derivatives

Terpenes and Terpene Derivatives

Editors

Pavel B. Drasar
Vladimir A. Khripach

MDPI • Basel • Beijing • Wuhan • Barcelona • Belgrade • Manchester • Tokyo • Cluj • Tianjin

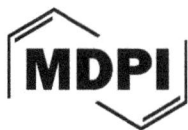

Editors
Pavel B. Drasar
University of Chemistry and
Technology
Czech Republic

Vladimir A. Khripach
The National Academy of
Sciences of Belarus
Belarus

Editorial Office
MDPI
St. Alban-Anlage 66
4052 Basel, Switzerland

This is a reprint of articles from the Special Issue published online in the open access journal *Molecules* (ISSN 1420-3049) (available at: https://www.mdpi.com/journal/molecules/special_issues/terpenes).

For citation purposes, cite each article independently as indicated on the article page online and as indicated below:

LastName, A.A.; LastName, B.B.; LastName, C.C. Article Title. *Journal Name* **Year**, *Volume Number*, Page Range.

ISBN 978-3-0365-2135-0 (Hbk)
ISBN 978-3-0365-2136-7 (PDF)

© 2021 by the authors. Articles in this book are Open Access and distributed under the Creative Commons Attribution (CC BY) license, which allows users to download, copy and build upon published articles, as long as the author and publisher are properly credited, which ensures maximum dissemination and a wider impact of our publications.

The book as a whole is distributed by MDPI under the terms and conditions of the Creative Commons license CC BY-NC-ND.

Contents

About the Editors vii

Preface to "Terpenes and Terpene Derivatives" ix

Pavel B. Drasar and Vladimir A. Khripach
Terpene Research Is Providing New Inspiration for Scientists
Reprinted from: *Molecules* **2021**, *26*, 5480, doi:10.3390/molecules26185480 1

Karolina A. Wojtunik-Kulesza
Approach to Optimization of FRAP Methodology for Studies Based on Selected Monoterpenes
Reprinted from: *Molecules* **2020**, *25*, 5267, doi:10.3390/molecules25225267 3

Julianderson Carmo, Polliane Cavalcante-Araújo, Juliane Silva, Jamylle Ferro,
Ana Carolina Correia, Vincent Lagente and Emiliano Barreto
Uvaol Improves the Functioning of Fibroblasts and Endothelial Cells and Accelerates the Healing of Cutaneous Wounds in Mice
Reprinted from: *Molecules* **2020**, *25*, 4982, doi:10.3390/molecules25214982 15

Gadah Abdulaziz Al-Hamoud, Raha Saud Orfali, Yoshio Takeda, Sachiko Sugimoto,
Yoshi Yamano, Nawal M. Al Musayeib, Omer Ibrahim Fantoukh, Musarat Amina,
Hideaki Otsuka and Katsuyoshi Matsunami
Lasianosides F–I: A New Iridoid and Three New Bis-Iridoid Glycosides from the Leaves of *Lasianthus verticillatus* (Lour.) Merr.
Reprinted from: *Molecules* **2020**, *25*, 2798, doi:10.3390/molecules25122798 31

Thuc-Huy Duong, Mehdi A. Beniddir, Nguyen T. Trung, Cam-Tu D. Phan, Van Giau Vo,
Van-Kieu Nguyen, Quynh-Loan Le, Hoang-Dung Nguyen and Pierre Le Pogam
Atypical Lindenane-Type Sesquiterpenes from *Lindera myrrha*
Reprinted from: *Molecules* **2020**, *25*, 1830, doi:10.3390/molecules25081830 43

Shagufta Perveen, Jawaher Alqahtani, Raha Orfali, Hanan Y. Aati, Areej M. Al-Taweel,
Taghreed A. Ibrahim, Afsar Khan, Hasan S. Yusufoglu, Maged S. Abdel-Kader and
Orazio Taglialatela-Scafati
Antibacterial and Antifungal Sesquiterpenoids from Aerial Parts of *Anvillea garcinii*
Reprinted from: *Molecules* **2020**, *25*, 1730, doi:10.3390/molecules25071730 53

Raktham Mektrirat, Terdsak Yano, Siriporn Okonogi, Wasan Katip and Surachai Pikulkaew
Phytochemical and Safety Evaluations of Volatile Terpenoids from *Zingiber cassumunar* Roxb. on Mature Carp Peripheral Blood Mononuclear Cells and Embryonic Zebrafish
Reprinted from: *Molecules* **2020**, *25*, 613, doi:10.3390/molecules25030613 63

Axelle Aimond, Kevin Calabro, Coralie Audoin, Elodie Olivier, Mélody Dutot,
Pauline Buron, Patrice Rat, Olivier Laprévote, Soizic Prado, Emmanuel Roulland,
Olivier P. Thomas and Grégory Genta-Jouvee
Cytotoxic and Anti-Inflammatory Effects of Ent-Kaurane Derivatives Isolated from the Alpine Plant *Sideritis hyssopifolia*
Reprinted from: *Molecules* **2020**, *25*, 589, doi:10.3390/molecules25030589 75

Hui Lyu, Wenjuan Liu, Bai Bai, Yu Shan, Christian Paetz, Xu Feng and Yu Chen
Prenyleudesmanes and A Hexanorlanostane from the Roots of *Lonicera macranthoides*
Reprinted from: *Molecules* **2019**, *24*, 4276, doi:10.3390/molecules24234276 85

H. D. Ponce-Rodríguez, R. Herráez-Hernández, J. Verdú-Andrés and P. Campíns-Falcó
Quantitative Analysis of Terpenic Compounds in Microsamples of Resins by Capillary Liquid Chromatography
Reprinted from: *Molecules* **2019**, *24*, 4068, doi:10.3390/molecules24224068 . . . . **95**

Kostas Ioannidis, Eleni Melliou and Prokopios Magiatis
High-Throughput ^{1}H-Nuclear Magnetic Resonance-Based Screening for the Identification and Quantification of Heartwood Diterpenic Acids in Four Black Pine (*Pinus nigra* Arn.) Marginal Provenances in Greece
Reprinted from: *Molecules* **2019**, *24*, 3603, doi:10.3390/molecules24193603 . . . . **107**

Magdalena Mizerska-Kowalska, Adrianna Sławińska-Brych, Katarzyna Kaławaj, Aleksandra Żurek, Beata Pawińska, Wojciech Rzeski and Barbara Zdzisińska
Betulin Promotes Differentiation of Human Osteoblasts In Vitro and Exerts an Osteoinductive Effect on the hFOB 1.19 Cell Line Through Activation of JNK, ERK1/2, and mTOR Kinases
Reprinted from: *Molecules* **2019**, *24*, 2637, doi:10.3390/molecules24142637 . . . . **121**

Chia-Cheng Lin, Jui-Hsin Su, Wu-Fu Chen, Zhi-Hong Wen, Bo-Rong Peng, Lin-Cyuan Huang, Tsong-Long Hwang and Ping-Jyun Sung
New 11,20-Epoxybriaranes from the Gorgonian Coral *Junceella fragilis* (Ellisellidae)
Reprinted from: *Molecules* **2019**, *24*, 2487, doi:10.3390/molecules24132487 . . . . **137**

Elwira Lasoń
Topical Administration of Terpenes Encapsulated in Nanostructured Lipid-Based Systems
Reprinted from: *Molecules* **2020**, *25*, 5758, doi:10.3390/molecules25235758 . . . . **145**

Synthesis, Modification and Biological Activity of Diosgenyl β-D-Glycosaminosides: An Overview
Reprinted from: *Molecules* **2020**, *25*, 5433, doi:10.3390/molecules25225433 . . . . **157**

Zhaobao Wang, JingXin Sun, Qun Yang and Jianming Yang
Metabolic Engineering *Escherichia coli* for the Production of Lycopene
Reprinted from: *Molecules* **2020**, *25*, 3136, doi:10.3390/molecules25143136 . . . . **183**

Maximilian Frey
Traps and Pitfalls—Unspecific Reactions in Metabolic Engineering of Sesquiterpenoid Pathways
Reprinted from: *Molecules* **2020**, *25*, 1935, doi:10.3390/molecules25081935 . . . . **197**

Uladzimir Bildziukevich, Zülal Özdemir and Zdeněk Wimmer
Recent Achievements in Medicinal and Supramolecular Chemistry of Betulinic Acid and Its Derivatives
Reprinted from: *Molecules* **2019**, *24*, 3546, doi:10.3390/molecules24193546 . . . . **207**

About the Editors

Pavel B. Drasar, professor, RNDr. D.S.; 2008 Chartered Scientist; 2004 Full professor of organic chemistry; 2004 D.S. in organic chemistry; 2002 associate professor (docent); 1997 EurChem; 1993 CChem, FRSC; 1972–1977 Ph.D. study, IOCB CAS, Prague; 1972 RNDr. (Rerum Naturalium Doctor); 1966–71 Charles University Prague; 2002 UCT Praha, educator, and research worker; 1972–2002, Institute of Organic Chemistry and Biochemistry (IOCB), CAS, Ph.D. research worker; 1971–1972 Charles University, assistant. Numerous board and committee memberships. Areas of the scientific interest include: synthesis and biological and physicochemical evaluation of steroids and their conjugates, steroidal and terpene lactones, alkaloids, brassinosteroids, carbohydrates and their conjugates, ion channel modifiers, synthesis of natural products, targeting of biologically active compounds by peptide vectors, etc. Publication activity: 274 documents and 1601/1187 citations in WoS, h-index 18, over 160 conferences, 16 books, and 38 patents.

Vladimir A. Khripach, professor, D.S., member of the BAS. M.S. (Chemistry); 1971, BSU, Minsk, Ph.D.; 1978, Inst. of Phys. Org. Chem., BSSR AS, Minsk, Dr.Sc. (Chemistry); 1990, Zelinsky Inst. Org. Chem., USSR AS, Moscow. Researcher, Zelinsky Inst. of Org. Chem., USSR AS, Moscow (1970–1971). Research worker, Inst. Bioorg. Chem., BAS (1971–1982). Head of the Lab. Steroid Chem., IBC BAS (1982–date). Areas of the scientific interest include: synthesis of biologically important natural substances and structure–activity relationships plant physiology, immunochemistry, medicinal chemistry, and supramolecular chemistry. Prize of the Mendeleev Chemical Society (1985). Gold Medals from All-Russian Exhibition Center, Moscow (1993, 1995, and 1996). State Prize Winner (1996). Jubilee Medal of the ASB (2009). Hanus Medal of Czech Chemical Society (2009). Medal of the Ukrainian State Foundation for Fundamental Research (2009). Publication activity: 500 publications (397 WoS, 2405/1476 citations, h-index 20), 5 books, and more than 50 patents.

Preface to "Terpenes and Terpene Derivatives"

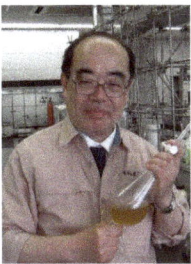

This Special Issue of *Molecules* "Terpenes and Terpene Derivatives" aims to underline current developments in all fields that are connected to terpene research and utilization and was set to commemorate the heritage of the great terpene scientist, Prof. Kenji Mori, who passed away in April 2019.

Kenji Mori developed his chemistry skills at the University of Tokyo where he in 1957 obtained a bachelor degree in agricultural chemistry. Finally, he mastered his Ph.D. thesis in 1962, under the supervision of Professor M. Matsui already on the topic of the total synthesis of plant terpenes–gibberellins. Then, until 1978 he was the Associate Professor at the Department of Agricultural Chemistry of the University of Tokyo, when he became Full Professor at the same department. After his retirement in 1995, he continued until 2001 at the Department of Chemistry of the Science University of Tokyo and worked with several Japanese companies and institutes as a consultant, especially at Riken Co.

Interestingly, he worked in the lab, as he stressed, "using his own hands" until the very end of his fruitful chemistry career. In addition, despite of his age he tirelessly lectured at numerous scientific meetings. One of the conferences where he was very active since the second half of the 20th century is the Conference on Isoprenoids. In 2018, he presented a lecture on his "Recent results in pheromone synthesis".

His activity at Isoprenoid conferences was the inspiration for the Isoprenoid Society to establish the Kenji Mori Prize and Medal. The first two medals were awarded to Takayoshi Awakawa (JP; 2020) and Miroslav Kvasnica (CZ, 2021).

The Special Issue of *Molecules* "Terpenes and Terpene Derivatives" was a sequel to successful Special Issue "Synthesis, Study and Utilization of Natural Products" and shall be followed by the new SI on "Terpenes, Steroids and their Derivatives" which started in 2021.

As the guest editors of the SIs we trust that intensive research in chemistry and all other aspects

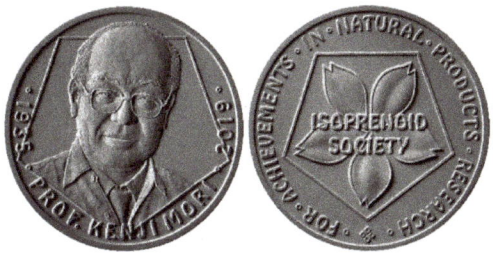

of isoprenoids brings new important information, not only in the field of medicinal drugs, but also in supramolecular, food, material, environmental sciences, and contributes to an ever-living exploration of Natural Products—an invaluable gift to people from Mother Nature (the expression "Mother Nature" Kenji used very often in his lectures).

Pavel B. Drasar, Vladimir A. Khripach
Editors

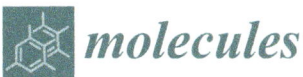

Editorial

Terpene Research Is Providing New Inspiration for Scientists

Pavel B. Drasar [1,*] and Vladimir A. Khripach [2]

[1] Department of Chemistry of Natural Compounds, University of Chemistry and Technology, Technicka 5, 166 28 Prague, Czech Republic
[2] Institute of Bioorganic Chemistry, National Academy of Sciences of Belarus, 5/2 Academician V. F. Kuprevich Street, BY-220141 Minsk, Belarus; khripach@iboch.by
* Correspondence: drasarp@vscht.cz

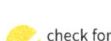

Citation: Drasar, P.B.; Khripach, V.A. Terpene Research Is Providing New Inspiration for Scientists. *Molecules* 2021, 26, 5480. https://doi.org/10.3390/molecules26185480

Received: 2 September 2021
Accepted: 8 September 2021
Published: 9 September 2021

Publisher's Note: MDPI stays neutral with regard to jurisdictional claims in published maps and institutional affiliations.

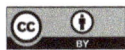

Copyright: © 2021 by the authors. Licensee MDPI, Basel, Switzerland. This article is an open access article distributed under the terms and conditions of the Creative Commons Attribution (CC BY) license (https://creativecommons.org/licenses/by/4.0/).

This current Special Issue of *Molecules* gathers selected communications on terpenes and terpene derivatives, clearly demonstrating the sustained interest in and importance of natural products in this field; fields connected to secondary metabolites; and renewable resources of plant and animal compounds for medicinal, material, supramolecular, and general chemistry research.

This issue gathers 17 papers, 5 review articles, and 12 research communications with a vast range of topics with different perspectives, such as the optimization of FRAP methodology for studies based on selected monoterpenes [1], and the improved functioning of fibroblasts and endothelial cells and accelerated healing of cutaneous wounds in mice caused by uvaol [2]. It presents a new iridoid and three new bis-iridoid glycosides from the leaves of *Lasianthus verticillatus*, lasianosides F–I [3], and atypical lindenane-type sesquiterpenes from *Lindera myrrha* [4]. It comprises a study of antibacterial and antifungal sesquiterpenoids from the aerial parts of *Anvillea garcinii* [5] and phytochemical and safety evaluations of volatile terpenoids from *Zingiber cassumunar* on mature carp peripheral blood mononuclear cells and embryonic zebrafish [6]. Similarly, it presents the cytotoxic and anti-inflammatory effects of *ent*-kaurane derivatives isolated from the alpine plant *Sideritis hyssopifolia* [7]. The issue also lists the prenyleudesmanes and a hexanorlanostane from the roots of *Lonicera macranthoides* [8]. There is discussion on the quantitative analysis of terpenic compounds in microsamples of resins by capillary liquid chromatography [9] and high-throughput ^{1}H-NMR-based screening for the identification and quantification of heartwood diterpenic acids in four black pine *Pinus nigra* marginal provenances in Greece [10]. This Special Issue presents the naturally occurring pentacyclic triterpene betulin, which promotes differentiation of human osteoblasts in vitro and exerts an osteoinductive effect on the hFOB 1.19 cell line through activation of JNK, ERK1/2, and mTOR kinases [11]. Two new 11,20-epoxybriaranes are described from the gorgonian coral *Junceella fragilis* from Ellisellidae [12].

The review articles describe the issue of topical administration of terpenes encapsulated in nanostructured lipid-based systems [13]; an overview of the synthesis, modification, and biological activity of diosgenyl β-D-glycosaminosides [14]; metabolic engineering of *Escherichia coli* for the production of lycopene [15]; traps and pitfalls—unspecific reactions in metabolic engineering of sesquiterpenoid pathways [16]; and the recent achievements in medicinal and supramolecular chemistry of betulinic acid and its derivatives [17].

The Special Issue also aims to commemorate the great work and legacy of Prof. Kenji Mori, providing important material not only to many chemists but also to the specialists in several other fields.

Funding: This research received no external funding.

Acknowledgments: The Guest Editor wishes to thank all the authors for their contributions to this Special Issue, all the reviewers for their work in evaluating the submitted articles, and the editorial staff of *Molecules* for their kind assistance.

Conflicts of Interest: The author declares no conflict of interest.

References

1. Wojtunik-Kulesza, K.A. Approach to Optimization of FRAP Methodology for Studies Based on Selected Monoterpenes. *Molecules* **2020**, *25*, 5267. [CrossRef] [PubMed]
2. Carmo, J.; Cavalcante-Araújo, P.; Silva, J.; Ferro, J.; Correia, A.C.; Lagente, V.; Barreto, E. Uvaol Improves the Functioning of Fibroblasts and Endothelial Cells and Accelerates the Healing of Cutaneous Wounds in Mice. *Molecules* **2020**, *25*, 4982. [CrossRef] [PubMed]
3. Al-Hamoud, G.A.; Orfali, R.S.; Takeda, Y.; Sugimoto, S.; Yamano, Y.; Al Musayeib, N.M.; Fantoukh, O.I.; Amina, M.; Otsuka, H.; Matsunami, K. Lasianosides F–I: A New Iridoid and Three New Bis-Iridoid Glycosides from the Leaves of *Lasianthus verticillatus* (Lour.) Merr. *Molecules* **2020**, *25*, 2798. [CrossRef] [PubMed]
4. Duong, T.-H.; Beniddir, M.A.; Trung, N.T.; Phan, C.-T.D.; Vo, V.G.; Nguyen, V.-K.; Le, Q.-L.; Nguyen, H.-D.; Pogam, P.L. Atypical Lindenane-Type Sesquiterpenes from *Lindera myrrha*. *Molecules* **2020**, *25*, 1830. [CrossRef] [PubMed]
5. Perveen, S.; Alqahtani, J.; Orfali, R.; Aati, H.Y.; Al-Taweel, A.M.; Ibrahim, T.A.; Khan, A.; Yusufoglu, H.S.; Abdel-Kader, M.S.; Taglialatela-Scafati, O. Antibacterial and Antifungal Sesquiterpenoids from Aerial Parts of Anvillea garcinia. *Molecules* **2020**, *25*, 1730. [CrossRef] [PubMed]
6. Mektrirat, R.; Yano, T.; Okonogi, S.; Katip, W.; Pikulkaew, S. Phytochemical and Safety Evaluations of Volatile Terpenoids from *Zingiber cassumunar* Roxb. on Mature Carp Peripheral Blood Mononuclear Cells and Embryonic Zebrafish. *Molecules* **2020**, *25*, 613. [CrossRef] [PubMed]
7. Aimond, A.; Calabro, K.; Audoin, C.; Olivier, E.; Dutot, M.; Buron, P.; Rat, P.; Laprévote, O.; Prado, S.; Roulland, E.; et al. Cytotoxic and Anti-Inflammatory Effects of Ent-Kaurane Derivatives Isolated from the Alpine Plant Sideritis hyssopifolia. *Molecules* **2020**, *25*, 589. [CrossRef] [PubMed]
8. Lyu, H.; Liu, W.; Bai, B.; Shan, Y.; Paetz, C.; Feng, X.; Chen, Y. Prenyleudesmanes and A Hexanorlanostane from the Roots of Lonicera macranthoides. *Molecules* **2019**, *24*, 4276. [CrossRef] [PubMed]
9. Ponce-Rodríguez, H.D.; Herráez-Hernández, R.; Verdú-Andrés, J.; Campíns-Falcó, P. Quantitative Analysis of Terpenic Compounds in Microsamples of Resins by Capillary Liquid Chromatography. *Molecules* **2019**, *24*, 4068. [CrossRef] [PubMed]
10. Ioannidis, K.; Melliou, E.; Magiatis, P. High-Throughput 1H-Nuclear Magnetic Resonance-Based Screening for the Identification and Quantification of Heartwood Diterpenic Acids in Four Black Pine (*Pinus nigra* Arn.) Marginal Provenances in Greece. *Molecules* **2019**, *24*, 3603. [CrossRef] [PubMed]
11. Mizerska-Kowalska, M.; Sławińska-Brych, A.; Kałwaj, K.; Żurek, A.; Pawińska, B.; Rzeski, W.; Zdzisińska, B. Betulin Promotes Differentiation of Human Osteoblasts In Vitro and Exerts an Osteoinductive Effect on the hFOB 1.19 Cell Line Through Activation of JNK, ERK1/2, and mTOR Kinases. *Molecules* **2019**, *24*, 2637. [CrossRef] [PubMed]
12. Lin, C.-C.; Su, J.-H.; Chen, W.-F.; Wen, Z.-H.; Peng, B.-R.; Huang, L.-C.; Hwang, T.-L.; Sung, P.-J. New 11,20-Epoxybriaranes from the Gorgonian Coral Junceella fragilis (Ellisellidae). *Molecules* **2019**, *24*, 2487. [CrossRef]
13. Lasoń, E. Topical Administration of Terpenes Encapsulated in Nanostructured Lipid-Based Systems. *Molecules* **2020**, *25*, 5758. [CrossRef]
14. Grzywacz, D.; Liberek, B.; Myszka, H. Synthesis, Modification and Biological Activity of Diosgenyl β-d-Glycosaminosides: An Overview. *Molecules* **2020**, *25*, 5433. [CrossRef]
15. Wang, Z.; Sun, J.X.; Yang, Q.; Yang, J. Metabolic Engineering *Escherichia coli* for the Production of Lycopene. *Molecules* **2020**, *25*, 3136. [CrossRef] [PubMed]
16. Frey, M. Traps and Pitfalls—Unspecific Reactions in Metabolic Engineering of Sesquiterpenoid Pathways. *Molecules* **2020**, *25*, 1935. [CrossRef] [PubMed]
17. Bildziukevich, U.; Özdemir, Z.; Wimmer, Z. Recent Achievements in Medicinal and Supramolecular Chemistry of Betulinic Acid and Its Derivatives. *Molecules* **2019**, *24*, 3546. [CrossRef] [PubMed]

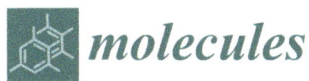

Article

Approach to Optimization of FRAP Methodology for Studies Based on Selected Monoterpenes

Karolina A. Wojtunik-Kulesza

Department of Inorganic Chemistry, Medical University of Lublin, 20-059 Lublin, Poland; karolina.wojtunik@umlub.pl

Academic Editors: Pavel B. Drasar and Vladimir A. Khripach
Received: 20 October 2020; Accepted: 10 November 2020; Published: 12 November 2020

Abstract: Terpenes, wide-spread secondary plant metabolites, constitute important parts of many natural compounds that hold various biological activities, including antioxidant, calming, antiviral, and analgesic activities. Due to their high volatility and low solubility in water, studies of compounds based on terpenes are difficult, and methodologies must be adjusted to their specific characteristics. Considering the significant influence of iron ions on dementia development, the activity of terpenes in reducing Fe^{3+} represents an important area to be determined. Previously obtained results were unreliable because ferric-reducing antioxidant power (FRAP) methodology was not adjusted regarding studying terpenes. Taking this fact into account, the aim of this study was to optimize the method for monoterpene assessment. The study included three modifications, namely, (1) slightly adjusting the entire FRAP procedure, (2) replacing methanol with other solvents (heptane, butanone, or ethyl acetate), and (3) adding Tween 20. Additionally, a thin layer chromatography (TLC) -FRAP assay was performed. The obtained results revealed significant improvement in the reduction activity of selected terpenes (linalool, α-phellandrene, and α-terpinene) in studies with Tween 20, whereas replacing methanol with other solvents did not show the expected effects.

Keywords: FRAP; terpenes; antioxidant

1. Introduction

The antioxidant effect is a well-studied, natural-compound bioactivity which can be determined by numerous methods, including spectrophotometry, chromatography, and theoretical consideration to account for in vitro and in vivo conditions [1,2]. Assays are based on scavenging free radicals (e.g., hydroxyl, superoxide), performing typical reduction reactions (e.g., reduction Fe^{3+} to Fe^{2+}), or inhibiting pro-oxidant enzymes (e.g., xantine oxydase), etc.

From a medical point of view, Fe^{3+} plays important roles in several harmful oxidation processes within the human organism. This results from the fact that the ion is responsible for the aggregation of hyperphosphorylated tau, and is associated with neurofibrillary tangles, as well as progressive supranuclear palsy (PSP). Reduction of Fe^{3+} to Fe^{2+} can reverse this process and solubilize tau species characteristic of neurodegeneration [3]. Among methods used to determine the reduction ability of Fe^{3+} to Fe^{2+} is ferric-reducing antioxidant power (FRAP), a colorimetric method which uses the ability of antioxidants to reduce the colorless $[Fe^{3+}\text{-}(2,4,6\text{-Tris}(2\text{-pirydyl})\text{-}s\text{-triazine})_2]^{3+}$ complex to the intensively blue-colored complex $[Fe^{2+}\text{-}(TPTZ)_2]^{2+}$ in acidic medium [4]. Such color changes are spectrophotometrically measured at 593 nm. Results are calculated based on using ferrous ion standard solution and certain antioxidant standards (in most cases, trolox). The outcome is considered in FRAP units, where one FRAP unit can be defined as the reduction of 1 M ferric ion to one ferrous ion [5]. This method is widely used to determine the antioxidant activity of plants, foods extracts, biological fluids, spices, vegetables, fruits, and many extracts and essential oils.

A FRAP assay requires specific conditions, including, among others, an acidic medium (pH 3.6) to facilitate iron solubility and a temperature of 37 °C. The low pH decreases the ionization potential that drives electron transfer and increases the redox potential, causing a shift in the dominant reaction mechanism [6,7]. Similarly to other assays, FRAP has limitations. The most important is the redox potential of the pair Fe^{3+}/Fe^{2+}, because any compound with redox potential lower than this can induce falsely high Fe^{3+} reduction results. Additionally, FRAP assay results depend on the timescale of analysis. The assay is based on the assumption that the redox reaction proceeds rapidly and that all reactions are complete between four and six minutes. This is not always the case [7].

An important feature to be considered at this point is the pro-oxidant character of the assay. Research established that one of the reaction products is Fe^{2+}, a pro-oxidant molecule that takes part in a Fenton reaction, leading to the formation of a hydroxyl radical. Nevertheless, numerous scientists explained that this problem can be resolved automatically in the reaction environment by using highly active antioxidants (e.g., polyphenols), which, despite activity toward Fe^{3+}, reveal an ability to scavenge free radicals [8].

The described method is widely used in biological activity studies. At this point, it is worth stating that the reaction environment is hydrophilic; an acetate buffer serves as base for the reaction, while HCl solution is applied to prepare the TPTZ solution and water is supplied for the Fe^{3+} solution. The environment drives a situation wherein the reduction activity of tested compounds largely depends on their solubility in the measured mixture. The issue of an aqueous reaction environment is not a problem in the case of alcoholic extracts because of their high solubility in water. The problem appears when dealing with hydrophobic compounds (e.g., terpenes), which are hydrocarbons and derivatives of hydrocarbons with low hydrosolubility.

The aim of this study was to evaluate diverse FRAP reaction conditions (e.g., Tween 20 addition, replacement of methanol with solvents of various polarity) in order to optimize a method for application with a selected group of terpenes (γ-terpinene, citral, citronellal, carvone, α-phellandrene, α-terpinene, α-pinene, farnesene, eucalyptol, terpinene-4-ol, β-myrcene, p-cymene, linalool, β-myrcene, isopulegol, menthol). An additional aim of this study was to ascertain the effect of combining FRAP with thin-layer chromatography (TLC). This is pioneering work, as previous literature data did not provide information about the TLC-FRAP method. The presented study is based on assessing terpenes possessing numerous biological activities, including antioxidant, acetylcholinesterase (AChE) inhibitory, anti-inflammatory, sedative, analgesic, etc. [9,10]. Among the tested compounds were terpenes diverse in terms of structure and chemical properties (e.g., ketone–carvone, alcohol–menthol, and hydrocarbon–farnesene).

2. Results

2.1. Spectrophotometric Studies

The first step of the performed studies was to ascertain the effect of only slightly modifying the basic methodology [11]. This involved replacing part of the water component with methanol to better dissolve the terpene content. This approach appeared to be ineffective. First, measurements based on the aqueous reaction environment caused clouding, in many cases without the combination of the FRAP solution with the studied terpene and, as a consequence, false-positive assay results were obtained. For the most part, the blue color as the result of $[Fe^{2+}\text{-}(TPTZ)_2]^{2+}$ creation was not observed and the clouding induced an increase in absorbance value. A slight modification based on terpene dilution in methanol before combination with FRAP solution, however, led to a positive effect. A 0.1 M terpene concentration revealed high citral, carvone, and γ-terpinene activity levels, and the reaction progression showed a deepening blue color without clouding (Table 1). In the case of α-phellandrene and α-terpinene, the blue color was also observed but alongside the appearance of clouding. In this case, the results were considered to be false-positive. The remaining terpenes, namely terpinene-4-ol, linalool, p-cymene, β-myrcene, citronellal, isopulegol, menthol, menthone, farnesene, and eucalyptol did not exhibit Fe^{3+} reduction activity, with no blue color and observation of clouding. The active three terpenes were analyzed in detail, with the activity considered in FRAP units, trolox, and gallic acid equivalents (Figure 1).

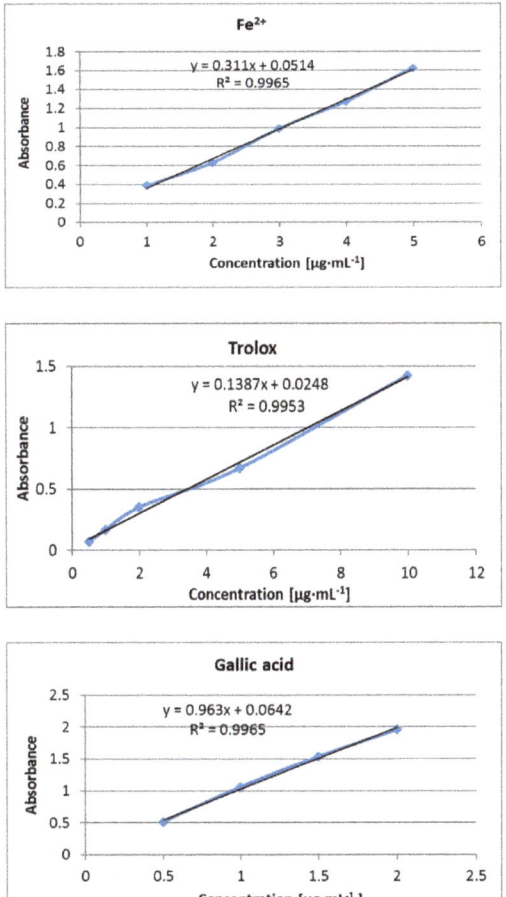

Figure 1. Calibration curves prepared for Fe^{2+}, trolox, and gallic acid.

Table 1. Ferris-reduced antioxidant power (FRAP) units, trolox equivalent, and gallic acid equivalent obtained for a selected group of terpenes during nonmodified FRAP assay.

Terpenes	FRAP Units (Fe^{2+} µg·mL^{-1})		Trolox Equivalent (µg·mL^{-1})		Gallic Acid Equivalent (µg·mL^{-1})	
	0.1 M	1 mg·mL^{-1}	0.1 M	1 mg·mL^{-1}	0.1 M	1 mg·mL^{-1}
γ-terpinene *	-	4.97	-	11.34	-	1.59
citral	3.45	4.30	7.93	9.85	1.10	1.38
carvone	3.58	0.44	8.24	1.19	1.15	1.13
α-phellandrene			\multicolumn{4}{c}{False-positive effect}			
α-terpinene			False-positive effect			
α-pinene			clouding/lack of color			
farnesene			clouding/lack of color			
eucalyptol			clouding/lack of color			
terpinene-4-ol			clouding/lack of color			
p-cymene			clouding/lack of color			
linalool			clouding/lack of color			
β-myrcene			clouding/lack of color			
citronellal			clouding/lack of color			
isopulegol			clouding/lack of color			
menthol			clouding/lack of color			

* Due to the high activity of γ-terpinene, the assay was determined for a concentration of 0.5 mg·mL^{-1}. In the case of a concentration of 0.1 M, absorbance was >>3.400.

The second step of the experiment intended to modify the method to enhance terpene solubility and avoid clouding. One possible way of obtaining a clear, non-clouded solution is to supplant methanol with another solvent. Taking into account that previous studies [12] revealed the positive influence of chloroform, ethyl acetate, and 2-butanone on the antioxidant activity of the selected group of terpenes, these solvents were applied in the FRAP assay. The basis of this modification was to replace the methanol component (used to dissolve the terpenes) with the three listed organic solvents. However, this minor modification did not bring the expected improvement in quality of the studied solution. In most cases, the clouding was stronger, probably resulting from high differences in polarity between the water/acetate buffer and the organic solvents. Hence, while the terpene solvents are effective, when added to the FRAP solution the outcome was extensive clouding.

In order to obtain a clear solution and reliable assay results, the addition of the surfactant Tween 20 to standard FRAP solution was investigated. This particular surfactant was chosen because it is characterized by very low toxicity, and is therefore often used in various branches of chemistry and pharmacy [13]. The outcome of this experiment was that, in a few cases, Tween 20 addition improved the solubility and study potential of certain investigated terpenes, as indicated by the appearance of the blue color and the reduction or disappearance of clouding. Among these were isopulegol, linalool, α-phellandrene, and α-terpinene (for which clouding was observed previously). Unfortunately, in many cases, Tween 20 augmentation resulted in clouding. These results are presented in Table 2.

The obtained results revealed that Tween 20 addition influenced the reduction activity of the analyzed terpenes. As indicated in Tables 1 and 2, the figures for FRAP units, trolox equivalent and gallic acid equivalents were reduced with regard to γ-terpinene, α-terpinene, citral, carvone, and α-phellandrene after assay modification when compared to the unmodified assay. In contrast, isopulegol, linalool (for all factors), carvone (0.5 mg·mL^{-1}) (for gallic acid equivalent), and α-phellandrene (1 mg/mL) (for FRAP units) exhibited higher reduction activity for the FRAP/surfactant solution. The remaining group of studied terpenes did not reveal a positive response after the modification. A slight difference was observed, however, α-pinene exhibited color appearance, albeit with simultaneously clouding.

Table 2. FRAP units, trolox equivalent, and gallic acid equivalent obtained for a selected group of terpenes via FRAP assay modified by the addition of Tween 20.

Terpenes	FRAP Units (Fe²⁺ µg·mL⁻¹)		Trolox Equivalent (µg·mL⁻¹)		Gallic Acid Equivalent (µg·mL⁻¹)	
	0.1 M	1 mg·mL⁻¹	0.1 M	1 mg·mL⁻¹	0.1 M	1 mg·mL⁻¹
γ-terpinene *	-	1.38 (for 0.25 mg·mL⁻¹)	-	7.51	-	1.04
citral	3.21	1.04	7.43	2.52	1.03	0.32
Carvone **	False-positive results	0.28	False-positive results	0.83	False-positive results	0.08
α-phellandrene	2.47	1.45	5.74	3.45	0.79	0.45
α-terpinene ***	-	5.75 (for 0.1 mg·mL⁻¹)	-	13.09	-	1.84
isopulegol	0.38	0.01	1.06	0.05	0.11	0.01
linalool	0.34	0.09	0.96	0.40	0.09	0.01
α-pinene			False-positive results ****			
farnesene			clouding/lack of color			
eucalyptol			clouding/lack of color			
terpinene-4-ol			clouding/lack of color			
p-cymene			clouding/lack of color			
β-myrcene			clouding/lack of color			
citronellal			clouding/lack of color			
menthol			clouding/lack of color			

* γ-Terpinene: This terpene revealed high activity at a concentration of 0.1 M and 1 mg·mL⁻¹, for which absorbance was >3.000. The measurements were performed at a concentration of 0.25 mg·mL⁻¹. ** Carvone: Measurements were performed at a concentration of 0.5 mg·mL⁻¹. *** α-Terpinene: This terpene exhibited high activity at a concentration of 0.1 M and 1 mg·mL⁻¹, for which absorbance was >3.000. The measurements were performed at a concentration of 0.1 mg·mL⁻¹. **** False-positive results: This effect was observed for probes with the blue color but clouding appeared simultaneously.

2.2. TLC–FRAP Assay

The approach to combining thin layer chromatography with FRAP assay required some small modification of the originally intended method. The first attempt to accomplish this was based on the basic methodology with Tween 20 augmentation at standard ratio, but the obtained results were not satisfactory. In order to improve the method, the ratio of the FRAP solution component was changed to 10:2:2. This improved spot contrast and facilitated results analysis. The obtained results are presented in Figure 2.

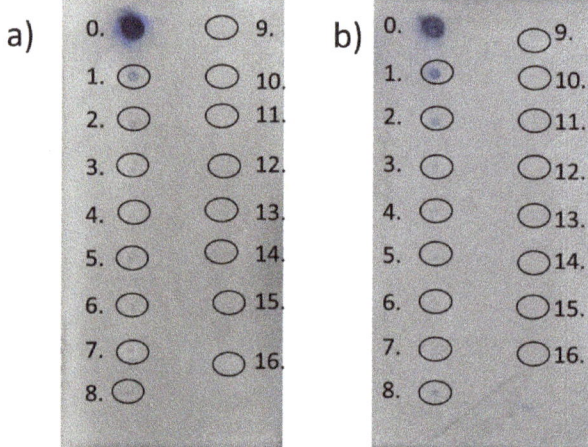

Figure 2. Results obtained for TLC–FRAP assay: (**a**) FRAP assay without modification; (**b**) FRAP with Tween 20. Active compounds appeared as dark spots on the light background. The compounds are numbered as follows: 0—gallic acid; 1—p-cymene; 2—eucalyptol; 3—farnesene; 4—carvone; 5—pulegone; 6—citronellal; 7—terpinene-4-ol; 8—γ-terpinene; 9—citral; 10—α-phellandrene; 11—menthone; 12—α-pinene; 13—linalool; 14—α-terpinene; 15—β-myrcene; 16—isopulegol.

The obtained results revealed a slightly positive impact of Tween 20 addition on terpene activity. When comparing the two TLC plates, the surfactant augmentation brought about a situation wherein p-cymene, eucalyptol, and γ-terpinene exhibited better reducing activity, although much less than gallic acid, a standard antioxidant. None of the remaining terpenes showed reduction activity in the proposed test.

3. Discussion

One possible way of counteracting the action of free radicals is to reduce trace metal ions able to generate reactive forms. Previous papers, however, presented few methods based on metal ion reduction. The reduction process in our organism is important because of its contribution to neurodegeneration [3,14]. Among the methods to investigate this reduction effect is FRAP, which is based on reducing Fe^{3+} to Fe^{2+}. An important limitation of the FRAP assay is the fact that it is based on an aqueous solution (acetate buffer), hence, the method is limited to dealing with hydrophilic substances, whereas plant essential oils and their antioxidant constituents (i.e., terpenes) are hydrophobic. Considering this, modification of the method is essential.

As mentioned previously, the presented studies that researched the antioxidant properties of terpenes revolved around investigating the effect of modifying the standard FRAP method by adding methanol (in order to resolve the analyzed terpenes) and then replacing methanol with various solvents, as well as augmenting the basic FRAP recipe with surfactant Tween 20. The results are discussed below.

The first modification, a methanol–terpene mixture, showed a positive influence in comparison to standard procedure (adding the analyzed compound to the standard FRAP mixture of acetate buffer, $FeCl_3$ in distilled water and TPTZ in HCl). The unmodified assay could not be undertaken due to the very low solubility of terpenes in the prepared solution. Regarding standard FRAP procedure, in almost all samples, clouding and/or insoluble substances were observed. The FRAP and methanol combination significantly improved the solubility and allowed determination of the antioxidant activity of the analyzed secondary plant metabolites.

In order to improve the solubility, the methanol component was replaced by various solvents that previous studies (details in [12]) found positively influenced terpene antioxidant activity. Among these were ethyl acetate and chloroform. While these are good terpene solvents, they negatively influence the prepared FRAP solution due to weak ability to mix with the aqueous solution.

One possible way to improve solubility is surfactant addition. All surfactants are characterized by displaying critical micelle concentration (CMC), the concentration above which surfactants can form micelles and aggregate with solutes, potentially leading to changes in their observed activity [15]. In the case of this type of modification, the CMC criteria must be considered because micelle formation can lead to changes in obtained results. In our work, in order to avert this phenomenon, the surfactant concentration was below the CMC. As shown in Tables 1 and 2, both positive and negative influences of Tween 20 addition were observed. A positive influence was noted for isopulegol and linalool, as their solubility improved in the studied solution. The other terpenes showed weaker reducing activity after Tween 20 addition. Analysis of the obtained results indicated that the differences may have resulted from the low solubility of substances in the nonmodified assay. Despite the solutions not appearing cloudy to the naked eye, detailed spectrophotometry analysis registered slight clouding, thus higher absorbance and false-positive results. Considering the positive influence of surfactants on solubility, as well as adherence to the CMC value, the reduction of biological activity of the studied compounds was not considered to be linked with the impact of surfactant on micelle creation. This fact was shown by two of the analyzed terpenes, (isopulegol and linalool), which revealed higher activity with surfactant addition, observed as blue color appearance as opposed to white clouding, as demonstrated in the previous stage of the experiment. The positive influence of Tween 20 addition was also observed for α-terpinene, which revealed a false-positive effect in the non-surfactant assay, while the activity significantly increased with a concentration of 0.1 M after surfactant addition. In this case, absorbance measurement was possible for smaller concentrations equal to 0.1 $mg \cdot mL^{-1}$, whereas for 0.1 M, absorbance measurement was impossible due to too high absorbance resulting from the deep blue color of the sample.

Detailed analysis of the obtained results revealed some structure–antioxidant activity relationships related to certain antioxidant mechanisms. In accordance with Sadeer et al. [16], FRAP is based on an electron transfer mechanism in which aryloxyl radicals are formed. In the presented studies, the highest reduction activity was observed for cyclic hydrocarbon terpenes with conjugated double bonds without single electron transfer (SET) moiety characteristics (with the exception of γ-terpinene without the moiety) (Figure 3).

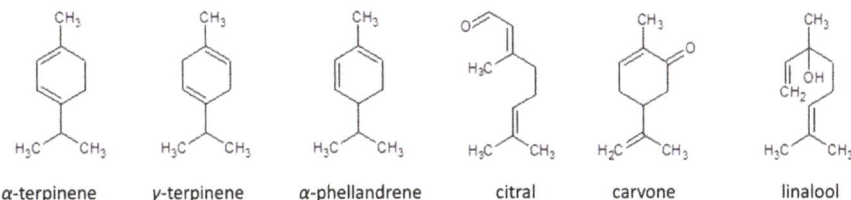

Figure 3. Structures of the most active terpenes in assay modified by Tween 20 addition.

In accordance with Spiegel et al. [17], lower FRAP assay activity was observed for methylated compounds compared to their nonmethylated counterparts. The authors explained this phenomenon by stating that the methylation process decreases the activity of electron- and hydrogen-donating groups. Simultaneously, they noticed that along with decreasing distance between carboxylic groups and ring formation, the influence of methylation increased. In a study of the terpene structure, it was noticeable that the most active did not include moieties characteristic for the single electron transfer (SET) mechanism (e.g., –OH). This effect could signal higher activity in relation to the remaining compounds. In our work, only citral, carvone, and linalool contained moieties, however, these compounds turned out to be weaker Fe^{3+} reducing agents. This phenomenon could be explained by the presence of conjugated double bonds and greater bond dissociation energy for allylic, alkylic, and vinylic hydrogen atoms. In accordance with [12], similar studies were obtained for reactions with 2,2-diphenyl-1-picrylhydrazyl (DPPH). While the reaction mechanism was different, the obtained results revealed explicit dependency between the terpene conjugated double bonds and their ability to reduce Fe(III). In our work, the high activity of γ-terpinene was noted. Despite lacking conjugated double bonds, γ-terpinene showed high reducing activity resulting from the resonance stabilization of the compound. Hence, in accordance with [18], allylic hydrogen transference from the discussed terpenes leads to resonance-stabilized radicals that are able to terminate the chain reaction. Considering terpene activity and their structure-activity relationship, it is highly probable that the hydrogen atom transfer (HAT) mechanism, along with SET, play crucial roles in antioxidant reaction mechanisms.

As indicated by the TLC–FRAP assay, the analyzed terpenes did not exhibit high antioxidant activity. Indeed, only three (p-cymene, eucalyptol, and γ-terpinene) turned out to be more active in the FRAP–Tween 20 solution analysis. The main problem in the determination of the reducing activity of terpenes via TLC–FRAP assay is their low water solubility. While the terpenes did not indicate the expected activity in the test, gallic acid (a standard antioxidant) appeared as a dark spot on a light background, demonstrating that combining FRAP analysis with TLC is possible. Taking into account the good hydrosolubility of alcoholic extracts, the combination of TLC and FRAP could be used as a fast method to determine the reducing activity of extracts and ascertain their most active ingredients.

4. Materials and Methods

4.1. Materials

The terpenes (−)-isopulegol (≥99%), menthol (≥99%), p-cymene (≥99%), eucalyptol (≥99%), (R)-(+)-pulegone (97%), γ-terpinene (97%), α-terpinene (≥95%), linalool (≥97%), (S)-(+)-carvone (≥96%), citronellal (≥95%), (−)-terpinene-4-ol (≥95%), citral (≥95%), menthone (≥90%), farnesene (mixtures of isomers, ≥90%), α-phellandrene (≥90%), β-myrcene (≥90%), and TPTZ (2,4,6-Tri(2-pyridyl)-s-triazine)) were obtained from Sigma-Aldrich (St. Louis, MO, USA). Acetic acid (ACS), $FeCl_3 \times 6H_2O$, $FeSO_4 \times 7H_2O$, phosphoric acid (ACS), hydrochloric acid (ACS), chloroform (ACS), ethyl acetate (ACS), 2-butanone (ACS), and methanol (analytic purity grade) were obtained from Polish Reagents (Gliwice, Poland). The standards trolox ((±)-6-hydroxy-2,5,7,8-tetramethylchromane-2-carboxylic acid, 97%) and gallic acid (>98%) were purchased from Sigma-Aldrich (St. Louis, MO, USA).

4.2. Methods

4.2.1. Basic FRAP Assay Methodology with Some Modifications

FRAP solution was prepared freshly each time by mixing (10:1:1 $v/v/v$) 0.3 M acetate buffer (pH 3.6) and 0.01 M TPTZ in 0.04 M HCl and 0.02 M $FeCl_3 \times 6H_2O$ and kept in the dark. Appropriate amounts of studied terpenes (final concentration of 0.1 M) were dissolved in a calculated small volume of methanol and then mixed with 2.4 mL of FRAP solution. The final volume of mixture was 2.8 mL. The prepared samples were vortexed and incubated at 37 °C by 20 min away from light. Absorbance was then measured at 593 nm using a Genesys 20 UV–vis spectrophotometer (Thermo FisherScientific, Waltham,

MA, USA) in a 1 cm quartz cell. FRAP working solution with deionized water instead of a sample was used as a blank. All measurements were carried out in triplicate. The results were calculated into µg·mL^{-1} Fe^{2+} on the calibration curve, which was prepared analogically using an aqueous solution of FeSO$_4$ at the concentration 1–5 µg·mL^{-1} (y = 0.311x + 0.0514, R^2 = 0.9965). Additionally, trolox and gallic acid were used as standards.

The assay was modified in order to determine the most beneficial reaction conditions for terpenes.

(a) Preparation of a terpene–methanol mixture that was added to the basic FRAP solution.
(b) Replacement of methanol (to terpenes dissolution) with other solvents (chloroform, ethyl acetate, or 2-butanone), in which terpenes revealed higher antioxidant activity in previous studies [12].
(c) Addition of Tween 20: The studied terpenes revealed weak solubility in aqueous conditions, which significantly influenced their reducing activity. Additionally, despite the blue color of the samples, the obtained results were falsified due to opacification. In order to resolve this problem, Tween 20 was added to the FRAP solution. The amount of the surfactant was kept below critical micelle concentration (CMC), which, for Tween 20, is equal 0.06 mM. The assay was conducted in two mixing orders, i.e., (1) mixing terpene and methanol, then FRAP and Tween 20, and (2) FRAP and Tween 20, then adding terpene and methanol to 2.8 mL.

4.2.2. FRAP-TLC

The experiment was performed with use of chromatographic HPTLC silica gel 60 (F254) plates (10 cm × 5 cm). Firstly, the studied terpenes were dissolved in methanol in order to facilitate application of the compounds onto the plates. In the first step, appropriate volumes of terpenes and gallic acid solution (as a standard compound), corresponding to 0.1 mg of each compound, were applied onto the plates. Afterward, the plates were sprayed with FRAP solution in a ratio of 10:2:2 (acetate buffer:FeCl$_3$:TPTZ). The plates were then scanned at time 0 and after 20 min. In the second step, the procedure was analogous to the first, but the FRAP solution was enriched with Tween 20 addition. The amount of the surfactant was kept below CMC. Active compounds were identified as blue spots on a white background.

5. Conclusions

The presented study results revealed that the most promising optimization for FRAP assay among those proposed was augmentation with surfactant. In this experiment, activity changes were observed both through spectrophotometric analysis, as well as by TLC–FRAP assay. In the case of spectrophotometric assay, only two terpenes (isopulegol and linalool) demonstrated higher reducing activities compared to the standard, but the positive influence of surfactant was observed by reduced clouding in the studied solutions, as well as by a reduced false-positive effect (e.g., α-terpinene, α-phellandrene). Despite the solution not showing a spectacular impact on antioxidant activity improvement, the obtained results were more reliable and reproducible. Similarly, the positive effect of Tween 20 was observed for the TLC–FRAP procedure, where adding surfactant to the FRAP solution brought about a situation wherein the active compounds appeared as dark spots in comparison to the nonmodified assay. Moreover, through Tween 20 addition, it was evident that γ-terpinene was active in comparison to the nonmodified assay where the terpene was observed to be inactive. Additionally, the obtained results allowed better insight into the mechanism of antioxidation and confirmed the significant influence of conjugated double bonds in the free radical scavenger and metal ion reduction process. Considering the antioxidant and AChE inhibitory activities of the analyzed terpenes, as well as their Fe(III) reduction abilities, the compounds could be considered as possible anti-neurodegenerative agents. However, more investigation is necessary.

Funding: This research received no external funding.

Acknowledgments: In this section you can acknowledge any support given which is not covered by the author contribution or funding sections. This may include administrative and technical support, or donations in kind (e.g., materials used for experiments).

Conflicts of Interest: The author declares no conflict of interest.

References

1. Thaipong, K.; Boonprakob, U.; Crosby, K.; Cisneros-Zevallosc, L.; Hawkins Byrne, D. Comparison of ABTS, DPPH, FRAP, and ORAC assays for estimating antioxidant activity from guava fruit extracts. *J. Food Compos. Anal.* **2006**, *19*, 669–675. [CrossRef]
2. Anbazhakan, K.; Sadasivam, K.; Praveena, R.; Salgado, G.; Cardona, W.; Glossman-Mitnik, D.; Gerli, L. Theoretical assessment of antioxidant property of polyproponoid and its derivatives. *Struct. Chem.* **2020**, *31*, 1089–1094. [CrossRef]
3. Wojtunik-Kulesza, K.; Oniszczuk, A.; Waksmundzka-Hajnos, M. An attempt to elucidate the role of iron and zinc ions in development of Alzheimer's and Parkinson's diseases. *Biomed. Pharmacother.* **2019**, *111*, 1277–1289. [CrossRef]
4. Benzie, I.F.F.; Strain, J.J. Ferric reducing/antioxidant power assay: Direct measure of total antioxidant activity of biological fuids and modifed version for simultaneous measurement of total antioxidant power and ascorbic acid concentration. *Methods Enzymol.* **1999**, *299*, 15–27. [CrossRef]
5. MacDonald-Wicks, L.K.; Wood, L.G.; Garg, M.L. Methodology for the determination of biological antioxidant capacity in vitro: A review. *J. Sci. Food Agric.* **2016**, *86*, 2046–2056. [CrossRef]
6. Gulcin, I. Antioxidants and antioxidant methods: An updated overview. *Arch. Toxicol.* **2020**, *94*, 651–715. [CrossRef] [PubMed]
7. Hagerman, A.E.; Riedl, K.M.; Jones, G.A.; Sovik, K.N.; Ritchard, N.T.; Hartzfeld, P.W.; Reichel, T.L. High molecular weight plant phenolics (tannins) as biological antioxidants. *J. Agric. Food Chem.* **1998**, *46*, 1887–1892. [CrossRef] [PubMed]
8. Umeno, A.; Horie, M.; Murotomi, K.; Nakajima, Y.; Yoshida, Y. Antioxidative and antidiabetic effects of natural polyphenols and isoflavones. *Molecules* **2016**, *21*, 708. [CrossRef] [PubMed]
9. Wojtunik-Kulesza, K.A.; Targowska-Duda, K.; Klimek, K.; Ginalska, G.; Jóźwiak, K.; Waksmundzka-Hajnos, M.; Cieśla, Ł. Volatile terpenoids as potential drug leads in Alzheimer's disease. *Open Chem.* **2017**, *15*, 332–343. [CrossRef]
10. Zhao, D.-D.; Jiang, L.-L.; Li, H.-Y.; Yan, P.-F.; Zhang, Y.-L. Chemical components and pharmacological activities of terpene natural products from the genus *Paeonia*. *Molecules* **2016**, *21*, 1362. [CrossRef] [PubMed]
11. Biskup, I.; Golonka, I.; Gamian, A.; Sroka, Z. Antioxidant activity of selected phenols estimated by ABTS and FRAP methods. *Postepy Hig. Med. Dosw.* **2013**, *67*, 958–963. [CrossRef]
12. Wojtunik, K.A.; Ciesla, L.M.; Waksmundzka-Hajnos, M. Model studies on the antioxidant activity of common terpenoid constituents of essential oils by means of the 2,2-diphenyl-1-picrylhydrazyl method. *J. Agric. Food Chem.* **2014**, *62*, 9088–9094. [CrossRef] [PubMed]
13. Wojtunik-Kulesza, K.; Cieśla, Ł.; Oniszczuk, A.; Waksmundzka-Hajnos, M. The influence of micellar system on antioxidant activity of common terpenoids measured by UV-Vis spectrophotometry. *Acta Pol. Pharm.* **2018**, *75*, 321–328. Available online: https://ptfarm.pl/wydawnictwa/czasopisma/acta-poloniae-pharmaceutica/110/-/27365 (accessed on 26 April 2018).
14. Sethi, S.; Joshi, A.; Arora, B.; Bhowmik, A.; Sharma, R.R.; Kumar, P. Significance of FRAP, DPPH, and CUPRAC assays for antioxidant activity determination in apple fruit extracts. *Eur. Food Res. Technol.* **2020**, *246*, 591–598. [CrossRef]
15. Chat, O.A.; Najar, M.H.; Mir, M.A.; Rather, G.M.; Dar, A.A. Effects of surfactant micelles on solubilization and DPPH radical scavenging activity of Rutin. *J. Colloid Interface Sci.* **2011**, *355*, 140–149. [CrossRef] [PubMed]
16. Sadeer, N.B.; Montesano, D.; Albrizio, S.; Zengin, G.; Mahomoodally, M.F. The versatility of antioxidant assays in food science and safety—Chemistry, applications, strengths, and limitations. *Antioxidants* **2020**, *9*, 709. [CrossRef] [PubMed]

17. Spiegel, M.; Kapusta, K.; Kołodziejczyk, W.; Saloni, J.; Zbikowska, B.; Hill, G.A.; Sroka, Z. Antioxidant activity of selected phenolic acids-ferric reducing antioxidant power assay and QSAR analysis of the structural features. *Molecules* **2020**, *25*, 3088. [CrossRef] [PubMed]
18. Wojtunik-Kulesza, K.A.; Cieśla, Ł.; Waksmundzka-Hajnos, M. Approach to determination a structure—Antioxidant activity relationship of selected common terpenoids evaluated by ABTS$^{\bullet+}$ radical cation assay. *Nat. Prod. Commun.* **2018**, *13*, 295–298. [CrossRef]

Sample Availability: Samples of the compounds are not available from the authors.

Publisher's Note: MDPI stays neutral with regard to jurisdictional claims in published maps and institutional affiliations.

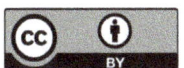

© 2020 by the author. Licensee MDPI, Basel, Switzerland. This article is an open access article distributed under the terms and conditions of the Creative Commons Attribution (CC BY) license (http://creativecommons.org/licenses/by/4.0/).

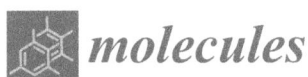

Article

Uvaol Improves the Functioning of Fibroblasts and Endothelial Cells and Accelerates the Healing of Cutaneous Wounds in Mice

Julianderson Carmo [1], Polliane Cavalcante-Araújo [1], Juliane Silva [1], Jamylle Ferro [1], Ana Carolina Correia [2], Vincent Lagente [3] and Emiliano Barreto [1,*]

1. Laboratory of Cell Biology, Federal University of Alagoas, 57072-900 Maceió, Brazil; julianderson.oliveira.bio@hotmail.com (J.C.); pollianearaujo@hotmail.com (P.C.-A.); juliane.silva@icbs.ufal.br (J.S.); jamylle.ferro@icbs.ufal.br (J.F.)
2. Garanhuns College of Science, Education and Technology, University of Pernambuco, 55294-902 Garanhuns, Brazil; ana.correia@upe.br
3. NuMeCan Institute (Nutrition, Metabolism and Cancer), Université de Rennes, INSERM, INRA, F-35000 Rennes, France; vincent.lagente@univ-rennes1.fr
* Correspondence: emilianobarreto@icbs.ufal.br; Tel.: +55-82-3214-1704

Received: 11 October 2020; Accepted: 27 October 2020; Published: 28 October 2020

Abstract: Uvaol is a natural pentacyclic triterpene that is widely found in olives and virgin olive oil, exerting various pharmacological properties. However, information remains limited about how it affects fibroblasts and endothelial cells in events associated with wound healing. Here, we report the effect of uvaol in the in vitro and in vivo healing process. We show the positive effects of uvaol on migration of fibroblasts and endothelial cells in the scratch assay. Protein synthesis of fibronectin and laminin (but not collagen type I) was improved in uvaol-treated fibroblasts. In comparison, tube formation by endothelial cells was enhanced after uvaol treatment. Mechanistically, the effects of uvaol on cell migration involved the PKA and p38-MAPK signaling pathway in endothelial cells but not in fibroblasts. Thus, the uvaol-induced migratory response was dependent on the PKA pathway. Finally, topical treatment with uvaol caused wounds to close faster than in the control treatment using experimental cutaneous wounds model in mice. In conclusion, uvaol positively affects the behavior of fibroblasts and endothelial cells, potentially promoting cutaneous healing.

Keywords: uvaol; terpenes medicinal; wound healing; fibroblasts; endothelial cells

1. Introduction

Wound healing is a dynamic and complex biological process that involves different types of cells working in concert to restore damaged tissues [1]. In this process, coordinated biological events, including phagocytosis, migration, proliferation, angiogenesis, and the synthesis of the extracellular matrix, culminates in the repair of injured tissue [2]. Indeed, wound healing begins at the moment of injury and progresses over three basic, highly integrated, and overlapping phases: (1) inflammation, which is associated with the recruitment of neutrophils and macrophages to the wound bed to clean the lesioned tissue; (2) tissue proliferation and formation, which involves the migration and proliferation of fibroblasts and the development of new blood vessels (angiogenesis); and (3) tissue remodeling, which involves the remodeling of the extracellular matrix to an architecture that approaches normal tissue [3,4].

Among biological processes involved in wound closure, the ability for cells to migrate to the wound bed is important. During the inflammatory phase, macrophages facilitate the non-phlogistic removal of various cell debris and secrete chemical mediators that promote the recruitment and activation of other cell types, including fibroblasts [5]. In turn, fibroblasts are responsible for producing the extracellular matrix, which ultimately forms the granulation tissue [6]. This matrix functions as a tissue support system, facilitating the migration of more fibroblasts and other cells, such as endothelial cells [7]. Endothelial cells require extracellular matrix (ECM) for migration to promote the formation of new blood vessels from the existing vasculature [2]. The formation of new blood vessels is a critical component of wound healing, with any impairment in the angiogenic response negatively impacting wound repair [8]. Therefore, fibroblasts and endothelial cells must function properly during the proliferation phase to prepare the foundation for the remodeling phase, which ensures tissue healing. Thus, improving the activity of these cells might help promote proper tissue repair and improve impaired healing. Therefore, it is important to identify compounds able to regulate the biological events of cells involved in healing, to develop new drugs aimed towards accelerated wound healing.

Plant-derived products have been used through the ages to treat various pathological processes, including wound healing [9,10]. These compounds induce healing and tissue regeneration through multiple connected mechanisms that often have synergistic effects on the overall efficiency of healing [11]. Amongst the many active components isolated from plants that have healing effects, pentacyclic triterpenes exhibit wound healing properties, mainly because they affect the production and activity of inflammatory mediators and growth factors [12,13].

Uvaol is a pentacyclic triterpene (Figure 1) that is abundant in olives and the leaves of olive trees (*Olea europaea*) [14]. It possesses a wide spectrum of pharmacological effects, including antioxidant [15] and anti-inflammatory activity [12]. In particular, uvaol interferes with allergic inflammatory responses by affecting the recruitment of leukocytes and production of cytokines at the site of inflammation [16]. It also has a vasodilator effect [17], inducing changes to the expression of surface proteins associated with cell adhesion [18]. The broad spectrum of pharmacological properties associated with this compound has resulted in it being targeted as a novel therapeutic agent for various pathological conditions. This broad range of actions indicates that uvaol interacts with diverse targets to achieve its therapeutic effects. However, the mechanism of how uvaol affects cells involved in the wound healing process has yet to be delineated. Here, we evaluated how uvaol affects biological responses of fibroblasts and endothelial cells involved in wound healing, as well its healing potential for cutaneous wounds, in mice.

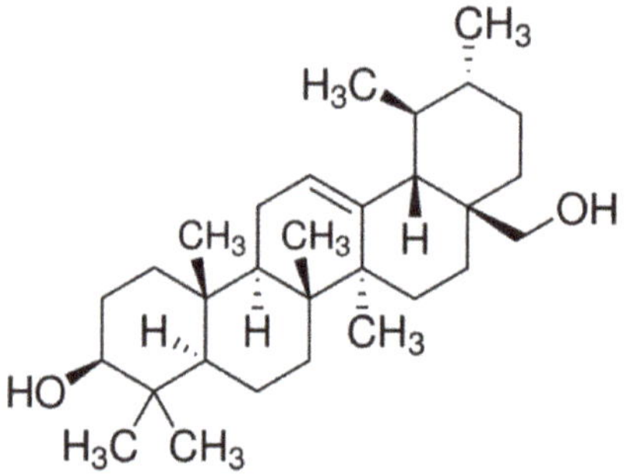

Figure 1. Chemical structure of uvaol.

2. Results

2.1. Effect of Uvaol on Cell Viability

MTT assays were used to evaluate how uvaol affects cell viability, and to ascertain the non-toxic concentration ranges of uvaol to treat cells. There were no significant changes in the viability of fibroblasts and endothelial cells after uvaol treatment with any of the tested doses for 24 h (Figure 2). Thus, we selected the doses of 10 or 50 mM to proceed to the next step, and evaluated their respective effects on cell migration.

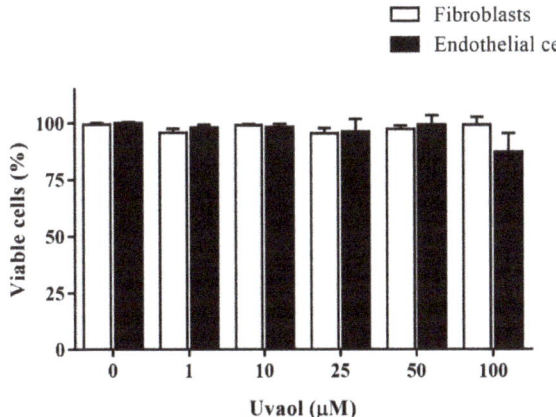

Figure 2. Effect of uvaol on the viability of fibroblast and endothelial cells. Cells were plated and treated with uvaol (1–100 µM) for 24 h. Cell viability was measured by MTT assay. The bars represent the mean ± standard deviation (SD) of three experiments performed in triplicate.

2.2. Effects of Uvaol Treatment on Fibroblast and Endothelial Cell Motility

Scratch assays were used to evaluate how uvaol affected fibroblast and endothelial cell migratory activity. Scratches were made on the monolayer of confluent cells, and were then treated with the respective culture medium (control) or uvaol at concentrations of 10 or 50 µM. Cell migration to the scratch area was evaluated at 0 and 24 h. Compared to DMEM-treated cells (control), only uvaol only at 50 mM concentration accelerated the migration of fibroblasts towards the scratched area (Figure 3A), with a significant wound closure rate of 22% (Figure 3B). Compared to RPMI-treated cells (control), uvaol at both tested concentrations (10 and 50 µM) significantly increased the migration of endothelial cells towards the scratched area (Figure 3C), with significant wound closure rates of 36% and 40%, respectively (Figure 3D). Thus, uvaol directly affects fibroblast and endothelial cells by enhancing their migration.

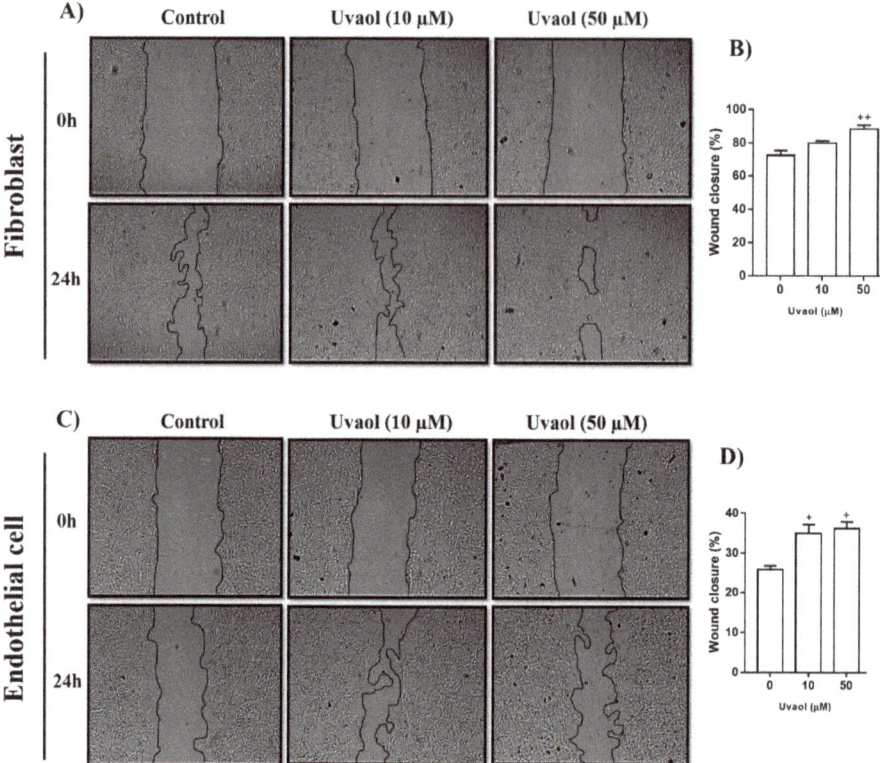

Figure 3. Effect of uvaol on the cell migration of fibroblasts and endothelial cells in the scratch assay. Cells were treated with 10 or 50 µM uvaol, and images were captured to calculate the scratch closure. Representative photomicrography images showing the scratched area of fibroblasts (**A**) and endothelial cells (**B**) treated with medium (control) or uvaol, and cell migration towards the cell-free area after 24 h (magnification 40×). The percentage of the scratch covered was measured by quantifying the total distance that cells moved from the edge of the scratch towards the center of the scratch, using ImageJ software, followed by conversion to a percentage of the wound that was covered (**C,D**). Values represent mean ± SD from three independent experiments. (+) $p < 0.05$ and (++) $p < 0.01$ compared with medium-treated cells after 24 h.

2.3. Effect of Uvaol on ECM Deposition by Fibroblasts

ECM contributes to various functions of cells, including migration. Thus, we evaluated whether uvaol treatment affects ECM protein synthesis. Fibroblasts were exposed for 24 h to uvaol, after which fibronectin, laminin, and collagen type I production was assessed by immunofluorescence analysis. Cells treated with DMEM (control) showed a basal level of fibronectin protein production organized around the cell nucleus (Figure 4A). Treatment with 50 µM uvaol increased the immunofluorescence staining of cytoplasmic fibronectin. Image analysis showed a 30% increase in intracytoplasmic fluorescence, reflecting fibronectin levels after treatment (Figure 4B). A similar phenomenon was observed in the production of laminin. Cells treated with DMEM (control) showed a basal level of laminin production in the cell cytoplasm (Figure 4C). Treatment with 50 µM uvaol increased the immunofluorescence staining of cytoplasmic laminin. Image analysis showed a 36% increase in laminin levels after treatment (Figure 4D). Unlike the proteins laminin and fibronectin, basal collagen type I expression in fibroblasts did not change after treatment with 50 µM uvaol for 24 h (Figure 4E,F).

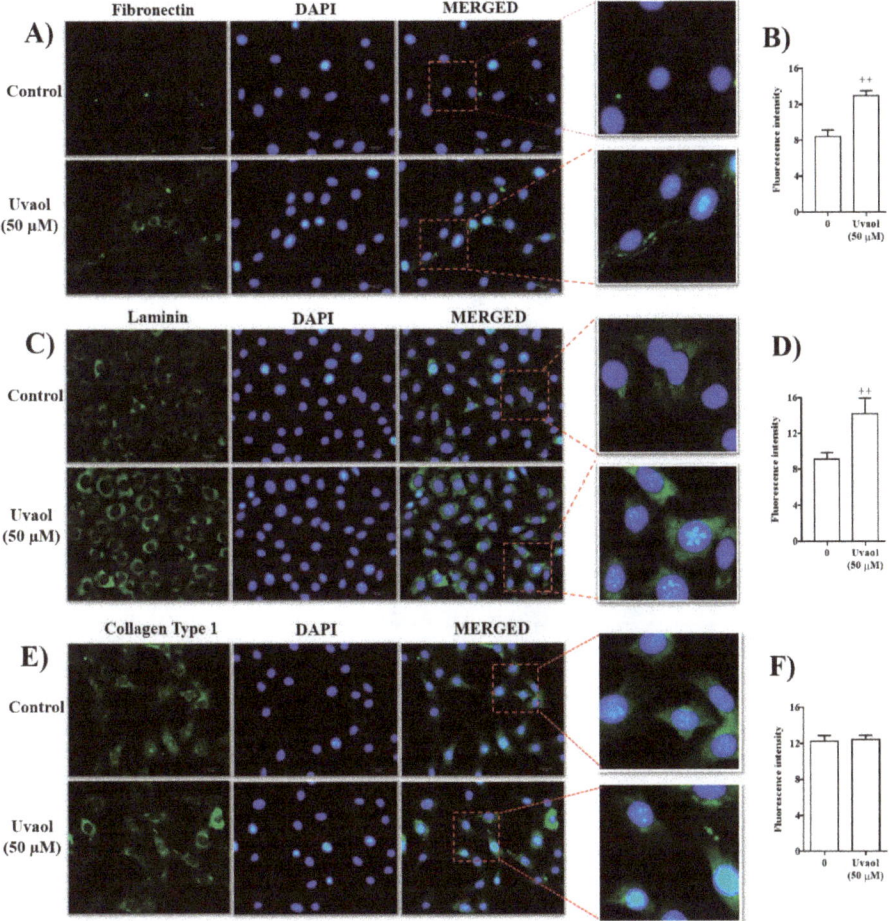

Figure 4. Effect of uvaol on the levels of fibronectin, laminin, and collagen type I in fibroblasts using immunofluorescence analysis. Fibroblasts were cultured with and without 50 μM uvaol. After 24 h, the cells were fixed and the extracellular matrix was immuno-stained using antibodies against fibronectin (**A**), laminin (**C**), and collagen type I (**E**). Nuclei were stained with DAPI. Each panel shows an image of one representative field from three independent experiments. Graph showing the results of the quantification of extracellular matrix synthesis of images from the respective panel (**B,D,F**). The image is displayed at × 400 original magnification and the red box indicates the region acquired for the quantification of extracellular matrix. Bars represent mean ± SD of three independent experiments. Statistical significance between groups was determined by ANOVA followed by Bonferroni's test. (++) $p < 0.01$ compared with respective medium-treated group.

2.4. Uvaol Stimulates Tube-Like Structure Formation In Vitro

To investigate whether uvaol affects endothelial morphogenesis, we employed an in vitro model of tube formation in which t.End1 cells assemble into vessel-like tubes containing lumens. Compared with the medium-treated cells (control), endothelial cells exposed to uvaol (10 μM) for 6 h exhibited an approximately 1.8-fold increase in tube-like structure formation (control) (Figure 5A,B).

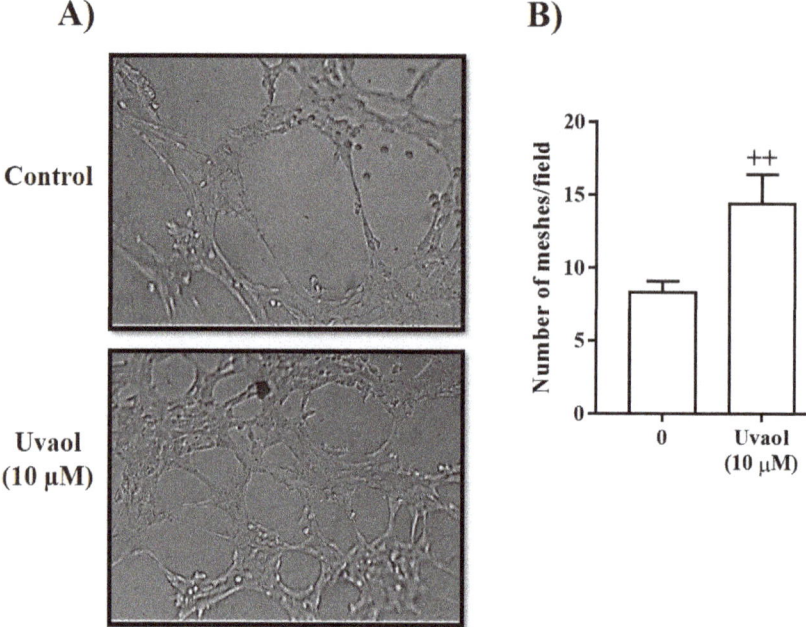

Figure 5. Effect of uvaol on the formation of the tubular network in endothelial cells on Matrigel after 16 h. (**A**) Representative images of tubule-like structures on Matrigel by endothelial cells following 16 h of treatment. The tubes were photographed under the microscope at 200× magnification. (**B**) Analysis of the number of meshes formed after medium or uvaol treatment. Bars represent mean ± SD of three independent experiments. Statistical significance between groups was determined by Student's test. (++) $p < 0.01$ compared with medium-treated cells after 16 h.

2.5. Involvement of the PKA and p38-MAPK Signaling Pathways in Uvaol Induced both Fibroblast and Endothelial Cell Motility

Because PKA and p38-MAPK cellular signaling pathways are associated with cell motility, we evaluated whether the effects of uvaol on motility of fibroblast and endothelial cells involved these protein kinases by using specific inhibitors of intracellular signaling. Compared to DMEM-treated cells (control), uvaol accelerated the migration of fibroblasts towards the scratched area after 24 h, with PKA inhibitor (PKI-(6-22)-amide (10 µM) treatment inhibiting this phenomenon by 25% (Figure 6A,B). Compared to medium-treated cells (control), uvaol accelerated the migration of endothelial cells towards the scratched area after 24 h (Figure 6C). Similar to that observed for fibroblasts, treatment with the PKA inhibitor (PKI-(6-22)-amide (10 µM) inhibited uvaol-induced endothelial cells' migration by 27% (Figure 6D).

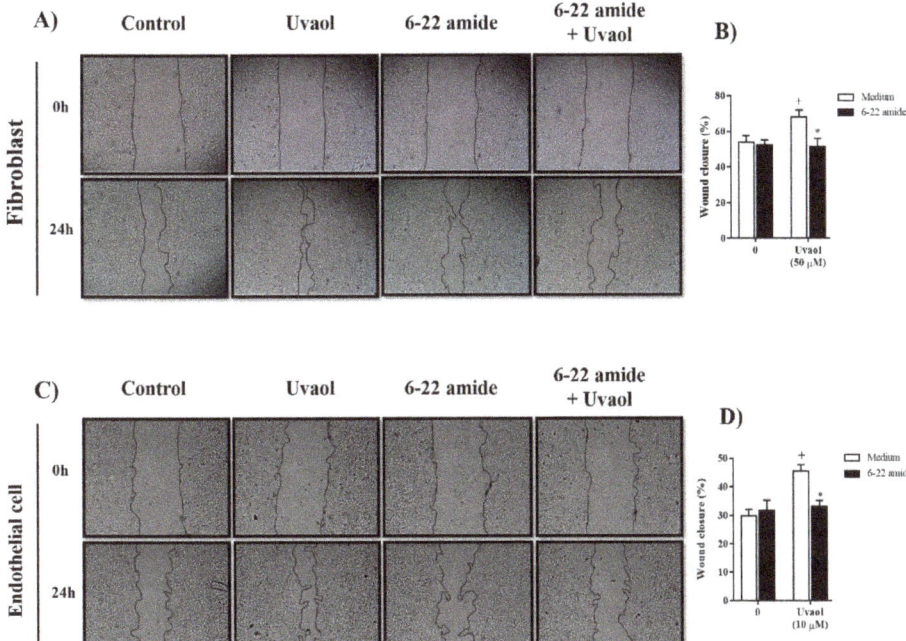

Figure 6. Inhibition of the PKA signaling pathway attenuates the migration of fibroblast and endothelial cells induced by uvaol. Scratch wounds were created in cell monolayers of cells using a sterile pipette tip. Representative photomicrography images showing the scratched area of fibroblasts (**A**) and endothelial cells (**C**) cultured with medium, uvaol or (6-22)-amide (a PKA inhibitor, 10 µM) in the presence of uvaol for 24 h (magnification 40×). The percentage of the scratch covered was measured by quantifying the total distance that cells moved from the edge of the scratch towards the center of the scratch, using ImageJ software, followed by conversion to a percentage of the wound that was covered (**B,D**). The bars represent mean ± SD of three independent experiments. Statistical differences were detected with two-way ANOVA followed by the Bonferroni test. (+) $p < 0.01$ compared to medium-treated cells, (*) $p < 0.05$ compared to uvaol-treated cells.

Compared to medium-treated cells (control), uvaol accelerated the migration of fibroblasts towards the scratched area after 24 h (Figure 7A). Treatment with the p38-MAPK inhibitor (SB203580, 10 µM) did not cause any significant alteration in uvaol-induced fibroblast migration (Figure 7B). However, the accelerated migration of endothelial cells in response to uvaol treatment was significantly inhibited in 37% by the inhibitor for p38-MAPK (Figure 7C,D). Thus, the enhanced migration of endothelial caused by uvaol is associated with both PKA and p38-MAPK signaling pathways. However, uvaol-induced migration in fibroblasts seemed to be dependent on the PKA pathway but not the p38-MAPK signaling pathway.

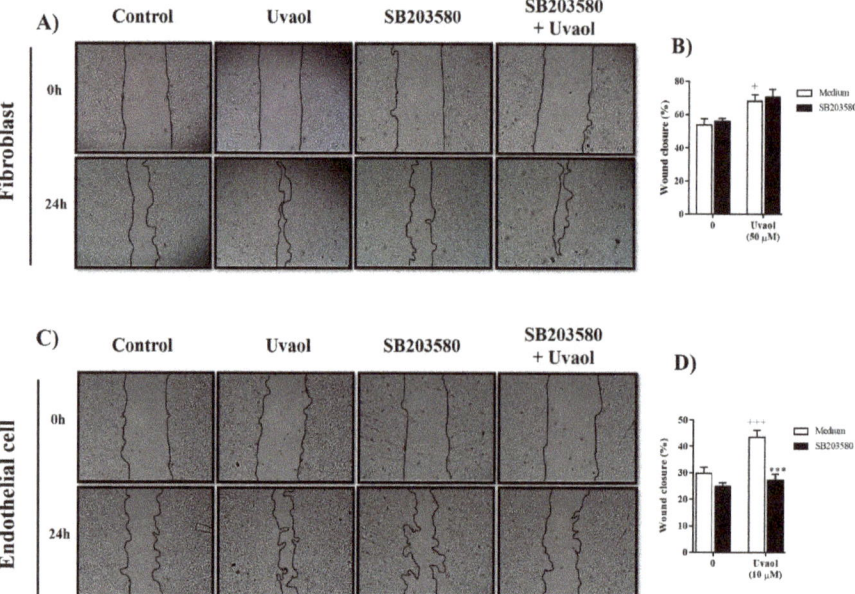

Figure 7. Inhibition of the p38-MAPK signaling pathway suppressed uvaol-improved migration in endothelial cells but not in fibroblasts. Scratch wounds were created in monolayers of cells using a sterile pipette tip. Representative photomicrography images showing the scratched area of fibroblasts (**A**) and endothelial cells (**C**) cultured with medium, uvaol or SB203580 (a p38-MAPK inhibitor, 10 µM) in the presence of uvaol for 24 h (magnification 40×). The percentage of the scratch covered was measured by quantifying the total distance that cells moved from the edge of the scratch towards the center of the scratch, using ImageJ software, followed by conversion to a percentage of the wound that was covered (**B,D**). Bars represent mean ± SD of three independent experiments. Statistical differences were detected with two-way ANOVA followed by the Bonferroni test. (+) $p < 0.01$ and (+++) $p < 0.001$ compared to medium-treated cells, (***) $p < 0.001$ compared to uvaol-treated cells.

2.6. Effects of Uvaol on the In Vivo Wound Healing Assay

During the wound healing process, deposition of the extracellular matrix and angiogenesis are necessary to form a new tissue and accelerate wound closure. Thus, we used the excision wound model to evaluate how uvaol affects wound healing in mice. The progression of healing was evaluated on days 3, 7, and 10 post wounding. The progression of wound closure after topical treatment with vehicle or uvaol (0.1% or 1%) was evaluated. In vehicle-treated animals, the wounded area reduced by 9% (day 3), 19% (day 7), and 35% (day 10) (Figure 8A). After application of 0.1% and 1% uvaol topically, wound area declined by 10% and 18% on day 3, 39% and 40% on day 7, and 59% and 60% on day 10, respectively (Figure 8B). During the healing period, the presence of infections that could extend the time of wound contraction was not detected. Thus, uvaol exhibited healing properties in vivo, in parallel to directly affecting the functioning of fibroblasts and endothelial cells in vitro.

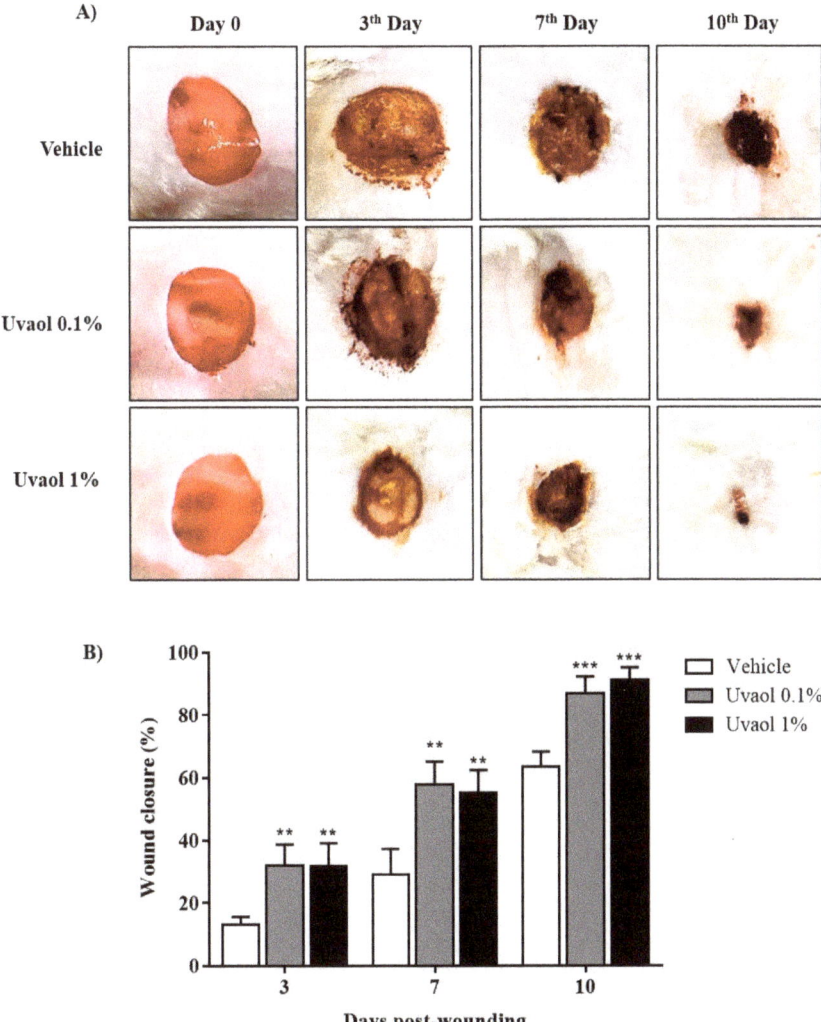

Figure 8. Effect of the topical application of uvaol in the excisional wounds of mice. (**A**) Representative photographs of wounds on days post wounding of animals treated with vehicle (PBS) and uvaol (0.1% or 1%). (**B**) Wound closure kinetics. The bars represent mean ± SD, $n = 5$ for each time point and group. Statistical differences were detected with two-way ANOVA followed by the Bonferroni test. (**) $p < 0.01$ and (***) $p < 0.001$ compared to vehicle-treated cells on each respective day.

3. Discussion

Triterpenes constitute a class of natural compounds that originate from plants that have a wide range of pharmacological effects. Thus, these compounds might be useful for treating various pathological conditions, including cutaneous wounds. During the healing process, certain mechanisms promote the wound healing process, including the migration of cells towards the injury area, the production of the extracellular matrix by fibroblasts, and the formation of new blood vessels by endothelial cells [2,19]. Thus, identifying compounds that improve these processes could lead to the discovery of new and cost-effective drugs for treating wounds. However, to the best of our knowledge, published studies are not available on how uvaol affects the functions of fibroblast and endothelial cells in vitro. Additionally, information remains limited on how uvaol influences cutaneous wound healing. This study demonstrated in vitro that uvaol accelerates cell migration via signaling pathways dependent on both PKA and p38-MAPK. We also demonstrated that it stimulated the production of ECM from fibroblasts, and the formation of tube-like structures from endothelial cells. Moreover, we confirmed that uvaol topical treatment accelerated the healing of cutaneous wounds.

Wound healing is characterized by the production of the extracellular matrix, which is associated with angiogenesis, requiring both fibroblasts and endothelial cells to complete the proliferative and remodeling phases [20]. During the course of the wound healing process, fibroblasts secrete extracellular matrix proteins that help the underlying endothelial cells to proliferate rapidly and migrate to the wound bed to form new vessels and ensure sufficient nutrients and oxygen reach the wound area to form new tissue [21]. Of note, healing is hindered if these cells fail to function, as observed in various non-healing diseases, such as diabetes and chronic venous leg ulcers [22]. Yet, these observations reinforce that stimuli with the ability to improve fibroblast and endothelial cell functions have a positive effect on wound healing [23].

One possible effect of uvaol on the viability of fibroblast and endothelial cells was evaluated to avoid the use of cytotoxic concentrations. We showed that uvaol does not have cytotoxic effects on fibroblasts or endothelial cells after 24 h of exposure at dose ranges of 1 to 100 µM. This result confirms previous studies that demonstrated the absence of toxicity of uvaol to distinct cell types [24]. Of note, uvaol prevents cell death caused by bacterial products [25], and has protector effects against heavy metal-induced cytotoxicity [26].

We subsequently assessed the influence of uvaol on cell migration using a scratch assay. Scratch assays are a standard in vitro methodology routinely used to identify substances that regulate cellular migration [27]. Our results showed that uvaol accelerated the migration of fibroblasts and endothelial cells. Thus, this triterpene directly affects these cells. These results were consistent with previous studies in which another triterpene also enhanced the motility of fibroblast and endothelial cells [28,29]. It is extremely important for these cells to migrate during the granulation tissue formation phase of wound healing [30].

We subsequently evaluated whether uvaol affects cellular events associated with wound healing, such as the deposition of ECM proteins and angiogenesis. Our study showed that the synthesis of fibronectin and laminin is enhanced in uvaol-treated fibroblasts, without impacting the production of type I collagen. Our results supported previous studies, which showed that other triterpenes and natural products, such as ginsenoside and propolis, enhance the synthesis of extracellular matrix proteins [31–33]. Furthermore, a pro-angiogenic effect of uvaol was observed in endothelial cells. In the tube formation assay, uvaol-treated cells clearly enhanced tube formation. This result indicates the potential of uvaol at inducing the formation of new blood vessels from existing vascular structures during angiogenesis. Our findings support previous studies that reported the pro-angiogenic effect of other triterpenes, such as asiaticoside [34], betulinic acid [35], astragaloside IV [36], and lupeol [29]. Overall, our results indicate that uvaol enhances the functions of fibroblasts and endothelial cells, which could be useful for wound healing.

The migration of fibroblast and endothelial cells is mediated by multiple intracellular signaling pathways, including protein kinase A (PKA) and p38-MAPK pathways [37]. Even knowing that uvaol downregulates the AKT/PI3K signaling pathway in cancer cells, such as HepG2 cells [38], knowledge remains limited about the effect of uvaol on signaling pathways of fibroblast and endothelial cells. Thus, to evaluate whether uvaol has an activating effect on these intracellular signaling pathways, we evaluated the migration of fibroblast and endothelial cells using the scratch assay in the presence of inhibitors of distinct signaling pathways. Our study demonstrated that the inhibitor PKI-(6-22)-amide prevented the migration of uvaol-provoked fibroblast and endothelial cells; thus, this PKA signaling pathway is likely involved in uvaol-induced migration. These findings support previous studies, which showed that other triterpenoids, such as ursolic acid [39], astragaloside [40], and fernenediol [41], induce the activation of the PKA pathway to generate their pharmacological effects. Of note, the activation of PKA intracellular signaling pathways upregulates ECM production by fibroblasts, contributing to tube formation and the motility of endothelial cells [42,43]. Our results revealed that the uvaol-induced migration of endothelial cells, but not fibroblasts, was inhibited by the inhibitor SB203580 in the p38-MAPK signaling pathway. Previous studies have already demonstrated that p38-MAPK pathway activity in endothelial cells is important for organizing cells into tube-like structures [44]. Thus, uvaol stimulates the activation of PKA and p38-MAPK signaling pathways in endothelial cells but only in the PKA signaling pathway for fibroblasts.

Wound healing is a dynamic process, composed of a cascade of interlocking biological events, in which the transition from inflammation to subsequent phases may be one of the most critical and defining steps. There is evidence to suggest that persistent inflammation results in upregulation of various proinflammatory cytokines and chemokines, which leads to delay in the wound closure [45]. Additionally, it has been reported that an excessive and prolonged inflammatory phase may be a factor in the conversion of acute wounds into non-healing chronic wounds [46]. Thus, active compounds able to reduce the intensity of the inflammatory response might accelerate the healing process by shortening the inflammatory phase. Previous studies reported that uvaol had shown anti-inflammatory activity by suppressing the secretion of inflammatory cytokines [16,47]. Inhibition of proinflammatory mediators may regulate the progress of cutaneous wound healing and thus represent a good therapeutic target [48]. Therefore, although speculative, the idea of uvaol accelerating wound closure by shortening the inflammatory phase cannot be dismissed. Further studies are necessary to investigate this concept.

This study showed that uvaol exhibits pharmacological effects that improve the functions of both fibroblasts and endothelial cells; thus, we evaluated whether uvaol accelerates the closing of cutaneous wounds. Our macroscopic analysis revealed that the topical application of uvaol promotes the healing of skin wounds by accelerating the closure of lesions from day 7 post-wounding. Based on our results and those of previous studies, uvaol might act by accelerating each phase of the healing process in the wound microenvironmetic of cells. This phenomenon might result in the faster closure of wounds.

In conclusion, the current study demonstrated that uvaol stimulates cellular events in fibroblast and endothelial cells that are critical for wound healing. This stimulatory activity supports the application of uvaol as a therapeutic agent in cutaneous wound healing.

4. Materials and Methods

4.1. Reagents

The following substances, purchased from Sigma Chemical Co. (St. Louis, MO, USA), were used: uvaol (Urs-12-ene-3,28-diol, ≥95% purity, PubChem CID: 92802; Figure 1), Tween-20, eosin, hematoxylin, Dulbecco's Modified Eagle Medium (DMEM), Roswell Park Memorial Institute medium (RPMI-1640), 3-[4,5-dimethylthiazol-2-yl]-2,5-diphenyltetrazolium bromide (MTT), phosphate-buffered saline (PBS) gentamicin, fetal bovine serum (FBS), trypsin, L-glutamine, 4′,6-diamidino-2′-phenylindole dihydrochloride (DAPI), SB203580 (p38-MAPK inhibitor), and (6-22)-amide (inhibitor of PKA). Xylazine (Anasedan®) and ketamine (Dopalen®) from Ceva (Paulínia, São Paulo, BRA), ethylenediaminetetraacetic acid (EDTA) and dimethyl sulfoxide (DMSO) from Synth (Diadema, SP, BRA). Antibodies against laminin, fibronectin, and collagen type I were purchased from Novotec (Bron, Lyon, France), while anti-goat IgG-fluorescein isothiocyanate (FITC) was from Santa Cruz Biotechnology (Dallas, TX, USA). Stock solution of uvaol was prepared in DMSO. The DMSO concentration applied to cells in culture never exceeded 0.1%. Neither the vehicle nor any of the compounds used in this study altered cell viability.

4.2. Cell Culture

The NIH3T3 fibroblast cell line and endothelioma tEnd.1 cell line were provided by Cell Bank of Rio de Janeiro, being maintained in DMEM and RPMI-1640, respectively. Both types of media were supplemented with 10% of heat-inactivated fetal bovine serum (FBS), L-glutamine (2 mM), and gentamicin (40 µg/mL) at 37 °C and in a humidified atmosphere containing 5% CO_2. The assays were performed using cells between three and six passages. In all experiments, untreated cells were used as negative controls.

4.3. Cell Viability Assay

The MTT assay was used to evaluate how uvaol affected cell viability [49]. In brief, NIH3T3 fibroblasts (7×10^3 cells/well) and tEnd.1 cells (10^4 cells/well) were seeded in 96-well plates and treated with uvaol at concentrations of 1, 10, 25, 50, and 100 µM for 24 h. Thereafter, the medium was replaced with fresh medium containing 5 mg/mL MTT (3-(4,5-dimethylthiazol-2-yl)-2,5-diphe-nyltetrazolium bromide). Following incubation (4 h) in a humidified CO_2 incubator at 37 °C and 5% CO_2, the supernatant was discarded and dimethyl sulfoxide solution (DMSO, 150 µL/well) was added to each well to solubilize the formazan crystals that had formed. After incubation at room temperature for 15 min, the optical density (OD) was measured at 540 nm using a spectrophotometer. Three separate wells were assayed for each treatment. The percentage viability relative to the control sample was determined as (OD of treated cells/OD of untreated cells) × 100.

4.4. Scratch Wound Healing Assay

To evaluate how uvaol affects fibroblast motility, we used the scratch assay, as described by [50]. Cells were cultured in a 24-well plate using medium containing 1% FBS, until 90% confluency was reached. Thereafter, a vertical stripe on the cell monolayer was made using a sterile pipette (200 µL) tip. The wells were washed twice with PBS to remove cell debris. Then, uvaol was added at concentrations of 1, 10, and 50 µM. As a control, the cells were treated with DMEM or RPMI containing 1% FBS. A low concentration of serum is the most common non-pharmaceutical method for minimizing proliferation in wound healing assays [51].

In a second set of experiments, the scratched monolayer was treated with the inhibitor of cAMP-dependent protein kinase A (PKA) (fragment (6-22)-amide, 10 µM) or with the inhibitor of p38 mitogen-activated protein kinase (p38-MAPK) (SB203580, 10 µM) 1 h before incubation with uvaol. After 24 h of treatment, the cells were photographed using invert microscopy (Olympus IX70, Tokyo, Japan) with a digital camera to measure wound closure (magnification, 40×). Cell migration was analyzed using ImageJ software (version 1.51k), and was expressed as the percentage of closure of the initial wound (scratch width at time zero) using the following formula: [(scratch width at time 0 − scratch width after an identified culture period)/(scratch width at time 0)] × 100%.

4.5. Immunofluorescence Staining

Fibroblasts (7×10^3) were cultured in 8-well Lab-Tek™ chamber glass slides (Thermo scientific) (Waltham, Massachusetts, USA) with complete medium (DMEM) for 24 h. The medium was then replaced, and the cells were treated with 50 µM uvaol for 24 h. Cells maintained in DMEM under the same conditions were used as controls. After treatment, the cultures were washed with PBS, fixed with 100% methanol for 10 min, and subjected to an indirect immunofluorescence assay, as previously described [52]. In brief, cells were rehydrated in PBS and incubated for 1 h with PBS containing 1% BSA to block non-specific binding. Next, samples were incubated with primary specific anti-fibronectin, anti-laminin, or anti-collagen type I antibodies (1:50) for 1 h in a humidified chamber. They were then washed with PBS, and incubated with appropriate FITC-conjugated secondary antibody (1:200) for 45 min at room temperature. DAPI staining was used to visualize the nuclei. Immuno-stained samples were analyzed by fluorescence microscopy. The staining of each section was analyzed to obtain the mean optical density value (MOD), which represented the fluorescence intensity per pixel [53].

4.6. Tube-Like Structure Formation Assay

The Matrigel-based tube formation assay was used to evaluate the angiogenic potential of uvaol. In brief, 80μL Matrigel solution (BD Biosciences) was applied to 98-well plates 2 h before cell seeding. After matrix formation, endothelial cells (104 cells) were placed on the matrix gel and cultured in the presence or absence of uvaol (10 μM) with RPMI medium containing 2% serum at 37 °C in a 5% CO_2 incubator. After 16 h, the formed network of tubes was visualized at 100× magnification by light microscopy. The number of tube-like structures per field was measured using angiogenesis Analyzer plugin in ImageJ. Each experiment was performed in triplicate. All data analyses were performed in a blinded manner.

4.7. Animals

Experiments were carried out on adult male Swiss mice (25–35 g) obtained from the Federal University of Alagoas (UFAL), Brazil, breeding unit. The animals were maintained with free access to food and water. They were kept at 22–28 °C, with a controlled 12 h light/dark cycle at the Institute of Biological and Health Sciences (UFAL). Experiments were performed during the light phase of the cycle. All experiments were carried out in accordance with institutional guidelines and ethics (License Number 016/2014).

4.8. Mouse Excisional Wound Model

The animals were anesthetized with an intraperitoneal (i.p.) injection of ketamine and xylazine (25 mg/kg, 25 mg/kg). They were shaved at the predetermined site before wounding. Subsequently, the dorsal region was shaved, wiped topically with distilled water, and circular wounds were made using a template of metal circle with a diameter of 1 cm. Animals were housed separately in disinfected cages after recovery from anesthesia. These conditions were maintained throughout the experiments [54]. The animals were then placed in separate cages to avoid any disturbance. Animals were topically treated with 50 μL of saline solution (vehicle, NaCl, 0.9%) or 50 μL of uvaol at 0.1% for 1% for once a day for 10 consecutive days starting from the day of wounding. All animals received topical treatment on the wounds once daily until the end of the experiments.

4.9. Wound Contraction Measurements

Macroscopic evaluation of the wounds was performed using a digital camera on day 0 (before the start of treatment) and on days 3, 7, and 10 after injury. The Optical SteadyShot DSC-W350 digital camera (14.1 megapixels) was positioned at a distance of 15 cm of wound. The data were analyzed using ImageJ software. The wound measurements on various days were expressed as the percentage of wound closure. The values were expressed as percentage values of day 0 measurements, and were calculated by the formula: $[(A0 - AI)/A0 \times 100]$, where A0 is the initial wound area (day 0) and AI is the wound area on days 3, 7, and 10 after the initial wound.

4.10. Statistical Analysis

Data were reported as mean ± standard deviation (SD), and were analyzed using GraphPad Prism software, version 5.0 (San Diego, CA, USA). One-way analysis of variance (ANOVA) followed by the post hoc Bonferroni test multiple comparison test was applied for the comparison among various groups and Student's t test to determine the significance of differences between two means. *p* values less than 0.05 were considered statistically significant.

Author Contributions: Conceptualization, J.C., P.C.-A. and E.B.; methodology, J.S. and A.C.C.; validation, J.F. and E.B.; writing—original draft preparation, J.C. and P.C.-A.; writing—review and editing, E.B. and V.L.; supervision, E.B.; funding acquisition, E.B. All authors have read and agreed to the published version of the manuscript.

Funding: This research was funded by Conselho Nacional de Desenvolvimento Científico e Tecnológico (CNPq), grant number 308898/2018-4.

Acknowledgments: This work was conducted during a scholarship supported by the International Cooperation Program CAPES/COFECUB Foundation at the University of Rennes-FR. Financed by CAPES–Brazilian Federal Agency for Support and Evaluation of Graduate Education within the Ministry of Education of Brazil.

Conflicts of Interest: The authors declare no conflict of interest.

References

1. Sorg, H.; Tilkorn, D.J.; Hager, S.; Hauser, J.; Mirastschijski, U. Skin wound healing: An update on the current knowledge and concepts. *Eur. Surg. Res.* **2017**, *58*, 81–94. [CrossRef]
2. Ammann, K.R.; DeCook, K.J.; Li, M.; Slepian, M.J. Migration versus proliferation as contributor to in vitro wound healing of vascular endothelial and smooth muscle cells. *Exp. Cell Res.* **2019**, *376*, 58–66. [CrossRef] [PubMed]
3. Kanji, S.; Das, H. Advances of stem cell therapeutics in cutaneous wound healing and regeneration. *Mediators Inflamm.* **2017**, *2017*, 5217967. [CrossRef] [PubMed]
4. Li, J.; Wang, J.; Wang, Z.; Xia, Y.; Zhou, M.; Zhong, A.; Sun, J. Experimental models for cutaneous hypertrophic scar research. *Wound Repair Regen.* **2019**, *1*, 126–144. [CrossRef] [PubMed]
5. Boniakowski, A.E.; Kimball, A.S.; Jacobs, B.N.; Kunkel, S.L.; Gallagher, K.A. Macrophage-mediated inflammation in normal and diabetic wound healing. *J. Immunol.* **2017**, *199*, 17–24. [CrossRef] [PubMed]
6. Tracy, L.E.; Minasian, R.A.; Caterson, E.J. Extracellular matrix and dermal fibroblast function in the healing wound. *Adv. Wound Care (New Rochelle)* **2016**, *5*, 119–136. [CrossRef]
7. Bainbridge, P. Wound healing and the role of fibroblasts. *J. Wound Care* **2013**, *22*, 407–408, 410–412.
8. DiPietro, L.A. Angiogenesis and wound repair: When enough is enough. *J. Leukoc. Biol.* **2016**, *100*, 979–984. [CrossRef]
9. Petrovska, B.B. Historical review of medicinal plants' usage. *Pharm. Rev.* **2012**, *6*, 1–5. [CrossRef]
10. Shukla, A.; Rasik, A.M.; Jain, G.K.; Shankar, R.; Kulshrestha, D.K.; Dhawan, B.N. In vitro and in vivo wound healing activity of asiaticoside isolated from Centella asiatica. *J. Ethnopharmacol.* **1999**, *65*, 1–11. [CrossRef]
11. Calixto, J.B. The role of natural products in modern drug discovery. *An. Acad. Bras. Cienc.* **2019**, *91*, e20190105. [CrossRef] [PubMed]
12. Agra, L.C.; Ferro, J.N.; Barbosa, F.T.; Barreto, E. Triterpenes with healing activity: A systematic review. *J. Dermatolog. Treat.* **2015**, *26*, 465–470. [CrossRef]
13. Hill, R.A.; Connolly, J.D. Triterpenoids. *Nat. Prod. Rep.* **2013**, *30*, 1028–1065. [CrossRef] [PubMed]
14. Sanchez-Quesada, C.; Lopez-Biedma, A.; Warleta, F.; Campos, M.; Beltran, G.; Gaforio, J.J. Bioactive properties of the main triterpenes found in olives, virgin olive oil, and leaves of Olea europaea. *J. Agric. Food Chem.* **2013**, *61*, 12173–12182. [CrossRef] [PubMed]
15. Allouche, Y.; Warleta, F.; Campos, M.; Sanchez-Quesada, C.; Uceda, M.; Beltran, G.; Gaforio, J.J. Antioxidant, antiproliferative, and pro-apoptotic capacities of pentacyclic triterpenes found in the skin of olives on MCF-7 human breast cancer cells and their effects on DNA damage. *J. Agric. Food Chem.* **2011**, *59*, 121–130. [CrossRef]
16. Agra, L.C.; Lins, M.P.; da Silva Marques, P.; Smaniotto, S.; Bandeira de Melo, C.; Lagente, V.; Barreto, E. Uvaol attenuates pleuritis and eosinophilic inflammation in ovalbumin-induced allergy in mice. *Eur. J. Pharmacol.* **2016**, *780*, 232–242. [CrossRef]
17. Luna-Vazquez, F.J.; Ibarra-Alvarado, C.; Rojas-Molina, A.; Romo-Mancillas, A.; Lopez-Vallejo, F.H.; Solis-Gutierrez, M.; Rojas-Molina, J.I.; Rivero-Cruz, F. Role of nitric oxide and hydrogen sulfide in the vasodilator effect of ursolic acid and uvaol from black cherry prunus serotina fruits. *Molecules* **2016**, *21*, 78. [CrossRef]
18. Martin, R.; Ibeas, E.; Carvalho-Tavares, J.; Hernandez, M.; Ruiz-Gutierrez, V.; Nieto, M.L. Natural triterpenic diols promote apoptosis in astrocytoma cells through ROS-mediated mitochondrial depolarization and JNK activation. *PLoS ONE* **2009**, *4*, e5975. [CrossRef]
19. Okamoto, T.; Akita, N.; Kawamoto, E.; Hayashi, T.; Suzuki, K.; Shimaoka, M. Endothelial connexin32 enhances angiogenesis by positively regulating tube formation and cell migration. *Exp. Cell Res.* **2014**, *321*, 133–141. [CrossRef]
20. Canedo-Dorantes, L.; Canedo-Ayala, M. Skin acute wound healing: A comprehensive review. *Int. J. Inflam.* **2019**, *2019*, 3706315. [CrossRef]

21. Li, J.; Zhang, Y.P.; Kirsner, R.S. Angiogenesis in wound repair: Angiogenic growth factors and the extracellular matrix. *Microsc. Res. Tech.* **2003**, *60*, 107–114. [CrossRef] [PubMed]
22. Lerman, O.Z.; Galiano, R.D.; Armour, M.; Levine, J.P.; Gurtner, G.C. Cellular dysfunction in the diabetic fibroblast: Impairment in migration, vascular endothelial growth factor production, and response to hypoxia. *Am. J. Pathol.* **2003**, *162*, 303–312. [CrossRef]
23. Hu, Y.; Rao, S.S.; Wang, Z.X.; Cao, J.; Tan, Y.J.; Luo, J.; Li, H.M.; Zhang, W.S.; Chen, C.Y.; Xie, H. Exosomes from human umbilical cord blood accelerate cutaneous wound healing through miR-21-3p-mediated promotion of angiogenesis and fibroblast function. *Theranostics* **2018**, *8*, 169–184. [CrossRef]
24. Somova, L.I.; Shode, F.O.; Mipando, M. Cardiotonic and antidysrhythmic effects of oleanolic and ursolic acids, methyl maslinate and uvaol. *Phytomedicine* **2004**, *11*, 121–129. [CrossRef]
25. Botelho, R.M.; Tenorio, L.P.G.; Silva, A.L.M.; Tanabe, E.L.L.; Pires, K.S.N.; Goncalves, C.M.; Santos, J.C.; Marques, A.L.X.; Allard, M.J.; Bergeron, J.D.; et al. Biomechanical and functional properties of trophoblast cells exposed to Group B Streptococcus in vitro and the beneficial effects of uvaol treatment. *Biochim. Biophys. Acta Gen. Subj.* **2019**, *1863*, 1417–1428. [CrossRef]
26. Miura, N.; Matsumoto, Y.; Miyairi, S.; Nishiyama, S.; Naganuma, A. Protective effects of triterpene compounds against the cytotoxicity of cadmium in HepG2 cells. *Mol. Pharmacol.* **1999**, *56*, 1324–1328. [CrossRef]
27. Jonkman, J.E.; Cathcart, J.A.; Xu, F.; Bartolini, M.E.; Amon, J.E.; Stevens, K.M.; Colarusso, P. An introduction to the wound healing assay using live-cell microscopy. *Cell. Adh. Migr.* **2014**, *8*, 440–451. [CrossRef]
28. Bernabe-Garcia, A.; Armero-Barranco, D.; Liarte, S.; Ruzafa-Martinez, M.; Ramos-Morcillo, A.J.; Nicolas, F.J. Oleanolic acid induces migration in Mv1Lu and MDA-MB-231 epithelial cells involving EGF receptor and MAP kinases activation. *PLoS ONE* **2017**, *12*, e0172574. [CrossRef]
29. Pereira Beserra, F.; Xue, M.; Maia, G.L.A.; Leite Rozza, A.; Helena Pellizzon, C.; Jackson, C.J. Lupeol, a pentacyclic triterpene, promotes migration, wound closure, and contractile effect in vitro: Possible involvement of PI3K/Akt and p38/ERK/MAPK pathways. *Molecules* **2018**, *23*, 2819. [CrossRef]
30. Liu, X.J.; Kong, F.Z.; Wang, Y.H.; Zheng, J.H.; Wan, W.D.; Deng, C.L.; Mao, G.Y.; Li, J.; Yang, X.M.; Zhang, Y.L.; et al. Lumican accelerates wound healing by enhancing alpha2beta1 integrin-mediated fibroblast contractility. *PLoS ONE* **2013**, *8*, e67124.
31. Hashim, P. The effect of Centella asiatica, vitamins, glycolic acid and their mixtures preparations in stimulating collagen and fibronectin synthesis in cultured human skin fibroblast. *Pak. J. Pharm. Sci.* **2014**, *27*, 233–237.
32. Kim, W.K.; Song, S.Y.; Oh, W.K.; Kaewsuwan, S.; Tran, T.L.; Kim, W.S.; Sung, J.H. Wound-healing effect of ginsenoside Rd from leaves of Panax ginseng via cyclic AMP-dependent protein kinase pathway. *Eur. J. Pharmacol.* **2013**, *702*, 285–293. [CrossRef] [PubMed]
33. Maquart, F.X.; Chastang, F.; Simeon, A.; Birembaut, P.; Gillery, P.; Wegrowski, Y. Triterpenes from Centella asiatica stimulate extracellular matrix accumulation in rat experimental wounds. *Eur. J. Dermatol.* **1999**, *9*, 289–296. [PubMed]
34. Phaechamud, T.; Yodkhum, K.; Charoenteeraboon, J.; Tabata, Y. Chitosan-aluminum monostearate composite sponge dressing containing asiaticoside for wound healing and angiogenesis promotion in chronic wound. *Mater. Sci. Eng. C Mater. Biol. Appl.* **2015**, *50*, 210–225. [CrossRef]
35. Li, J.; Bao, G.; E, A.L.; Ding, J.; Li, S.; Sheng, S.; Shen, Z.; Jia, Z.; Lin, C.; Zhang, C.; et al. Betulinic acid enhances the viability of random-pattern skin flaps by activating autophagy. *Front. Pharmacol.* **2019**, *10*, 1017. [CrossRef]
36. Cheng, S.; Zhang, X.; Feng, Q.; Chen, J.; Shen, L.; Yu, P.; Yang, L.; Chen, D.; Zhang, H.; Sun, W.; et al. Astragaloside IV exerts angiogenesis and cardioprotection after myocardial infarction via regulating PTEN/PI3K/Akt signaling pathway. *Life Sci.* **2019**, *227*, 82–93. [CrossRef]
37. Huang, C.; Jacobson, K.; Schaller, M.D. MAP kinases and cell migration. *J. Cell Sci.* **2004**, *117*, 4619–4628. [CrossRef]
38. Bonel-Perez, G.C.; Perez-Jimenez, A.; Gris-Cardenas, I.; Parra-Perez, A.M.; Lupianez, J.A.; Reyes-Zurita, F.J.; Siles, E.; Csuk, R.; Peragon, J.; Rufino-Palomares, E.E. Antiproliferative and pro-apoptotic effect of uvaol in human hepatocarcinoma HepG2 cells by affecting G0/G1 cell cycle arrest, ROS production and AKT/PI3K signaling pathway. *Molecules* **2020**, *25*, 4254. [CrossRef]
39. Ramos-Hryb, A.B.; Cunha, M.P.; Pazini, F.L.; Lieberknecht, V.; Prediger, R.D.S.; Kaster, M.P.; Rodrigues, A.L.S. Ursolic acid affords antidepressant-like effects in mice through the activation of PKA, PKC, CAMK-II and MEK1/2. *Pharmacol. Rep.* **2017**, *69*, 1240–1246. [CrossRef]

40. Wang, Z.; Li, Q.; Xiang, M.; Zhang, F.; Wei, D.; Wen, Z.; Zhou, Y. Astragaloside alleviates hepatic fibrosis function via PAR2 signaling pathway in diabetic rats. *Cell. Physiol. Biochem.* **2017**, *41*, 1156–1166. [CrossRef]
41. Castro, A.J.G.; Cazarolli, L.H.; da Luz, G.; Altenhofen, D.; da Silva, H.B.; de Carvalho, F.K.; Pizzolatti, M.G.; Silva, F. Fern-9(11)-ene-2alpha,3beta-diol Action on insulin secretion under hyperglycemic conditions. *Biochemistry* **2018**, *57*, 3894–3902. [CrossRef]
42. Bodnar, R.J.; Yates, C.C.; Wells, A. IP-10 blocks vascular endothelial growth factor-induced endothelial cell motility and tube formation via inhibition of calpain. *Circ. Res.* **2006**, *98*, 617–625. [CrossRef]
43. Lv, T.; Du, Y.; Cao, N.; Zhang, S.; Gong, Y.; Bai, Y.; Wang, W.; Liu, H. Proliferation in cardiac fibroblasts induced by beta1-adrenoceptor autoantibody and the underlying mechanisms. *Sci. Rep.* **2016**, *6*, 32430. [CrossRef]
44. Ling, G.; Ji, Q.; Ye, W.; Ma, D.; Wang, Y. Epithelial-mesenchymal transition regulated by p38/MAPK signaling pathways participates in vasculogenic mimicry formation in SHG44 cells transfected with TGF-beta cDNA loaded lentivirus in vitro and in vivo. *Int. J. Oncol.* **2016**, *49*, 2387–2398. [CrossRef]
45. Barchitta, M.; Maugeri, A.; Favara, G.; Magnano San Lio, R.; Evola, G.; Agodi, A.; Basile, G. Nutrition and wound healing: an overview focusing on the beneficial effects of curcumin. *Int. J. Mol. Sci.* **2019**, *20*, 1119. [CrossRef]
46. Landen, N.X.; Li, D.; Stahle, M. Transition from inflammation to proliferation: A critical step during wound healing. *Cell. Mol. Life Sci.* **2016**, *73*, 3861–3885. [CrossRef]
47. Du, S.Y.; Huang, H.F.; Li, X.Q.; Zhai, L.X.; Zhu, Q.C.; Zheng, K.; Song, X.; Xu, C.S.; Li, C.Y.; Li, Y.; et al. Anti-inflammatory properties of uvaol on DSS-induced colitis and LPS-stimulated macrophages. *Chin. Med.* **2020**, *15*, 43. [CrossRef]
48. Nguyen, V.L.; Truong, C.T.; Nguyen, B.C.Q.; Vo, T.V.; Dao, T.T.; Nguyen, V.D.; Trinh, D.T.; Huynh, H.K.; Bui, C.B. Anti-inflammatory and wound healing activities of calophyllolide isolated from Calophyllum inophyllum Linn. *PLoS ONE* **2017**, *12*, e0185674. [CrossRef]
49. Da Silva, E.C.O.; Dos Santos, F.M.; Ribeiro, A.R.B.; de Souza, S.T.; Barreto, E.; Fonseca, E. Drug-induced anti-inflammatory response in A549 cells, as detected by Raman spectroscopy: A comparative analysis of the actions of dexamethasone and p-coumaric acid. *Analyst* **2019**, *144*, 1622–1631. [CrossRef]
50. Cardoso, S.H.; de Oliveira, C.R.; Guimaraes, A.S.; Nascimento, J.; de Oliveira Dos Santos Carmo, J.; de Souza Ferro, J.N.; de Carvalho Correia, A.C.; Barreto, E. Synthesis of newly functionalized 1,4-naphthoquinone derivatives and their effects on wound healing in alloxan-induced diabetic mice. *Chem. Biol. Interact.* **2018**, *291*, 55–64. [CrossRef]
51. Davis, P.K.; Ho, A.; Dowdy, S.F. Biological methods for cell-cycle synchronization of mammalian cells. *Biotechniques* **2001**, *30*, 1322–1331. [CrossRef]
52. Smaniotto, S.; de Mello-Coelho, V.; Villa-Verde, D.M.; Pleau, J.M.; Postel-Vinay, M.C.; Dardenne, M.; Savino, W. Growth hormone modulates thymocyte development in vivo through a combined action of laminin and CXC chemokine ligand 12. *Endocrinology* **2005**, *146*, 3005–3017. [CrossRef]
53. Dong, Z.; Zhao, X.; Tai, W.; Lei, W.; Wang, Y.; Li, Z.; Zhang, T. IL-27 attenuates the TGF-beta1-induced proliferation, differentiation and collagen synthesis in lung fibroblasts. *Life Sci.* **2016**, *146*, 24–33. [CrossRef] [PubMed]
54. Agra, I.; Pires, L.L.; Carvalho, P.S.; Silva-Filho, E.A.; Smaniotto, S.; Barreto, E. Evaluation of wound healing and antimicrobial properties of aqueous extract from Bowdichia virgilioides stem barks in mice. *An. Acad. Bras. Cienc.* **2013**, *85*, 945–954. [CrossRef]

Sample Availability: Samples of the compounds are not available from the authors.

Publisher's Note: MDPI stays neutral with regard to jurisdictional claims in published maps and institutional affiliations.

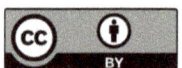

© 2020 by the authors. Licensee MDPI, Basel, Switzerland. This article is an open access article distributed under the terms and conditions of the Creative Commons Attribution (CC BY) license (http://creativecommons.org/licenses/by/4.0/).

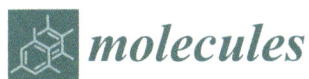

Article

Lasianosides F–I: A New Iridoid and Three New Bis-Iridoid Glycosides from the Leaves of *Lasianthus verticillatus* (Lour.) Merr.

Gadah Abdulaziz Al-Hamoud [1,2], Raha Saud Orfali [1], Yoshio Takeda [3], Sachiko Sugimoto [2], Yoshi Yamano [2], Nawal M. Al Musayeib [1], Omer Ibrahim Fantoukh [1], Musarat Amina [1], Hideaki Otsuka [4] and Katsuyoshi Matsunami [2,*]

1. Department of Pharmacognosy, College of Pharmacy, King Saud University, Riyadh 11495, Saudi Arabia; galhamoud@ksu.edu.sa (G.A.A.-H.); rorfali@ksu.edu.sa (R.S.O.); nalmusayeib@ksu.edu.sa (N.M.A.M.); ofantoukh@ksu.edu.sa (O.I.F.); mamina@ksu.edu.sa (M.A.)
2. Graduate School of Biomedical and Health Sciences, Hiroshima University, 1-2-3 Kasumi, Minami-ku, Hiroshima 734-8553, Japan; ssugimot@hiroshima-u.ac.jp (S.S.); yamano@hiroshima-u.ac.jp (Y.Y.)
3. Faculty of Integrated Arts and Sciences, The University of Tokushima, 1-1 Minamijosanjima-Cho, Tokushima 770-8502, Japan; takeda@ias.tokushima-u.ac.jp
4. Faculty of Pharmacy, Yasuda Women's University, 6-13-1 Yasuhigashi, Asaminami-ku, Hiroshima 731-0153, Japan; otsuka-h@yasuda-u.ac.jp
* Correspondence: matunami1@hiroshima-u.ac.jp; Tel.: +81-82-257-5735

Academic Editors: Pavel B. Drasar and Vladimir A. Khripach
Received: 12 May 2020; Accepted: 15 June 2020; Published: 17 June 2020

Abstract: A series of iridoid glycosides were isolated from the leaves of *Lasianthus verticillatus* (Lour.) Merr., belonging to family Rubiaceae. A new iridoid glycoside, lasianoside F (**1**), and three new bis-iridoid glycosides, lasianosides G–I (**2**–**4**), together with four known compounds (**5**–**8**) were isolated. The structures were established by spectroscopic methods, including 1D and 2D NMR experiments (^{1}H, ^{13}C, DEPT, COSY, HSQC, HMBC, and NOESY) in combination with HR-ESI-MS and CD spectra.

Keywords: Rubiaceae; iridoids; bis-iridoids; *Lasianthus verticillatus*; lasianoside

1. Introduction

Rubiaceae is the fourth-largest angiosperm family, comprising approximately 660 genera and 11,500 species and classified into 42 tribes [1]. Rubiaceae has a long history of investigation on the distribution of iridoid glycoside through its species. These investigations were started by isolation of asperuloside from six plants belonging to the family Rubiaceae, as a characteristic iridoid for this genus [2]. The classification of the occurrence of iridoid glucoside in Rubiaceae subfamilies was initiated by Kooiman 1969 [3]. Later, this classification was approved by investigation of 35 selected Rubiaceae plants by TLC, GC, and GC-MS; the result revealed that asperuloside and deacetylasperulosidic acid occur in most plants of the Rubioideae subfamily, especially in *Lasianthus* species [4]. Previous phytochemical studies on some *Lasianthus* species revealed the presence of iridoids, iridoid glycosides, anthraquinones, and terpenes [5–10]. In our previous study, we isolated a bis-iridoid glycoside from *L. wallichii* for the first time [11] and five undescribed iridane type glycosides, lasianosides A–E, from *L. verticillatus* [12]. These results indicated that the genus *Lasianthus* is a promising rich source in secondary metabolites; however, only limited numbers of *Lasianthus* species have been investigated until now. To continue research of this genus, we performed further phytochemical investigation of the leaves of *L. verticillatus*. As a result, a new iridoid glycoside, lasianoside F (**1**), and three new bis-iridoid glycosides, lasianosides G–I (**2**–**4**) were isolated in this study. The chemical structures were determined by spectroscopic (Figures S1–S41) and chemical analyses, as shown in Figure 1.

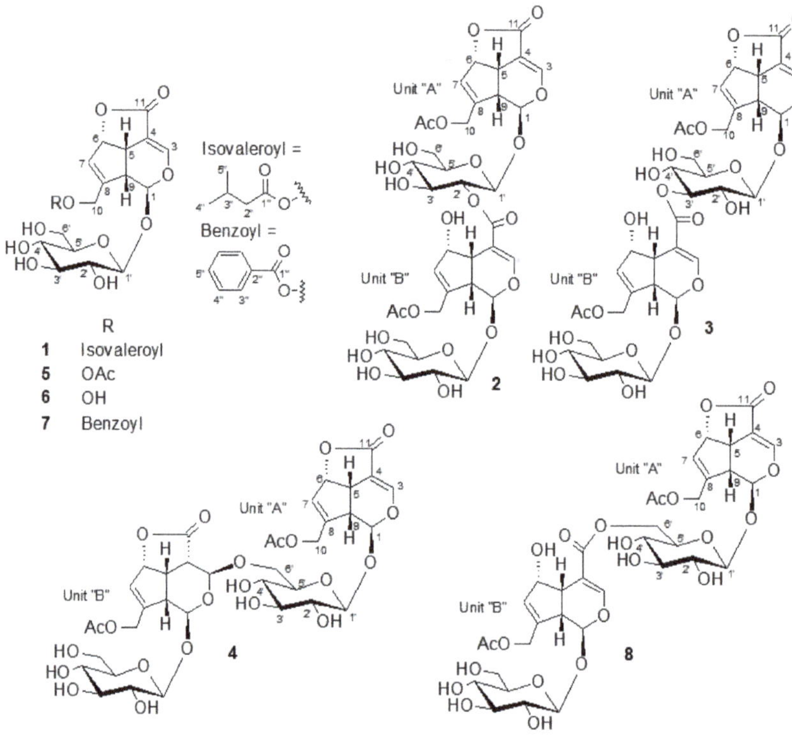

Figure 1. Isolated compounds from *L. verticillatus* (**1**–**8**).

2. Results

2.1. Isolation and Spectroscopic Analyses of the Compounds

The 1-BuOH and EtOAc fractions of methanolic extract of the leaves of *L. verticillatus* were subjected to fractionation by Diaion HP-20 and silica gel column chromatographies, respectively. The resulting fractions were separated on octadecylsilane (ODS) column chromatography, then purified by preparative high-performance liquid chromatography (HPLC) to obtain a new iridoid glycoside (**1**), three new bis-iridoid glycosides (**2**–**4**), in addition to five known compounds: asperuloside (**5**), deacetyl asperuloside (**6**) [13], besperuloside (**7**) [14], and iridoid glycoside dimer (**8**) [6] (Figure 1).

2.1.1. Chemical Structure of Compound 1

Compound (**1**) was obtained as a colorless amorphous powder with a specific optical rotation of $[\alpha]^{22}_D - 65.5$. The molecular formula was deduced to be $C_{21}H_{28}O_{11}$ from HR-ESI-MS (m/z 479.1521 $[M + Na]^+$, calcd for $C_{21}H_{28}O_{11}Na$, 479.1524), which suggested eight degrees of unsaturation. The UV spectrum showed absorption maxima at 234 nm, indicating the presence of an enone system, and IR absorption bands at 3406, 1733, 1658, and 1634 cm^{-1} that corresponded to hydroxy, carbonyl, and olefinic groups. The ^{1}H-NMR spectrum of **1** (Table 1) showed one oxymethylene at δ_H 4.69 and 4.81 ppm, two olefinic protons; one at δ_H 7.32 ppm assigned to conjugated enol ether and the other at δ_H 5.75 ppm, two methines at δ_H 3.70 and 3.31 ppm, two oxymethines at δ_H 5.59 and δ_H 5.98 ppm, one anomeric proton at δ_H 4.70, together with signals of isovaleroyl unit (one methylene at δ_H 2.27ppm, one methine at δ_H 2.09 ppm, and two equivalent methyl signals at δ_H 0.98 ppm). The ^{13}C-NMR spectrum of **1** showed 21 signals, of which six signals could be attributed to a glucopyranosyl unit (δc 100.0, 78.4, 77.9, 74.7, 71.6, and 62.8), ten signals for an iridoid skeleton (δc 37.5, 45.4, 61.7, 86.4, 93.3, 106.2, 129.1, 144.4, 150.4, and 172.6) which were similar to those reported for asperuloside (**5**) [13], and five other signals that contributed to the isovaleroyl unit (δc 22.8 (2C), 26.8, 44.0, 174.2).

Table 1. The ^{13}C and ^{1}H-NMR spectroscopic data for **1**.

Position	δc	δ_H Multi (J in Hz)
1	93.3	5.98 d (1.0)
3	150.4	7.32 d (2.0)
4	106.2	-
5	37.5	3.70 t-like (6.8)
6	86.4	5.59 br dt (6.5, 1.7)
7	129.1	5.75 br t (1.8)
8	144.4	-
9	45.4	3.31 m
10	61.7	4.69 dd (14.4, 1.0) 4.81 dd (14.4, 1.0)
11	172.6	-
1'	100.0	4.70 d (7.9)
2'	74.7	3.22 dd (9.1, 7.9)
3'	77.9	3.40 br t (8.9)
4'	71.6	3.30 m
5'	78.4	3.37 ddd (9.3, 6.0, 2.1)
6'	62.8	3.70 dd (11.8, 6.0) 3.94 dd (11.8, 2.1)
1''	174.2	-
2''	44.0	2.28, 2H, d (7.2)
3''	26.8	2.09 nonet-like (6.8)
4''/5''	22.8	0.98, 6H, d (6.6)

m: multiplet or overlapped signals. (175, 500 MHz, CD$_3$OD, δ in ppm).

The HMBC correlations (Figure 2) from H$_2$-10 (δ_H 4.69 and 4.81) to C-1'' (δc 174.1), and from anomeric proton H-1' (δ_H 4.70) to C-1 (δc 93.3) ascertained the presence of isovaleroyl moiety on C-10 and glucosyl moiety on C-1, respectively. The coupling constant of anomeric proton H-1' (J = 7.9 Hz) indicated β linkage for glucose moiety, while acid hydrolysis of **1** yielded D-glucose that was identified by HPLC analysis with a chiral detector in comparison with authentic D-glucose. The relative configuration of **1** was assigned on the basis of a NOESY experiment (Figure 3). The correlations observed between H-5/H-6 and H-9 suggested β-orientation of H-5, H-6, and H-9. The presence of the correlations of H-1/H-9 and H-1/H-10, and the absence of H-1/H-5 were in good agreement with the proposed structure. The chemical shift values and the coupling patterns of **1** were similar to those of asperuloside (**5**) [13]. The CD spectrum ($\Delta\varepsilon$ = −4.11 at 245 nm) confirmed the absolute configuration of **1** to be the same as asperuloside (**5**). Thus, compound **1** was identified as isovalerate of deacetyl asperuloside, designated as lasianoside F.

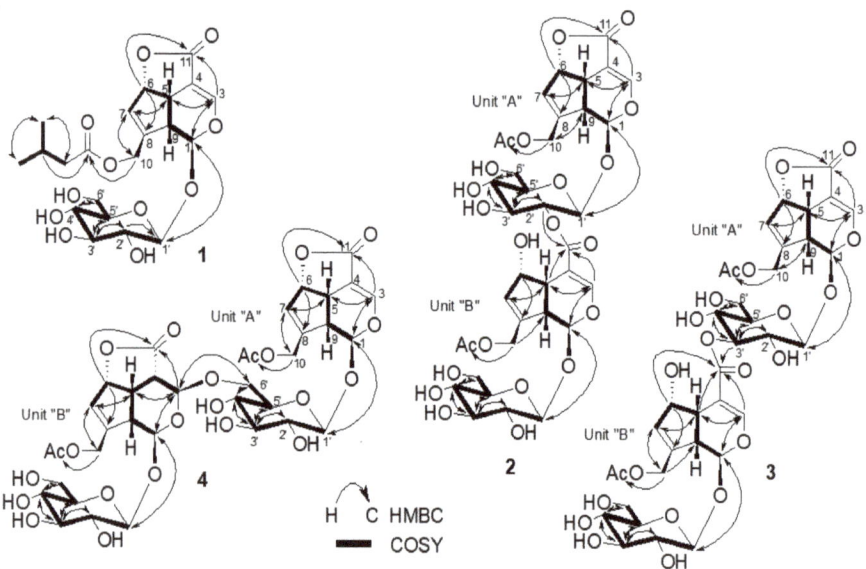

Figure 2. COSY and HMBC correlations of **1**–**4**.

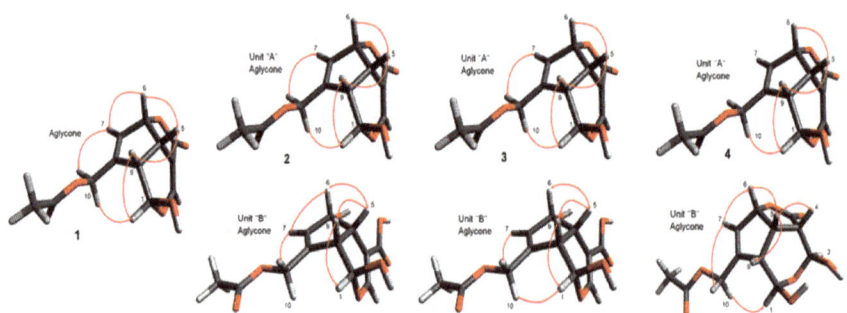

Figure 3. Key NOE correlations of **1**–**4**.

2.1.2. Chemical Structure of Compound 2

Compound (**2**) was isolated as a colorless amorphous powder with a specific optical rotation of $[\alpha]^{22}_D - 55.0$. Its molecular formula $C_{36}H_{44}O_{22}$, from its HR-ESI-MS (m/z 851.2214 [M + Na]$^+$ (calcd for $C_{36}H_{44}O_{22}$Na 851.2216), indicating 15 degrees of unsaturation. The UV spectra of **2** exhibited absorption maxima at 236 nm, characteristic of an enol ether system. Similarly, IR spectra displayed absorption bands corresponding to hydroxy, carbonyl, and olefinic groups at 3309, 1736, 1541 cm^{-1}, respectively. Duplication of the signals in both ^{1}H and ^{13}C-NMR spectra (Tables 2 and 3) of **2** clearly implied the dimeric nature of two iridoid glycosides. The proton signals arising in the region of δ_H 3.27–4.92 in ^{1}H-NMR spectrum including two anomeric protons at δ_H 4.70 (1H, d, J = 7.8 Hz) and 4.92 (1H, d, J = 8.2 Hz) supported the presence of two glucosyl units in **2** (Table 2). Furthermore, two sp^2 methine proton signals at δ_H 7.15 (1H, d, J = 1.9 Hz) and 7.70 (1H, d, J = 1.1 Hz), which are characteristic for C-3 protons confirmed the presence of two iridoid moieties having an enol ether function. Consistent with these observations, the ^{13}C-NMR spectrum showed 36 signals comprising four carbonyl carbons (δ_C 167.6, 172.2, 172.2 and 172.7), eight olefinic carbons (δ_C 106.3, 107.7, 129.1, 131.6, 143.9, 146.5, 150.1 and 156.3), six oxygenated carbons (four methines δ_C 75.2, 86.1, 94.1 and 101.8;

two methylenes δc 61.9 and 63.8), four sp³ methine carbons (δc 37.6, 42.9, 45.1 and 45.9) together with two anomeric carbons (δc 98.7, 100.9) and oxygenated carbons arising in the region of δc 62.7–78.6 belonging to two glucose moieties (Table 3). Thus, the two partial structures of **2** were referred to as units "A" and "B" and determined to be asperuloside (**5**) and asperulosidic acid [5,13], respectively. The 1D and 2D-NMR data of compound **2** were very similar to those of the bis-iridoid glucoside (**8**) that reported in [11]. The only evident difference was observed in the glycosyl part of unit "A", i.e., the lower field shifted H-2′ at δ_H 4.80, and upper field shifted H$_2$-6′, δ_H 3.69 and 3.94 ppm, indicating that **2** was a positional isomer of **8**, and the attachment site between "A" and "B" units was deduced to be at C-2′ of unit "A" via an ester linkage. This assumption was further verified by a correlation from H-2′ (δ_H 4.80) of unit "A" to C-11 (δ_C 167.6) of unit "B" in the HMBC spectrum (Figure 2). Moreover, acid hydrolysis of **2** gave D-glucose, which was identified by HPLC analysis with a chiral detector, while β-anomeric configurations were established from the coupling constant of anomeric protons, 8.2 and 7.8 Hz. The relative and absolute configurations of aglycone parts of **2** were determined to be identical to **5** by comparison of their chemical shift values, coupling constants, NOESY experiment (Figure 3), and CD data. Therefore, the structure of **2** was characterized as shown in Figure 1, named lasianoside G.

Table 2. ^{1}H-NMR data of compounds **2–3** (500 MHz, CD$_3$OD, δ in ppm, J in Hz).

Position	2		3	
	Unit A δ_H Multi (J in Hz)	Unit B δ_H Multi (J in Hz)	Unit A δ_H Multi (J in Hz)	Unit B δ_H Multi (J in Hz)
1	5.86 d (1.4)	5.05 d (9.1)	5.99 br s	5.07 d (9.2)
3	7.15 d (1.9)	7.70 d (1.1)	7.33 br d (1.7)	7.77 br d (1.3)
4	-	-	-	-
5	3.43 m	2.86 ddd (7.1, 5.7, 1.1)	3.69 m	3.12 br t (6.8)
6	5.51 br dt (6.6, 1.6)	4.80 m	5.59 br t (6.2)	4.89 m
7	5.69 br t (1.6)	6.00 br d (1.7)	5.76 br s	6.05 br d (1.9)
8	-	-	-	-
9	3.27 m	2.73 t-like (8.5)	3.36 m	2.72 t-like (8.1)
10	4.62 dd (14.6, 0.9) 4.74 m	4.82 m 4.95 dd (14.8, 0.6)	4.69 br d (14.4) 4.80 m	4.82 m 4.97 br d (15.8)
11	-	-	-	-
10-COCH$_3$	-	-	-	-
10-COCH$_3$	2.05 s	2.09 s	2.10 s	2.10 s
1′	4.92 d (8.2)	4.70 d (7.8)	4.84 m	4.75 d (7.9)
2′	4.80 m	3.27 m	3.44 dd (9.6, 8.1)	3.27 t-like (8.3)
3′	3.67 t-like (9.2)	3.38 m	5.08 t-like (8.6)	3.30 m
4′	3.38 m	3.29 m	3.59 t-like (9.4)	3.28 m
5′	3.45 m	3.29 m	3.51 ddd (9.8, 5.6, 1.9)	3.40 br d (8.8)
6′	3.69 dd (11.9, 6.7) 3.94 dd (11.9, 1.8)	3.61 dd (12.0, 5.6) 3.83 dd (12.0, 1.4)	3.74 m 3.95 dd (11.9, 1.9)	3.63 dd (11.9, 5.8) 3.87 dd (11.9, 1.7)

m: multiplet or overlapped signals.

Table 3. ^{13}C-NMR spectroscopic data for **2** and **3** (125, 175*) MHz, CD$_3$OD, δ in ppm).

Position	2		3 *	
	Unit A	Unit B	Unit A	Unit B
1	94.1	101.8	93.4	101.4
3	150.1	156.3	150.3	156.2
4	106.3	107.7	106.2	108.0
5	37.6	42.9	37.5	42.5
6	86.1	75.2	86.4	75.8
7	129.1	131.6	129.0	131.5
8	143.9	146.5	144.3	146.2
9	45.1	45.9	45.3	46.4
10	61.9	63.8	62.0	63.8
11	172.2	167.6	172.6	168.6
10-COCH$_3$	172.7	172.2	172.4	172.6
10-COCH$_3$	20.6	20.8	20.7	20.8
1′	98.7	100.9	100.0	100.6
2′	74.5	74.9	73.0	74.9
3′	75.6	77.8	78.7	77.9
4′	71.6	71.7	70.0	71.6
5′	78.5	78.6	78.6	78.6
6′	62.7	63.0	62.4	63.0

*: Measured by 175 MHz.

2.1.3. Chemical Structure of Compound 3

Compound (**3**) was obtained as a colorless amorphous powder, with a specific optical rotation of $[\alpha]^{22}_D$ − 59.9. The molecular formula was assigned as C$_{36}$H$_{44}$O$_{22}$ by HR-ESI-MS at *m/z* 851.2212 [M + Na]$^+$ (calcd for C$_{36}$H$_{44}$O$_{22}$ Na 851.2216), indicating that **3** was also another positional isomer of **8**. Comparison of ^{1}H and ^{13}C-NMR data (Tables 2 and 3) showed that the structure of **3** was similar to that of **8**. The significant change occurred in glucose moiety of unit "A", i.e., the chemical shift of H-3′ moved to downfield at δ$_H$ 5.08 ppm, and the chemical shift of H$_2$-6′ moved to upfield at δ$_H$ 3.74 and 3.95 ppm, which suggested that the position of esterification between unit "A" and "B" was changed from H-6′ to H-3′. This suggestion was supported by a correlation between the H-3′ (δ$_H$ 5.08) of unit "A" and C-11(δ$_c$ 168.6) of unit "B" in HMBC spectrum (Figure 2). The structure of this compound was verified by further analysis of 2D-NMR data, including COSY, HSQC, and HMBC spectra. The relative and absolute configurations of aglycone parts of **3** were identical to those of **2** by comparison of their chemical shift values, coupling constants, NOESY experiment (Figure 3), and CD analysis. From these data, the structure of **3** was characterized as shown in Figure 1, designated as lasianoside H.

2.1.4. Chemical Structure of Compound 4

Compound (**4**) was isolated as a colorless amorphous powder, with a specific optical rotation of $[\alpha]^{22}_D$ − 60.1. It has molecular formula of C$_{36}$H$_{44}$O$_{22}$ established from its ^{13}C-NMR data and positive mode HR-ESI-MS [*m/z* 851.2215 [M + Na]$^+$ (calcd for C$_{36}$H$_{44}$O$_{22}$ Na 851.2216)]. The ^{13}C-NMR data showed signals resembling those of **8**, except the presence of two sp^3 methines, C-4 at δc 44.4 and C-3 at 97.4 ppm in unit "B" of **4**, instead of resonances of two olefinic carbons at the same position of **8**, in addition to lower field shift of C-11 and C-6 to δc 176.9 and 87.9 ppm, respectively (Table 4). This change coincided with the disappearance of an enol ether proton signal and the appearance of methine proton at δ$_H$ 3.36 ppm together with oxymethine proton at δ$_H$ 5.27 ppm that correspond to H-4 and H-3 of unit "B", respectively (Table 4). The above data suggested the absence of a double bond between C-3 and C-4 and the presence of γ-lactone ring in the aglycone part of unit "B". The occurrence of γ-lactone was confirmed by HMBC correlation from H-6 (δ$_H$ 5.41) to C-11 (δc 176.9) (Figure 2). A detailed analysis of NMR data (COSY, HSQC, and HMBC) suggested two partial structures in **4**, i.e., asperuloside (**5**) [13] and 3,4-dihydro-3-oxy asperuloside [15]. The attachment between "A" and "B" units was found to be between C-6′ of unit "A" and C-3 of unit "B" via *O*-linkage due to a long-range correlation between H$_2$-6′ of unit "A" (δ_H 3.95 and 4.18) and C-3 of unit "B" (δ_C 97.4) in the HMBC spectrum (Figure 2). HPLC analysis after acid hydrolysis of **4** revealed that the glycosyl units were D-configurations. The relative and absolute configurations of unit "A" were the same as **5** by comparison of NOESY, chemical shifts, and coupling constants. On the other hand, the stereochemistry of part "B" was achieved by NOESY analysis, particularly for those of chiral centers H-4, H-5, H-6, and H-9. In the NOESY spectrum, the correlations between H-5/H-4, H-6, and H-9, indicated β-orientation of H-4, H-5, H-6, and H-9 (Figure 3). The stereochemistry of C-3 in unit "B" was also determined as Figure 1, because of the chemical shift similarity with 3,4-dihydro-3-methoxy asperuloside [15], coupling constants, and the absence of NOE correlation between H-3/H-4,5,9. The CD spectrum showed essentially the same cotton effect as asperuloside (**5**). Base on the above findings, the structure of **4** was assigned as shown in Figure 1, named lasianoside I.

Table 4. The ^{13}C and ^{1}H-NMR spectroscopic data for **4** (175 MHz, 500 MHz, CD$_3$OD, δ in ppm).

Position	Unit A		Unit B	
	δ_C	δ_H multi (J in Hz)	δ_C	δ_H multi (J in Hz)
1	93.5	5.91 d (1.1)	97.0	5.14 d (6.0)
3	150.3	7.33 d (1.9)	97.4	5.27 d (3.6)
4	106.3	-	44.4	3.36 m
5	37.5	3.69 td-like (6.8, 1.8)	37.5	3.47 m
6	86.4	5.59 dt (6.6, 1.4)	87.9	5.41 br d (6.5)
7	128.9	5.75 br s	125.9	6.01 br s
8	144.3	-	152.5	-
9	45.5	3.37 m	46.3	3.05 m
10	61.9	4.68 br dd (14.3, 1.0) 4.79 dd (14.6, 1.2)	62.8	4.68 dd-like (14.3, 1.0) 5.00 br d (15.9)
11	172.6	-	176.9	-
10-COCH$_3$	172.2	-	172.6	-
10-COCH$_3$	20.8	2.13 s	20.8	2.09 s
1′	100.2	4.75 d (8.1)	99.6	4.73 d (8.1)
2′	74.5	3.24 dd (8.9, 8.1)	75.0	3.24 dd (8.9, 8.1)
3′	77.8	3.42 m	77.9	3.43 m
4′	71.2	3.42 m	71.6	3.30 m
5′	76.6	3.57 br dd (9.4, 3.6)	78.4	3.32 m
6′	68.1	3.95 dd (11.7, 1.4) 4.18 dd (11.7, 5.0)	62.8	3.67 dd (11.7, 3.6) 3.88 br d (11.7)

m: multiplet or overlapped signals.

3. Materials and Methods

3.1. General Methods

Optical rotations and CD data were measured with JASCO P-1030 and Jasco J-720 polarimeters (Jasco, Tokyo, Japan), respectively. IR spectra were recorded on Horiba FT-710 Fourier transform infrared (Horiba, Kyoto, Japan), and UV spectra were obtained on Jasco V-520 UV/Vis spectrophotometers. NMR measurements were performed on Bruker Avance 500 and 700 spectrometers, with tetramethylsilane (TMS) as internal standard (Bruker Biospin, Rheinstetten, Germany). Stable conformations were calculated using a Merck Molecular Force Field (MMFF94s). HR-ESI-MS spectra were obtained using LTQ Orbitrap XL mass spectrometer (Thermo Fisher Scientific, Waltham, MA). Diaion HP-20 (Atlantic Research Chemical Ltd., UK), silica gel 60 (230–400 mesh, Merck, Germany), and octadecyl silica (ODS) gel (Cosmosil 75C$_{18}$–OPN (Nacalai Tesque, Kyoto, Japan; Φ = 35 mm, L = 350 mm) were used for column chromatography (CC). Analytical thin-layer chromatography (TLC) was performed on precoated silica gel plates 60 GF$_{254}$ (0.25 mm in thickness, Merck). For visualization of TLC plates, 10% sulfuric acid reagent was used. Isolated compounds were purified by HPLC using an ODS column (Cosmosil 10C$_{18}$-AR, Nacalai Tesque, Kyoto, 10 mm × 250 mm, flow rate 2.5 mL/min) with a mixture of H₂O and MeOH and the eluate was monitored by refractive index and/or a UV detector. After hydrolysis, the sugars were analyzed by HPLC using an amino column (Shodex Asahipak NH2P-50 4E (4.6 mm × 250 mm), CH_3CN-H_2O (3:1) 1mL/min) together with a chiral detector (Jasco OR-2090plus).

3.2. Plant Material

Leaves of *L. verticillatus* were collected in 2000 from Iriomote Island, Okinawa Prefecture, Japan. A voucher specimen of the plant was deposited in the herbarium of the Department of Pharmacognosy, Faculty of Pharmaceutical Sciences, Hiroshima University (IR0009-LT).

3.3. Extraction and Isolation

The air-dried and powdered leaves (7.0 kg) of *L. verticillatus* (Lour.) Merr. were extracted by maceration with MeOH (98 L × 2) and concentrated to 90% MeOH solution, then defatted with 3 L of *n*-hexane. The remaining solution was evaporated and resuspended in 1 L H_2O and extracted by EtOAc (1 L × 3, 46.5 g) and 1-BuOH (1 L × 3, 178.5 g), successively.

A portion of 1-BuOH fraction (124.5 g) was fractionated by Diaion HP-20 column (Φ = 10 cm, L = 60 cm, 2.5 kg), eluting with stepwise MeOH/H_2O gradient (0 to 60% MeOH, 15 L each); similar fractions were grouped together to give 20 fractions (Fr. Lt1–Lt20). The fraction Lt8 (18.8 g) was separated on silica gel CC (Φ = 4.5 cm, L = 50 cm, 400 g), eluting with $CHCl_3$ / MeOH gradient (100:0 to 70:30, 2.5 L each) to obtain 16 fractions (Fr. Lt8.1–Lt8.16). Fractions Lt8.13 (240 mg) was subjected to open reversed phase (ODS) CC with 10% aq. methanol (400 mL) to 100% methanol (400 mL), linear gradient, lead to six fractions (Frs. Lt8.13.1–Lt8.13.6). Purification of Lt8.13.2 (174 mg) by preparative HPLC, 5% aq. methanol, to give compound **6** (30.5 mg). Fraction Lt15 (7.22 g) was proceeded on silica gel CC (Φ = 5.2 cm, L = 38 cm, 350 g), using the gradient mixture of $CHCl_3$/MeOH (100:0 to 70:30, 2.5 L each), to obtain 12 fractions (Frs. Lt15.1–Lt15.12). The residue Lt15.8 (1.88 g) was separated by HPLC, 40% aq. methanol, to provide compounds **8** (42.0 mg) and **2** (31.0 mg). The fraction Lt17 (6.15 g) was further purified by silica gel CC (Φ = 5 cm, L = 40 cm, 380 g), eluting with stepwise $CHCl_3$/MeOH gradient (100:0 to 70:30, 2.4 L each), to obtain 11 fractions (Frs. Lt17.1–Lt17.11). The residue Lt17.5 (282 mg) was further purified by HPLC, 25% aq. acetone, to give compound **1** (13.4 mg), while the other residue Lt17.7 (839 mg) was separated by HPLC, 28% aq. acetone, to obtain compounds **3** (25.0mg) and **4** (13.0). A portion of EtOAc fraction (42.8 g) was chromatographed on silica gel CC (Φ = 5 cm, L = 40 cm, 400 g), eluting with $CHCl_3$ (2.5 L), followed by stepwise $CHCl_3$/MeOH (50:1, 20:1, 15:1, 10:1, 7:1, 5:1, 3:1, 1:1, 2.5 L each), then 100% MeOH (2.5 L), lead ten fractions (Frs. LtE1–LtE10). Each fraction of LtE4 (21.9 g) and LtE6 (22.0 g) was separated by open reversed phase (ODS) CC with 10% aq. methanol (400 mL) to 100% methanol (400 mL), linear gradient, lead eight fractions (Frs. LtE4.1–LtE4.8 and Frs. LtE6.1–LtE6.8, respectively). The residue LtE4.2 (199 mg) was further purified by HPLC, 20% aq. acetone, to provide compound **5** (7.60 mg), while the residue LtE6.4 (262 mg) was purified by HPLC, 35% aq. acetone, to give **7** (5.60 mg).

3.4. Spectroscopic Data of Compounds **1–4**

Lasianoside F (**1**): (2a*S*,4a*S*,5*S*,7b*S*)-4-[(3-methylbutanoyloxy)methyl]-5-(β-D-glucopyranosyloxy)-2a,4a,5,7b-tetrahydro-1H-2,6-dioxacyclopent[cd]inden-1-one. Colorless amorphous powder $[\alpha]^{22}_D$ − 65.5 (c 0.88, MeOH); HR-ESI-MS (positive ion mode): *m/z*: 479.1521 [M + Na]⁺ (calcd for $C_{21}H_{28}O_{11}Na$, 479.1524); CD λ_{max} (c 2.19 × 10⁻⁵ M, MeOH) nm ($\Delta\varepsilon$): 245 (−4.11); UV (MeOH) λ_{max} nm (log ε) 234 (4.04); IR (film) ν_{max}: 3406, 2960, 1733, 1658, 1634, 1292, 1183, 1164, 1077, 1017, 762 cm⁻¹; ¹H-NMR (500 MHz, CD_3OD) and ¹³C (175 MHz, CD_3OD): Table 1.

Lasianoside G (**2**): (2a*S*,4a*S*,5*S*,7b*S*)-4-[[2-*O*-[[(1*S*,4a*S*,5*S*,7a*S*)-7-[(acetyloxy)methyl]-1-(β-D-glucopyranosyloxy)-1,4a,5,7a-tetrahydro-5-hydroxycyclopenta[c]pyran-4-yl]carbonyl]-β-D-glucopyranosyl]oxy]-2a,4a,5,7b-tetrahydro-1H-2,6-dioxacyclopent[cd]inden-1-one. Colorless amorphous powder [α]^{22}$_D$ − 55.0 (c 0.10, MeOH); HR-ESI-MS (positive ion mode): *m/z*: 851.2214 [M + Na]$^+$ (calcd for C$_{36}$H$_{44}$O$_{22}$Na, 851.2216); CD λ$_{max}$ (c 2.35 × 10^{-5} M, MeOH) nm (Δε): 235 (−8.04); UV (MeOH) λ$_{max}$ nm (log ε) 236 (4.10); IR (film) ν$_{max}$: 3309, 2925, 1736, 1716, 1541, 1260, 1162, 1057, 1033, 669 cm^{-1}; ^{1}H-NMR (500 MHz, CD$_3$OD) and ^{13}C (175 MHz, CD$_3$OD): Tables 2 and 3.

Lasianoside H (**3**): (2a*S*,4a*S*,5*S*,7b*S*)-4-[(acetyloxy)methyl]-5-[[3-*O*-[[(1*S*,4a*S*,5*S*,7a*S*)-7-[(acetyloxy) methyl]-1-(β-D-glucopyranosyloxy)-1,4a,5,7a-tetrahydro-5-hydroxycyclopenta[c]pyran-4-yl]carbonyl]-β-D-glucopyranosyl]oxy]-2a,4a,5,7b-tetrahydro-1H-2,6-dioxacyclopent[cd]inden-1-one. Colorless amorphous powder [α]^{22}$_D$ − 59.9 (c 1.38, MeOH); HR-ESI-MS (positive ion mode): *m/z*: 851.2212 [M + Na]$^+$ (calcd for C$_{36}$H$_{44}$O$_{22}$Na, 851.2216); CD λ$_{max}$ (c 1.41 × 10^{-5} M, MeOH) nm (Δε): 245 (−5.73); UV (MeOH) λ$_{max}$ nm (log ε) 235 (4.31); IR (film) ν$_{max}$: 3388, 2932, 1730, 1658, 1632, 1261, 1158, 1075, 1044, 788 cm^{-1}; ^{1}H-NMR (500 MHz, CD$_3$OD) and ^{13}C (175 MHz, CD$_3$OD): Tables 2 and 3.

Lasianoside I (**4**): (2a*S*,4a*S*,5*S*,7b*S*)-4-[(acetyloxy)methyl]-5-[[6-*O*-[[(2a*R*,4a*S*,5*R*,7*S*,7a*S*,7b*S*)-4-[(acetyloxy)methyl]-5-(β-D-glucopyranosyloxy)-2a,4a,5,7,7a,7b-hexahydro-1H-2,6-dioxacyclopenta [cd]inden-1-one-7-yl]]-β-D-glucopyranosyl]oxy]-2a,4a,5,7b-tetrahydro-1H-2,6-dioxacyclopent[cd]inden-1-one. Colorless amorphous powder [α]^{22}$_D$ − 60.1 (c 1.38, MeOH); HR-ESI-MS (positive ion mode): *m/z*: 851.2215 [M + Na]$^+$ (calcd for C$_{36}$H$_{44}$O$_{22}$Na, 851.2216); CD λ$_{max}$ (c 1.14 × 10^{-5} M, MeOH) nm (Δε): 245 (−3.48); UV (MeOH) λ$_{max}$ nm (log ε) 234 (4.23); IR (film) ν$_{max}$: 3407, 2927, 1739, 1658, 1254, 1175, 1070, 1052, 1017, 758 cm^{-1}; ^{1}H-NMR (500 MHz, CD$_3$OD) and ^{13}C (175 MHz, CD$_3$OD): Table 4.

Asperuloside (**5**): Colorless amorphous powder, [α]^{24}$_D$ − 170.6 (c 0.32, MeOH); HR-ESI-MS (positive ion mode): *m/z*: 437.1053 [M + Na]$^+$ (calcd for C$_{18}$H$_{22}$O$_{11}$Na, 437.1054); ^{13}C-NMR (175 MHz, CD$_3$OD) δ$_C$: 20.6 (CH$_3$-CO-), 37.4 (C-5), 45.3 (C-9), 61.9 (C-10), 62.8 (C-6′), 71.6 (C-4′), 74.6 (C-2′), 77.9 (C-5′), 78.4 (C-3′), 86.3 (C-6), 93.3 (C-1), 100.0 (C-1′), 106.2 (C-4), 128.9 (C-7), 144.3 (C-8), 150.3 (C-3), 172.3 (C-11), 172.6 (CH$_3$-CO-).

Deacetyl asperuloside (**6**): Colorless amorphous powder, [α]^{24}$_D$ − 125.4 (c 0.62, MeOH); HR-ESI-MS: *m/z*: 395.0946 [M + Na]$^+$ (calcd for C$_{16}$H$_{20}$O$_{10}$Na 395.0948); ^{13}C-NMR (175 MHz, CD$_3$OD) δ$_C$: 37.5 (C-5), 45.0 (C-9), 60.1 (C-10), 62.8 (C2-6′), 71.6 (C-4′), 74.6 (C-2′), 77.9 (C-5′), 78.4 (C-3′), 86.7 (C-6), 93.3 (C-1), 99.3 (C-1′), 106.5 (C-4), 125.7 (C-7), 149.8 (C-8), 150.3 (C-3), 172.9 (C-11).

Besperuloside (**7**): Colorless amorphous powder, [α]^{25}$_D$ − 109.8 (c 0.38, MeOH); HR-ESI-MS: *m/z*: 499.1210 [M + Na]$^+$ (calcd for C$_{23}$H$_{24}$O$_{11}$Na 499.1211); ^{13}C-NMR (175 MHz, CD$_3$OD) δ$_C$: 37.4 (C-5), 45.0 (C-9), 62.6 (C-10), 62.7 (C-6′), 71.5 (C-4′), 74.6 (C-2′), 77.9 (C-5′), 78.4 (C-3′), 86.3 (C-6), 93.4 (C-1), 100.0 (C-1′), 106.2 (C-4), 129.4 (C-7), 129.7 (C-3″, 5″), 130.7 (C-2″, 6″), 130.9 (C-1″), 134.6 (C-4″), 144.3 (C-8), 150.3 (C-3), 165.9 (C-7″), 172.9 (C-11).

Compound (**8**): Colorless amorphous powder, [α]^{24}$_D$ − 52.5 (c 0.58, MeOH); HR-ESI-MS: *m/z*: 851.2216 [M + Na]$^+$ (calcd for C$_{36}$H$_{44}$O$_{22}$Na 851.2216); ^{13}C-NMR (175 MHz, CD$_3$OD) δ$_C$: 20.8, 20.8 (each CH$_3$-CO-), 37.4 (C-5A), 42.8 (C-5B), 45.2 (C-9A), 46.3 (C-9B), 61.9 (C-10A), 62.9 (C-6′B), 63.8 (C-10B), 64.4 (C-6′A), 71.5 (C-4′A), 71.7 (C-4′B), 74.6 (C-2′A), 74.9 (C-2′B), 75.5 (C-6B), 75.8 (C-5′A), 77.6 (C-5′B), 77.8 (C-3′A), 78.5 (C-3′B), 86.4 (C-6A), 93.2 (C-1A), 99.9 (C-1′A), 100.5 (C-1′B), 101.4 (C-1B), 106.3 (C-4A), 108.1 (C-4B), 129.2 (C-7A), 131.8 (C-7B), 144.1 (C-8A), 146.0 (C-8B), 150.2 (C-3A), 155.8 (C-3B), 168.6 (C-11B), 172.2 (C-11A), 172.6 (2 × CH$_3$-CO-).

3.5. Acid Hydrolysis

Each compound (2 mg) was refluxed individually in 1 M HCL (1.0 mL) at 80 °C for 3 h. The solution was neutralized with Amberlite IRA96SB (OH$^-$ form), then it was filtered. The filtrate was evaporated and partitioned between EtOAc: H$_2$O mixture (1:1). The aqueous layer was analyzed by HPLC with an amino column [Ashipak NH2P-50 4E, CH$_3$CN-H$_2$O (3:1), 1mL/min] and a chiral detector (JASCO OR-2090plus). The peak that appeared at t_R 8.15 min (positive optical sign) supported the presence of D-glucose in the structures of iridoid glucosides (**1**–**4**) [12].

4. Conclusions

In summary, the chemical composition of the leaves of *L. verticillatus* was further investigated to lead the isolation of a new iridoid glycoside, lasianoside F (**1**) and three new bis-iridoid glycosides, lasianosides G–I (**2**–**4**), together with four known compounds (**5**–**8**). The structures of isolated compounds (**1**–**8**) were characterized by physical and spectroscopic data analyses, including one-dimensional (1D) and two-dimensional (2D) NMR, IR, UV, and high-resolution electrospray ionization mass spectra (HR-ESI-MS). The absolute configuration of the new compounds was determined by acid hydrolysis and the analysis of the CD cotton effect.

Supplementary Materials: Supplementary Materials are available online, Figures S1–S41: HR-ESI-MS, ^{1}H, ^{13}C-NMR, DEPT, COSY, HSQC, HMBC, UV, and IR spectra of **1**–**4**.

Author Contributions: Conceptualization, Y.T., H.O., and K.M.; Data curation, G.A.A.-H. and R.S.O.; Funding acquisition, H.O. and K.M.; Investigation, G.A.A.-H. and Y.T.; Methodology, S.S. and Y.Y.; Project administration, R.S.O., M.A., and K.M.; Resources, Y.T. and H.O.; Supervision, K.M.; Validation, S.S., N.M.A.M. and O.I.F.; Writing—original draft, G.A.A.-H.; Writing—review and editing, G.A.A.-H., R.S.O., N.M.A.M., O.I.F., M.A. and K.M. All authors have read and agreed to the published version of the manuscript.

Funding: This work was supported in part by the King Saud University External Joint Supervision Program (EJSP), Kingdom of Saudi Arabia, and by Grants-in-Aid from the Ministry of Education, Culture, Sports, Science and Technology of Japan, and the Japan Society for the Promotion of Science (Nos. 17K15465, 17K08336, and 18K06740).

Acknowledgments: The measurements of HR-ESI-MS and NMR were performed with LTQ Orbitrap XL spectrometer and JEOL ECA500 at the Natural Science Center for Basic Research and Development (N-BARD), Hiroshima University. The other experimental facilities and useful suggestions for publication of this work was kindly supported by a grant from the 'Research Center of the Female Scientific and Medical Colleges', Deanship of Scientific Research, King Saud University.

Conflicts of Interest: The authors report no conflicts of interest.

References

1. Robbrecht, E.; Manen, J.F. The major evolutionary lineages of the coffee family (Rubiaceae, angiosperms). Combined analysis (nDNA and cpDNA) to infer the position of Coptosapelta and Luculia, and supertree construction based on rbcL, rps16, trnLtrnF and atpB-rbcL data. A new classification in two subfamilies, Cinchonoideae and Rubioideae. *Syst. Geogr. Plants* **2006**, *76*, 85–146.
2. Briggs, L.H.; Nicholls, G.A. Chemistry of the coprosma genus VIII. The occurrence of asperuloside. *J. Chem. Soc.* **1954**, *1954*, 3940–3943. [CrossRef]
3. Kooiman, P. The occurrence of asperulosidic glycosides in the Rubiaceae. *Acta Bot. Neerl.* **1969**, *18*, 124–137. [CrossRef]
4. Inouye, H.; Takeda, Y.; Nishimura, H.; KANOMI, A.; Okuda, T.; Puff, C. Chemotaxonomic studies of Rubiaceous plant containing iridoid glycosides. *Phytochemistry* **1988**, *27*, 2591–2598. [CrossRef]
5. Yang, D.; Zhang, C.; Liu, X.; Zhang, Y.; Wang, K.; Ceng, Z. Chemical constituents and antioxidant activity of *Lasianthus hartii*. *Chem. Nat. Compd.* **2017**, *53*, 390–393. [CrossRef]
6. Li, B.; Lai, X.W.; Xu, X.H.; Yu, B.W.; Zhu, Y. A new anthraquinone from the root of *Lasianthus acuminatissimus*. *Yao Xue Xue Bao* **2007**, *42*, 502–504. [PubMed]
7. Li, B.; Zhang, D.M.; Luo, Y.M.; Chen, X. Three new antitumor anthraquinone glycosides from *Lasianthus acuminatissimus* Merr. *Chem. Pharm. Bull.* **2006**, *54*, 297–300. [CrossRef] [PubMed]
8. Li, B.; Zhang, D.M.; Luo, Y.M. A new sesquiterpene lactone from roots of *Lasianthus acuminatissimus*. *Yao Xue Xue Bao* **2006**, *41*, 426–430. [PubMed]
9. Li, B.; Zhang, D.M.; Luo, Y.M. Chemical constituents from root of *Lasianthus acuminatissimus* I. *Zhongguo Zhong Yao Za Zhi* **2006**, *31*, 133–135. [PubMed]
10. Dallavalle, S.; Jayasinghe, L.; Kumarihamy, B.M.M.; Merlini, L.; Musso, L.; Scaglioni, L. A new 3,4-*seco*-lupane derivative from *Lasianthus gardneri*. *J. Nat. Prod.* **2004**, *67*, 911–913. [CrossRef] [PubMed]
11. Takeda, Y.; Shimidzu, H.; Mizuno, K.; Inouchi, S.; Masuda, T.; Hirata, E.; Shinzato, T.; Aramoto, M.; Otsuka, H. An iridoid glucoside dimer and a non-glycosidic iridoid from the leaves of *Lasianthus wallichii*. *Chem. Pharm. Bull.* **2002**, *50*, 1395–1397. [CrossRef] [PubMed]

12. Al-Hamoud, G.A.; Orfali, R.S.; Perveen, S.; Mizuno, K.; Takeda, Y.; Nehira, T.; Masuda, K.; Sugimoto, S.; Yamano, Y.; Otsuka, H.; et al. Lasianosides A–E: New iridoid glucosides from the leaves of *Lasianthus verticillatus* (Lour.) Merr. and their antioxidant activity. *Molecules* **2019**, *24*, 3995. [CrossRef] [PubMed]
13. Otsuka, H.; Yoshimura, K.; Yamasaki, K.; Cantoria, M.C. Isolation of 10-O-Acyl Iridoid glucosides from a Philippine medicinal plant, *Oldenlandia corymbose* L. (Rubiaceae). *Chem. Pharm. Bull.* **1991**, *39*, 2049–2052. [CrossRef]
14. Taskova, R.M.; Gotfredsen, C.H.; Jensen, S.R. Chemotaxonomy of Veroniceae and its allies in the Plantaginaceae. *Phytochemistry* **2006**, *67*, 286–301. [CrossRef] [PubMed]
15. Podanyi, B.; Kocsis, A.; Szabo, L.; Reid, R.S. An NMR study of the solution conformation of two asperuloside derivatives. *Phytochemistry* **1990**, *29*, 861–866. [CrossRef]

Sample Availability: Samples of the compounds **1–8** are available from the authors.

© 2020 by the authors. Licensee MDPI, Basel, Switzerland. This article is an open access article distributed under the terms and conditions of the Creative Commons Attribution (CC BY) license (http://creativecommons.org/licenses/by/4.0/).

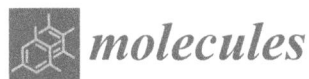

Article

Atypical Lindenane-Type Sesquiterpenes from *Lindera myrrha*

Thuc-Huy Duong [1], Mehdi A. Beniddir [2], Nguyen T. Trung [3], Cam-Tu D. Phan [3], Van Giau Vo [4,5], Van-Kieu Nguyen [6,7], Quynh-Loan Le [8], Hoang-Dung Nguyen [8,9,*] and Pierre Le Pogam [2,*]

1. Department of Chemistry, University of Education, 280 An Duong Vuong Street, District 5, Ho Chi Minh City 700000, Vietnam; huydt@hcmue.edu.vn
2. Équipe "Pharmacognosie-Chimie des Substances Naturelles", BioCIS, Université Paris-Sud, CNRS, Université Paris-Saclay, 5 Rue J.-B. Clément, 92290 Châtenay-Malabry, France; mehdi.beniddir@universite-paris-saclay.fr
3. Laboratory of Computational Chemistry and Modelling (LCCM), Quy Nhon University, Quy Nhon City 55100, Vietnam; nguyentientrung@qnu.edu.vn (N.T.T.); phandangcamtu@qnu.edu.vn (C.-T.D.P.)
4. Bionanotechnology Research Group, Ton Duc Thang University, Ho Chi Minh City 700000, Vietnam; vovangiau@tdtu.edu.vn
5. Faculty of Pharmacy, Ton Duc Thang University, Ho Chi Minh City 700000, Vietnam
6. Institute of Fundamental and Applied Sciences, Duy Tan University, Ho Chi Minh City 700000, Vietnam; nguyenvankieu2@duytan.edu.vn
7. Faculty of Natural Sciences, Duy Tan University, Da Nang 550000, Vietnam
8. Institute of Tropical Biology, Vietnam Academy of Science and Technology, Ho Chi Minh City 700000, Vietnam; lqloan@itb.ac.vn
9. NTT-High tech Institute, Nguyen Tat Thanh University, Ho Chi Minh City 700000, Vietnam
* Correspondence: dung0018034@yahoo.com (H.-D.N.); pierre.le-pogam-alluard@universite-paris-saclay.fr (P.L.P.)

Academic Editors: Pavel B. Drasar and Vladimir A. Khripach
Received: 30 March 2020; Accepted: 13 April 2020; Published: 16 April 2020

Abstract: Two new lindenane sesquiterpenes were obtained from the roots of *Lindera myrrha*. These compounds were structurally elucidated by HRMS data, extensive NMR analyses, and comparison between experimental and theoretical ^{13}C-NMR data. Myrrhalindenane A is the first monomeric seco-D lindenane displaying a non-rearranged, cyclohexanic C-ring. Myrrhalindenane B is the second occurrence of an angular lindenane-sesquiterpene related to a C_6-C_7 lactonization.

Keywords: *Lindera*; sesquiterpene; lindenane; DFT-NMR

1. Introduction

Lindera is a core genus of the Litseeae tribe of the Lauraceae family [1]. Many *Lindera* plants are of salient economical interest for soap and lubricant manufacturing (especially *Lindera communis* and *Lindera glauca*) owing to their elevated fatty oil content, while others are used to produce fragrances, species, and even building timber. As to ethnopharmacological claims, *Lindera aggregata* is included in various preparations of the Chinese Pharmacopoeia for treating urinary system diseases and inflammatory-related health hazards [2]. Other plants are also used in folk medicine such as *Lindera umbellate*, which is endowed with antispasmodic properties and has beneficial effects on gastric ulcers, cholera, and beriberi [3]. Fueled by the diverse interests lying in these plants, a wealth of skeletons were reported to have occurred in this well-studied family, the most represented of which include sesquiterpenes (mainly lindenanes, eudesmanes, and germacranes), and aporphine alkaloids, along with some typical α-methylene-γ-butyrolactones collectively known as butanolides, and a few emblematic polysubstituted cyclopentanediones designated as lucidones [2]. Within this thoroughly studied genus, *Lindera myrrha* (Lour.) Merr., a small shrub common in central Vietnam, long remained unstudied. Conducted in 1994, the first phytochemical investigation dedicated to this species led to the isolation of a suite of aporphine alkaloids, including a new noraporphine, oduocine; and a new oxaporphine, oxoduocine [4]. A novel dihydroisocoumarin, lindermyrrhin, was further described from *L. myrrha* [5], but as far as can be ascertained, its terpene content remained unstudied. With this in mind, our study focused on the sesquiterpenes of *L. myrrha* roots, leading to the isolation of two new structures: myrrhalindenanes A and B. The structures of the isolated compounds **1** and **2** were elucidated by the interpretation of their spectroscopic data and by comparison with those described in the literature.

2. Results and Discussion

Compounds **1** and **2** were isolated from the methanol extract of *L. myrrha* by repeated chromatographic fractionations, including column chromatography, size-exclusive column chromatography, and preparative TLC.

Compound **1** was isolated as a white, amorphous solid. Its molecular formula was determined to be $C_{15}H_{18}O_4$ from its HRESIMS ion at *m/z* 285.1090 [M + Na]$^+$ (calculated for $C_{15}H_{18}O_4Na$, 285.1097). The ^{13}C-NMR spectrum, along with HSQC data, exhibited 15 signals for carbons consisting of one carbonyl, one carboxyl, two olefinic quaternaries, an oxygenated tertiary carbon, an olefinic methine, an exo-methylene, three methines, and a quaternary carbon (Table 1). These functionalities accounted for 4 indices of H deficiency, defining the tricyclic scaffold of **1** (Figure 1). The ^{1}H-^{1}H correlation spectroscopy spectrum of **1** showed a proton spin system of a 1,2-disubstituted cyclopropane ring (δ_H 1.46 (H-1); δ_H 0.71/1.52 (H$_2$-2); and δ_H 2.00 (H-3)) (Supplementary Materials). These structural features were evocative of a lindenane-type sesquiterpene [6]. The cautious analysis of the 2D-NMR spectra revealed a polycyclic framework embedded with a sterically congested cyclopentane, as deduced from the HMBC correlations from the angular methyl group at δ_H 1.13 (H$_3$-14) to the carbons resonating at δ_C 31.1 (C-1), δ_C 76.5 (C-5), and δ_C 51.2 (C-9), and from the exo-methylene that was located at C-4 based on long-range heteronuclear crosspeaks between the olefinic protons at δ_H 4.99/5.17 (H$_2$-15) to C-3 (δ_C 23.4) and C-5 (δ_C 76.5). The chemical shift of the isolated diastereotopic methylene group at δ_H 2.31/2.39 (each 1H, d, *J* = 15.5 Hz) hinted at it being vicinal to a carbonyl function. This tentative assignment was supported by the HMBC crosspeak from H$_2$-9 to the carbon resonating at δ_C 197.7 (C-8). Altogether, these spectroscopic data left no choice but to introduce a $\Delta^{6,7}$ moiety. The C-6 location of the olefinic proton was validated based on the HMBC correlations from H-6 to C-5, the quaternary olefinic carbon resonating at δ_C 163.1 (C-7), and to C-8. In the end, the C-9 location of the side chain was established owing to the HMBC correlations from the methine at δ_H 3.50 (H-11) to both C-7 and C-8. This methine was deduced to have been substituted by a methyl and a carboxylic acid group based on (i) the COSY crosspeak between this and the methyl protons at δ_H 1.13 (CH$_3$-14), and (ii) the HMBC correlation from these methyl protons to both C-7 and the carbon resonating at δ_C 174.0 (C-12). These spectroscopic features determined the planar structure of **1**, namely myrrhalindenane A, as indicated in Figure 2. The NOESY correlations between H$_2$-2 and H$_3$-14 determined their synfacial orientation. Aside from the doubts regarding C-5 configuration, the absolute configuration assignment of C-11 represented a vexing problem in its achiral environment. These spectroscopic features led us to consider four different stereochemical arrangements, as indicated in Figure 3. DFT-NMR chemical shift calculations and the subsequent DP4 probability method [7] were performed on these different candidates. This DP4 application demonstrated the structural equivalence of **1** with diastereoisomer 1C with 88.8% probability (Figure 3).

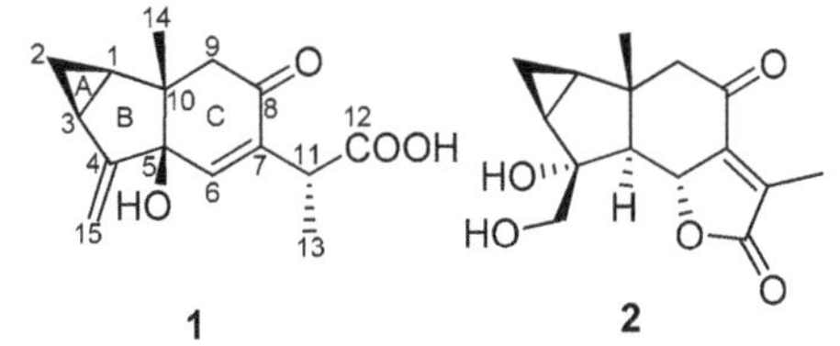

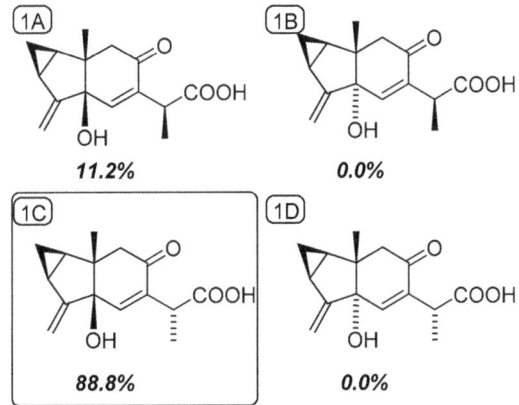

Figure 1. Chemical structures of compounds 1 and 2.

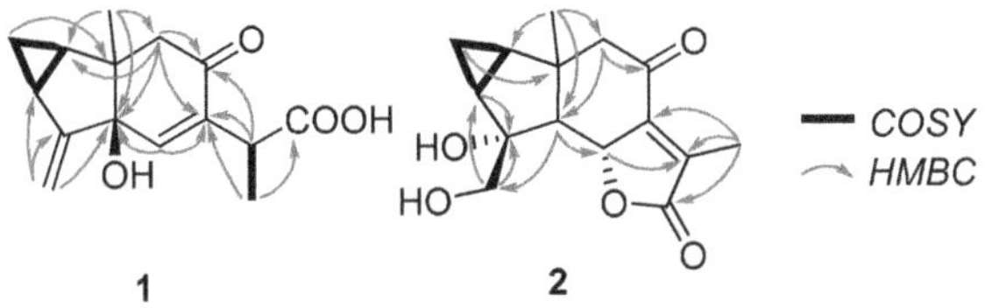

Figure 2. COSY and key HMBC correlations of compounds 1 and 2.

Figure 3. Chemical structures of the four possible diastereoisomers of compound 1 along with their respective DP4 probabilities.

Table 1. ^{13}C- and ^{1}H-NMR spectroscopic data (125/500 MHz) for 1–2 in acetone-d_6 (δ in ppm).

	1		2	
	δ_C	δ_H (J, Hz)	δ_C	δ_H (J, Hz)
1	31.1	1.46, 1H, m	29.1	1.49, 1H, m
2	13.3	1.52, 1H, m 0.71, 1H, m	12.3	1.36, 1H, m 0.70, 1H, m
3	23.4	2.00, 1H, m	28.7	1.87, 1H, m
4	155.9	-	80.1	-
5	76.5	-	63.8	2.27, 1H, d, 12.0
6	145	6.65, 1H, s	78.4	5.03, 1H, dq, 12.0, 2.0
7	136.1	-	154.6	-
8	197.7	-	197.7	-
8	150	-	148.7	-
9	51.2	2.39, 1H, d, 15.5 2.31, 1H, d, 15.5	56.5	2.67, 1H, d, 16.0 2.62, 1H, d, 16.0
10	50.8	-	41.4	-

Table 1. Cont.

	1		2	
	δ_C	δ_H (J, Hz)	δ_C	δ_H (J, Hz)
11	38.9	3.50, 1H, q, 7.0	132.1	-
12	174	-	173.9	-
13	16.6	1.26, 3H, d, 7.0	9.8	1.92, 3H, s
14	18.3	1.13, 3H, s	21.9	1.11, 3H, s
15	109	5.17, 1H, s 4.99, 1H, s	68.2	3.67, 1H, d, 10.5 3.80, 1H, d, 10.5

Compound **2** was obtained as a white, amorphous solid. Its molecular formula, $C_{15}H_{18}O_5$, was established from the sodiated ion peak at *m/z* 301.1047 (calculated for $C_{15}H_{18}O_5Na$), differing from compound **1** by an additional oxygen atom. Notwithstanding their common lindenane core, the NMR data revealed some salient structural differences between these compounds. The ^{13}C-NMR data revealed the lack of the exo-methylene moiety and the loss of the olefinic proton although a tetrasubstituted double bond could be identified. In line with this latter point, the downfield ^{1}H chemical shift of the signal related to the methyl CH_3-13 (δ_H 1.92 vs. 1.26), combined with the shielding of the corresponding carbon (δ_C 9.8 vs. 16.6) were evocative of its location on a double bond [8]. Conversely, the ^{1}H-NMR spectrum displayed further signals corresponding to a tertiary methine at δ_H 2.27 (1H, d, *J* = 12.5 Hz), coupled with an oxygenated methine at δ_H 5.03 (1H, d, *J* = 12.5 Hz). Likewise, an additional set of oxygenated diastereotopic methylene at δ_H 3.80/3.67 could be identified, as well as a new tertiary oxygenated methine at δ_C 80.1. Along with the unchanged carbonyl moieties at δ_C 197.7 and 173.9, these functionalities represented three indices of hydrogen deficiency, determining the tetracyclic appendage of **2**. The oxygenated methylene could be located at C-4 based on the long-range heteronuclear correlations from these protons to C-3 (δ_C 28.7), C-4 (δ_C 80.1), and C-5 (δ_C 63.8). The joint HMBC correlations from the methyl protons at δ_H 1.11 and of the diastereotopic methylene signals at δ_H 2.62/2.67 (each 1H, d, *J* = 16 Hz) to the carbon resonating at δ_C 63.8, validated the occurrence of a methine at this specific position (C-5). The chemical shift of C-4 (δ_C 80.1) defined the presence of a hydroxy group on it. Such B-ring structures are recurrent within lindenane sesquiterpenes, falling into the third subtype defined by Du [9]. The tetracyclic core of **2**, and the unchanged chemical shifts of both C-8 and C-9 left no possibility but to introduce an additional α-methyl-$\Delta^{\alpha,\beta}$-γ lactone fused ring at C-6/C-7. This assumption was validated by the correlations from the olefinic-located methyl at δ_H 2.27 to the quaternary carbons C-7 (δ_C 154.6) and C-11 (δ_C 132.1), to the carbonyl-type carbon C-12 (δ_C 173.9), and from the oxymethine proton H-6 to C-11. These spectroscopic data were fully consistent with those of formerly reported sesquiterpene lactones [10,11]. The antiperiplanar orientation of H-5 and H-6 could be determined from the magnitude of the coupling constant value (*J* = 11.5 Hz) [11]. Having in mind, i) the consensual trans arrangement of the hydrindane system in lindenane sesquiterpenes, and ii) the antifacial orientations of H-5 and H-6, only left the configuration of C-4 pending assignment [12,13]. A preferred configuration for C-4 prevails with a β-OH group and an α-oxygenated methylene moiety, so that Du's lindenane sesquiterpene subtypes define the absolute configuration of this stereocenter [9]. Nevertheless, exceptions were reported throughout literature [11,14,15], so assigning the configuration of these positions based solely on biosynthetic considerations is not a relevant approach to reliably establish the configuration of such compounds. To remedy this, DFT-NMR calculations and subsequent ^{13}C-NMR data comparison of the two possible epimers against the experimental data set, resulted in the prediction of diastereoisomer **2A** with 100% probability (Figure 4).

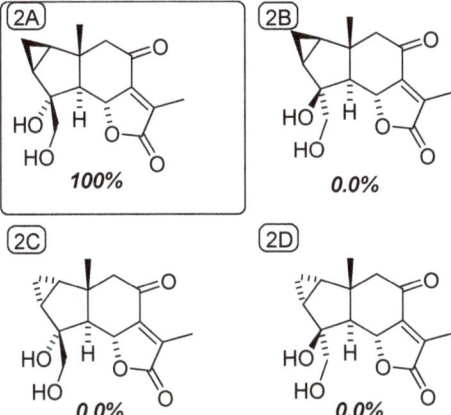

Figure 4. Chemical structures of the four possible diastereoisomers of compound 2 along with their respective DP4 probabilities.

Compounds **1** and **2** were found to be unstable on storage. After three days at room temperature, both had undergone ca. 70% decomposition to yield a mixture of products. The minute amounts of compound precluded any further repurification attempt. In these conditions, the recorded ECD spectra provided no clear-cut match, irrespective of the absolute configuration used in TDDFT. This observation is in line with precedents having outlined the inherent instability of lindenane ring system [16,17], which was occasionally reported in the course of former phytochemical investigations [18]. Despite the lack of spectroscopic evidence, the consensual β-orientation of both the methyl and cyclopropyl functions not only in *Lindera* species [2], but also within the Chloranthaceae plants that produce a much higher number of these sesquiterpenes [19,20], gave strong support to the preferred absolute configuration depicted in Figure 1.

The determined A/B ring substitution pattern of myrrhalindenane A is common among lindenane sesquiterpenes, falling into the lindenane sesquiterpenoid subtype I, as defined by Du and co-workers [9]. Conversely, the occurrence of oxygenated substituents at C-5 is rather uncommon among lindenane sesquiterpenes, since this position is often substituted by an α-disposed hydrogen atom, or is unsaturated due to either a $\Delta^{4,5}$ or a $\Delta^{5,6}$ function [13]. A few structures were however reported to contain an oxygenated substituent at C-5 such as sarcandralactone A, which revealed a 5β-OH group [21] or the dimeric sarcandrolide F that exhibits a 5β-OOH group [22]. The side chain located at C-7 can be assumed to arise from the hydrolysis of a 2-methyl-2-butyrolactone or a 2-methylbutyrolactone D ring related to the canonical lindenane skeleton. Only a few seco-D lindenanes have been reported to date. Some such compounds were formerly described in the *Lindera* species as strychnilactone [23], lindenanolide G [24], and linderagalactones B and C [25]. Nevertheless, all these structures undergo later rearrangement to afford a α-pyrone C-ring, therefore differing from the currently reported carbon skeleton. These compounds also differ from **1** by the constant occurrence of a $\Delta^{7,11}$ moiety. Remarkably, a wealth of seco D-lindenanes were reported within lindenane sesquiterpenoid [4 + 2] dimers, especially from the *Sarcandra* species, e.g., sarcandrolides [22,26]; and various *Chloranthus* plant species such as shizukaol species [27–29], chlorahololides [30,31], spicachloranthins E and F [32], and chlorajaponilides [33], among many others. The biosynthesis of dimeric lindenane sesquiterpenes is deemed to proceed via a Diels–Alder reaction with $\Delta^{4,15}$ and $\Delta^{5,6}$ representing the diene reactive unit [34]. Furyldiene lindenanes and, more generally speaking, molecules displaying these structural features rendering them prone to undergoing Diels–Alder addition, seem to be too unstable to be isolable [9]. This inherent reactivity towards dimerization most likely accounts for **1** being the first reported seco D-lindenane monomer, which can be readily related to its $\Delta^{6,7}$ function that prevents it from dimerizing. Lindermyrrhin B (**2**) is the second example of a 3/5/6/5 tetracyclic lindenane-type sesquiterpene lactone formed at C-6 and C-7, with the first such occurrence being reported from *Xanthium sibericum* (Asteraceae) [11].

3. Materials and Methods

3.1. General

The NMR spectra were measured on a Bruker Avance III (500 MHz for ^{1}H-NMR and 125 MHz for ^{13}C-NMR, Bruker, Bremen, Germany) spectrometer with TMS as internal standard. Chemical shifts are expressed in ppm with reference to the residual protonated solvent signals (acetone-d6 with δ_H 2.05, δ_C 206.26, and 29.84) or the internal TMS (0.00). The HR–ESI–MS were recorded on a HR–ESI–MS Bruker microOTOF Q-II (Bremen, Germany). TLC was carried out on precoated silica gel 60 F254 or silica gel 60 RP-18 F254S (Merck, Darmstadt, Germany), and spots were visualized by spraying with 10% H_2SO_4 solution followed by heating. Gravity column chromatography was performed with silica gel 60 (0.040–0.063 mm, Himedia, Mumbai, India).

3.2. Plant Material

The roots of *Lindera myrrha* were collected from Cu Chi District, Ho Chi Minh City, in July 2016. The botanical sample was authenticated by Dr. Pham Van Ngot, Department of Botany, Faculty of Biology, Ho Chi Minh University of Pedagogy. A voucher specimen (No UP-B05) was deposited in the herbarium of the Department of Organic Chemistry, Faculty of Chemistry, Ho Chi Minh University of Education.

3.3. Extraction and Isolation

Roots of *Lindera myrrha* (7.5 kg) were extracted by maceration with MeOH (3 × 20 L) at ambient temperature for 4 h each. The filtrated solution was evaporated to dryness under reduced pressure to obtain a crude extract (420 g). This extract was subsequently reextracted using solvents of increasing polarities, *n*-hexane-EtOAc (1:1) (HA, 72.1 g), and EtOAc (EA, 125.8 g). The latter was applied to normal phase silica gel CC, and isocratically eluted with a solvent system of *n*-hexane-EtOAc-acetone (1:1:1) to afford fraction EA1 (8.1 g). Continuous elution of the column with EtOAc-acetone (1:1), EtOAc-MeOH (8:2), and EtOAc-MeOH (5:5) afforded four fractions, namely EA2 (4.2 g), EA3 (13.6 g), EA4 (7.8 g), and EA5 (40.4 g), respectively.

Fraction EA1 (8.1 g) was rechromatographed on column chromatography, to be isocratically eluted with a $CHCl_3$-EtOAc-acetone-AcOH (100:40:25:1) solvent system to afford subfractions EA1.1 (2.03 g), EA1.2 (2.53 g), EA1.3 (1.22 g), and EA1.4 (1.8 g). Among these, subfraction EA1.3 was submitted to Sephadex LH-20 column chromatography, eluted with MeOH to afford three sub-fractions EA1.3.1 (0.7 g), EA1.3.2 (0.3 g), and EA1.3.3 (0.2 g). Fraction EA1.3.2 was further purified by preparative TLC using *n*-hexane-$CHCl_3$-EtOAc-acetone-AcOH (1:1:2:2:0.02) as eluent to afford compounds **1** (3.1 mg) and **2** (1.1 mg).

Myrrhalindenane A (**1**). White amorphous solid. ^{1}H- and ^{13}C-NMR (see Table 1); HRESIMS *m/z* 285.1090 [M + Na]$^+$ (calculated for $C_{15}H_{18}O_4Na$, 285.1103).

Myrrhalindenane B (**2**). White amorphous solid. ^{1}H- and ^{13}C-NMR (see Table 1); HRESIMS *m/z* 301.1047 [M + Na]$^+$ (calculated for $C_{15}H_{18}O_5Na$, 301.1052).

3.4. Computational Details

All DFT calculations were carried out using Gaussian 09 software package [35]. The stable conformations were optimized at B3LYP/6-311++G(2d,2p) level of theory, as confirmed by the absence of imaginary frequencies at the same level. Theoretical ^{13}C-NMR chemical shifts were deduced from the isotropic magnetic shielding tensors by using gauge-independent atomic orbital (GIAO) methodology at B3LYP/6-311+G(d,p) [36–38]. The DP4 probabilities were performed using online implementation available from http://www-jmg.ch.cam.ac.uk/tools/nmr/DP4/ [7].

4. Conclusions

The investigation of the so-far unstudied terpenic content of *Lindera myrrha* afforded two novel monomeric lindenanes. Despite the elevated number of such metabolites formerly reported to occur in Lauraceae and Chloranthaceae, these two compounds display unusual structural features. Among these, the combination of a native cyclohexanic C ring and of a seco-D cycle, unprecedented within monomeric lindenanes reported so far, is particularly worth being stressed out.

Supplementary Materials: The following are available online. ^{1}H- and ^{13}C-NMR spectra, HMBC spectra, and HRMS spectra for **1** and **2**; atomic coordinates of the lowest-energy conformers of the four candidate diastereoisomers of **1** and **2**.

Author Contributions: V.G.V. and T.-H.D. conceived and designed the experiments; V.G.V. and T.-H.D. performed the isolation work; T.-H.D., V.-K.N., and P.L.P. analyzed NMR data; N.T.T., C.-T.D.P., M.A.B., and P.L.P. designed and performed the DFT-NMR calculations; P.L.P., M.A.B., and T.-H.D. wrote the manuscript. All the authors reviewed and validated the present manuscript prior to its being submitted. All authors have read and agreed to the published version of the manuscript.

Funding: This research was funded by the Vietnam National Foundation for Science and Technology Development (NAFOSTED) under grant number 106-NN.02-2016.32.

Acknowledgments: We would like to thank Khanh-Binh Mai from the Department of Chemistry, University of Pittsburgh, for giving precious advice on DP4 probability.

Conflicts of Interest: The authors declare no conflict of interest.

References

1. Zhao, M.-L.; Song, Y.; Ni, J.; Yao, X.; Tan, Y.-H.; Xu, Z.-F. Comparative chloroplast genomics and phylogenetics of nine *Lindera* species (Lauraceae). *Sci. Rep.* **2018**, *8*, 8844. [CrossRef]
2. Cao, Y.; Xuan, B.; Peng, B.; Li, C.; Chai, X.; Tu, P. The genus *Lindera*: a source of structurally diverse molecules having pharmacological significance. *Phytochem. Rev.* **2016**, *15*, 869–906. [CrossRef]
3. Tanaka, H.; Ichino, K.; Ito, K. A novel flavanone, linderatone, from *Lindera umbellata*. *Chem. Pharm. Bull. (Tokyo)* **1985**, *33*, 2602–2604. [CrossRef]
4. Phan, B.-H.; Seguin, E.; Tillequin, F.; Koch, M. Aporphine alkaloids from *Lindera myrrha*. *Phytochemistry* **1994**, *35*, 1363–1365. [CrossRef]
5. Duong, T.-H.; Nguyen, V.-K.; Nguyen-Pham, K.-T.; Sichaem, J.; Nguyen, H.-D. Lindermyrrhin, a novel 3,4-dihydroisocoumarin from *Lindera myrrha* roots. *Nat. Prod. Res.* **2019**, 1–6. [CrossRef] [PubMed]
6. Hayashi, N.; Komae, H. Chemistry and distribution of sesquiterpene furans in Lauraceae. *Biochem. Syst. Ecol.* **1980**, *8*, 381–383. [CrossRef]
7. Smith, S.G.; Goodman, J.M. Assigning Stereochemistry to Single Diastereoisomers by GIAO NMR Calculation: The DP4 Probability. *J. Am. Chem. Soc.* **2010**, *132*, 12946–12959. [CrossRef] [PubMed]
8. Wu, B.; He, S.; Pan, Y. Sesquiterpenoid with new skeleton from *Chloranthus henryi*. *Tetrahedron Lett.* **2007**, *48*, 453–456. [CrossRef]
9. Du, B.; Huang, Z.; Wang, X.; Chen, T.; Shen, G.; Fu, S.; Liu, B. A unified strategy toward total syntheses of lindenane sesquiterpenoid [4 + 2] dimers. *Nat. Commun.* **2019**, *10*, 1892. [CrossRef]
10. Saito, Y.; Ichihara, M.; Okamoto, Y.; Gong, X.; Kuroda, C.; Tori, M. Twelve new compounds from *Ligularia melanothyrsa*; isolation of melanothyrsins A–E, normelanothyrsin A, and other eremophilane sesquiterpenoids. *Tetrahedron* **2014**, *70*, 2621–2628. [CrossRef]
11. Shi, Y.-S.; Liu, Y.-B.; Ma, S.-G.; Li, Y.; Qu, J.; Li, L.; Yuan, S.-P.; Hou, Q.; Li, Y.-H.; Jiang, J.-D.; et al. Bioactive Sesquiterpenes and Lignans from the Fruits of *Xanthium sibiricum*. *J. Nat. Prod.* **2015**, *78*, 1526–1535. [CrossRef] [PubMed]
12. Ishiyama, H.; Hashimoto, A.; Fromont, J.; Hoshino, Y.; Mikami, Y.; Kobayashi, J. Halichonadins A–D, new sesquiterpenoids from a sponge *Halichondria* sp. *Tetrahedron* **2005**, *61*, 1101–1105. [CrossRef]

13. Xu, Y.-J. Phytochemical and Biological Studies of *Chloranthus* Medicinal Plants. *Chem. Biodivers.* **2013**, *10*, 1754–1773. [CrossRef] [PubMed]
14. Kawabata, J.; Mizutani, J. Shizukanolides D, E and F, Novel Lindenanolides from *Chloranthus* spp. (Chloranthaceae). *Agric. Biol. Chem.* **1989**, *53*, 203–207. [CrossRef]
15. Hu, X.; Yang, J.; Xu, X. Three Novel Sesquiterpene Glycosides of *Sarcandra glabra*. *Chem. Pharm. Bull. (Tokyo)* **2009**, *57*, 418–420. [CrossRef] [PubMed]
16. Yue, G.; Yang, L.; Yuan, C.; Du, B.; Liu, B. Total syntheses of lindenane-type sesquiterpenoids: (±)-chloranthalactones A, B, F, (±)-9-hydroxy heterogorgiolide, and (±)-shizukanolide E. *Tetrahedron* **2012**, *68*, 9624–9637. [CrossRef]
17. Fenlon, T.W.; Jones, M.W.; Adlington, R.M.; Lee, V. Synthesis of *rac*-Lindenene via a thermally induced cyclopropanation reaction. *Org. Biomol. Chem.* **2013**, *11*, 8026–8029. [CrossRef]
18. Wu, B.; Chen, J.; Qu, H.; Cheng, Y. Complex Sesquiterpenoids with Tyrosinase Inhibitory Activity from the Leaves of *Chloranthus tianmushanensis*. *J. Nat. Prod.* **2008**, *71*, 877–880. [CrossRef]
19. Cao, C.-M.; Peng, Y.; Shi, Q.-W.; Xiao, P.-G. Chemical Constituents and Bioactivities of Plants of Chloranthaceae. *Chem. Biodivers.* **2008**, *5*, 219–238. [CrossRef]
20. Wang, A.-R.; Song, H.-C.; An, H.-M.; Huang, Q.; Luo, X.; Dong, J.-Y. Secondary Metabolites of Plants from the Genus *Chloranthus*: Chemistry and Biological Activities. *Chem. Biodivers.* **2015**, *12*, 451–473. [CrossRef] [PubMed]
21. He, X.-F.; Yin, S.; Ji, Y.-C.; Su, Z.-S.; Geng, M.-Y.; Yue, J.-M. Sesquiterpenes and Dimeric Sesquiterpenoids from *Sarcandra glabra*. *J. Nat. Prod.* **2010**, *73*, 45–50. [CrossRef] [PubMed]
22. Ni, G.; Zhang, H.; Liu, H.-C.; Yang, S.-P.; Geng, M.-Y.; Yue, J.-M. Cytotoxic sesquiterpenoids from *Sarcandra glabra*. *Tetrahedron* **2013**, *69*, 564–569. [CrossRef]
23. Kouno, I.; Hirai, A.; Fukushige, A.; Jiang, Z.-H.; Tanaka, T. New Eudesmane Sesquiterpenes from the Root of *Lindera strychnifolia*. *J. Nat. Prod.* **2001**, *64*, 286–288. [CrossRef]
24. Zhang, C.; Nakamura, N.; Tewtrakul, S.; Hattori, M.; Sun, Q.; Wang, Z.; Fujiwara, T. Sesquiterpenes and Alkaloids from Lindera chunii and Their Inhibitory Activities against HIV-1 Integrase. *Chem. Pharm. Bull.* **2002**, *50*, 6. [CrossRef] [PubMed]
25. Gan, L.-S.; Zheng, Y.-L.; Mo, J.-X.; Liu, X.; Li, X.-H.; Zhou, C.-X. Sesquiterpene Lactones from the Root Tubers of *Lindera aggregata*. *J. Nat. Prod.* **2009**, *72*, 1497–1501. [CrossRef] [PubMed]
26. Wang, L.-J.; Xiong, J.; Liu, S.-T.; Liu, X.-H.; Hu, J.-F. Sesquiterpenoids from *Chloranthus henryi* and Their Anti-neuroinflammatory Activities. *Chem. Biodivers.* **2014**, *11*, 919–928. [CrossRef] [PubMed]
27. Kawabata, J.; Fukushi, Y.; Tahara, S.; Mizutani, J. Shizukaol a, a sesquiterpene dimer from *Chloranthus japonicus*. *Phytochemistry* **1990**, *29*, 2332–2334. [CrossRef]
28. Kawabata, J.; Mizutani, J. Dimeric sesquiterpenoid esters from *Chloranthus serratus*. *Phytochemistry* **1992**, *31*, 1293–1296. [CrossRef]
29. Kawabata, J.; Fukushi, E.; Mizutani, J. Sesquiterpene dimers from *Chloranthus japonicus*. *Phytochemistry* **1995**, *39*, 121–125. [CrossRef]
30. Yang, S.-P.; Gao, Z.-B.; Wang, F.-D.; Liao, S.-G.; Chen, H.-D.; Zhang, C.-R.; Hu, G.-Y.; Yue, J.-M. Chlorahololides A and B, Two Potent and Selective Blockers of the Potassium Channel Isolated from *Chloranthus holostegius*. *Org. Lett.* **2007**, *9*, 903–906. [CrossRef]
31. Yang, S.-P.; Gao, Z.-B.; Wu, Y.; Hu, G.-Y.; Yue, J.-M. Chlorahololides C–F: a new class of potent and selective potassium channel blockers from *Chloranthus holostegius*. *Tetrahedron* **2008**, *64*, 2027–2034. [CrossRef]
32. Kim, S.-Y.; Kashiwada, Y.; Kawazoe, K.; Murakami, K.; Sun, H.-D.; Li, S.-L.; Takaishi, Y. Spicachlorantins C–F, hydroperoxy dimeric sesquiterpenes from the roots of *Chloranthus spicatus*. *Tetrahedron Lett.* **2009**, *50*, 6032–6035. [CrossRef]
33. Yan, H.; Ba, M.-Y.; Li, X.-H.; Guo, J.-M.; Qin, X.-J.; He, L.; Zhang, Z.-Q.; Guo, Y.; Liu, H.-Y. Lindenane sesquiterpenoid dimers from *Chloranthus japonicus* inhibit HIV-1 and HCV replication. *Fitoterapia* **2016**, *115*, 64–68. [CrossRef] [PubMed]
34. Yuan, C.; Du, B.; Deng, H.; Man, Y.; Liu, B. Total Syntheses of Sarcandrolide J and Shizukaol D: Lindenane Sesquiterpenoid [4+2] Dimers. *Angew. Chem. Int. Ed.* **2017**, *56*, 637–640. [CrossRef]
35. Frisch, M.J.; Trucks, G.W.; Schlegel, H.B.; Scuseria, G.E.; Robb, M.A.; Cheeseman, J.R.; Scalmani, G.; Barone, V.; Mennucci, B.; Petersson, G.A.; et al. *Gaussian09 Revision D.01*; Gaussian Inc.: Wallingford, CT, USA, 2013.

36. Konstantinov, I.A.; Broadbelt, L.J. Regression formulas for density functional theory calculated 1H and 13C NMR chemical shifts in toluene-d_8. *J. Phys. Chem. A* **2011**, *115*, 12364–12372. [CrossRef]
37. Ditchfield, R. Self-consistent perturbation theory of diamagnetism: I. A gauge-invariant LCAO method for NMR chemical shifts. *Mol. Phys.* **1974**, *27*, 789–807. [CrossRef]
38. Wolinski, K.; Hinton, J.F.; Pulay, P. Efficient implementation of the gauge-independent atomic orbital method for NMR chemical shift calculations. *J. Am. Chem. Soc.* **1990**, *112*, 8251–8260. [CrossRef]

Sample Availability: Samples of compounds **1** and **2** are not available from the authors.

© 2020 by the authors. Licensee MDPI, Basel, Switzerland. This article is an open access article distributed under the terms and conditions of the Creative Commons Attribution (CC BY) license (http://creativecommons.org/licenses/by/4.0/).

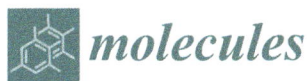

Article

Antibacterial and Antifungal Sesquiterpenoids from Aerial Parts of *Anvillea garcinii*

Shagufta Perveen [1,*], Jawaher Alqahtani [1,2], Raha Orfali [1], Hanan Y. Aati [1], Areej M. Al-Taweel [1], Taghreed A. Ibrahim [1], Afsar Khan [3], Hasan S. Yusufoglu [4], Maged S. Abdel-Kader [4,5] and Orazio Taglialatela-Scafati [2,*]

1. Department of Pharmacognosy, College of Pharmacy, King Saud University. P. O. Box 22452, Riyadh 11495, Saudi Arabia; jalqahtani@ksu.edu.sa (J.A.); rorfali@ksu.edu.sa (R.O.); hati@ksu.edu.sa (H.Y.A.); amaltaweel@ksu.edu.sa (A.M.A.-T.); tshehata@ksu.edu.sa (T.A.I.)
2. Department of Pharmacy, School of Medicine and Surgery, University of Naples Federico II, Via D. Montesano 49, 80131 Naples, Italy
3. Department of Chemistry, COMSATS University Islamabad, Abbottabad Campus, Abbottabad-22060, Pakistan; afsarhej@gmail.com
4. Department of Pharmacognosy, College of Pharmacy, Prince Sattam Bin Abdulaziz University, P.O. Box 173, Al-Kharj 11942, Saudi Arabia; h.yusufoglu@psau.edu.sa (H.S.Y.); mpharm101@hotmail.com (M.S.A.-K.)
5. Department of Pharmacognosy, Faculty of Pharmacy, Alexandria University, Alexandria 21215, Egypt
* Correspondence: shakhan@ksu.edu.sa (S.P.); scatagli@unina.it (O.T.-S.)

Academic Editors: Pavel B. Drasar and Valeria Patricia Sülsen
Received: 9 March 2020; Accepted: 7 April 2020; Published: 9 April 2020

Abstract: Two new sesquiterpenoids belonging to the guaiane, 4α,9α,10α-trihydroxyguaia-11(13)en-12,6α-olide (**1**), and germacrane, 9β-hydroxyparthenolide-9-*O*-β-D-glucopyranoside (**2**), classes have been isolated from the leaves of the Saudi medicinal plant *Anvillea garcinii* along with seven known compounds (**3–9**). The structures of the new metabolites were elucidated by spectroscopic analysis, including one-dimensional (1D) and two-dimensional (2D) Nuclear Magnetic Resonance (NMR) and high-resolution electrospray ionization mass spectrometry (HR-ESIMS). The antimicrobial properties of **1–9** were screened against seven different pathogenic microbes, and compounds **1–3** showed a potent antifungal activity.

Keywords: *Anvillea garcinii*; Saudi medicinal plants; sesquiterpene lactones; antifungal activity

1. Introduction

Traditional medicines are a powerful weapon for mankind and they have been used to treat several health disorders since ancient times. The last few decades have witnessed a renaissance in the use of natural products, and traditional medicine in general, to prevent or cure several ailments. While they are considered one of the possible options in several countries, they are practically the main therapeutic option in many developing countries, including those of the Arabian Peninsula.

Flora of Saudi Arabia is evidently and understandably not as rich and diverse as that of countries of the Mediterranean basin; however, it has a vital role for various ecosystems, especially in maintaining the environmental balance and stability [1]. The dominating plant family is Asteraceae, one of the largest plant families on the planet, which is a family that includes more than one thousand genera and twenty thousand species [2]. Asteraceae plants are well known for their biological and pharmacological effects, largely ascribable to the presence of phytochemicals belonging to polyphenol, flavonoid, and terpenoid classes [3].

Anvillea is probably the smallest genus of the Asteraceae family, since it includes only four species, distributed in a large area spanning from North Africa to Iran, including several Middle Eastern countries, such as Egypt, Palestine, and Saudi Arabia [4]. In Saudi Arabia, *Anvillea* genus is represented by the following two species: *A. garcinii* and *A. radiata*. *A. garcinii* DC (Arabic name Nuqd) is one of the most important ethnomedicinal plants used in the Arabian Peninsula region, indicated for symptomatic relief of various illnesses such as cold, gastrointestinal disorders, and respiratory system problems [3]. Traditionally, the dried plant is crushed, mixed with honey or date and olive oil, and used to treat cold symptoms [4].

Flavonoids and sesquiterpene lactones have been the predominant class of secondary metabolites obtained by phytochemical studies on *A. garcinii* [5–11]. Our previous investigations on this plant disclosed the presence of sesquiterpene lactones of the guaianolide- and germacranolide-types, including the corresponding amino acid adducts, as well as some flavonoids glycosides [11–13]. The class of *Anvillea* sesquiterpene lactones is dominated by derivatives with the parthenolide skeleton, germacranolides endowed with significant biological activities in cancer and inflammation, as well as in metabolic disorders [14]. Previous examination of the aerial parts of *A. garcinii* have afforded several members of the parthenolide class, such as 9α- and 9β-hydroxyparthenolide, 9α- and 9β-hydroxy-1β,10α-epoxyparthenolide, parthenolid-9-one, and its *cis*-isomer [15]. In addition, guaianolide-type sesquiterpenoids, a class of phytochemicals with a broad range of activities, including cytotoxic, antiprotozoal, and anti-inflammatory potential [16], also constitute prominent *A. garcinii* metabolites. Leucodin and zaluzanin C and their derivatives [17], as well as garcinamine E and other guaianes [13], have been isolated from this species.

This richness of bioactive secondary metabolites prompted us to continue our phytochemical and biological investigation of *A. garcinii*, with the final aim of obtaining a detailed picture of the metabolome of this plant, providing solid scientific grounds for its use in traditional medicines and possibly, to develop a new phytotherapeutic drug from this natural source. In this manuscript we report the isolation of two new sesquiterpenoids belonging to the guaiane (4α,9α,10α-trihydroxyguaia-11(13)en-12,6α-olide, (**1**)) and germacranolide (9β-hydroxyparthenolide-9-O-β-D-glucopyranoside, (**2**)) classes, along with seven known compounds (**3–9**) (Figure 1) and the results of screening for antimicrobial activity on the isolated metabolites.

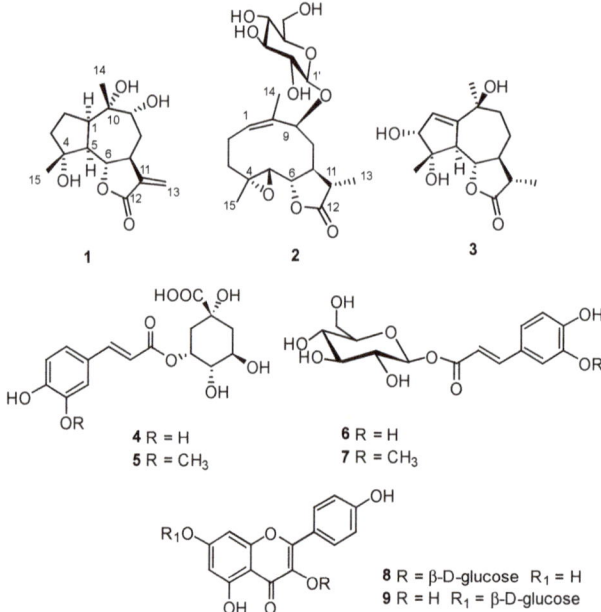

Figure 1. Chemical structures of metabolites isolated from *Anvillea garcinia*.

2. Results and Discussion

Previous investigations on *A. garcinii* aerial parts selected the *n*-butanol fraction of the methanol extract as the richest in polar sesquiterpenoids. Its chromatographic separation was achieved using a combination of Sephadex LH-20, silica gel, and RP-18 column chromatography, and yielded two new (**1–2**) and seven known compounds (**3–9**) (Figure 1). The structures of these metabolites were elucidated by spectroscopic analysis, mainly one-dimensional (1D) and two-dimensional (2D) NMR and electrospray ionization mass spectrometry (ESIMS). Compounds **3–9** were identified as 3α,4α,10β-trihydroxy-11β-guai-1-en-12,6α-olide (**3**) [18], chlorogenic acid (**4**) [19], 3-*O*-feruloylquinic acid (**5**) [20], 1-*O*-caffeoyl-β-D-glucopyranose (**6**) [21], 1-*O*-feruloyl-β-D-glucopyranose (**7**) [22], kaempferol-3-*O*-glucopyranoside (**8**) [23], and kaempferol-7-*O*-glucopyranoside (**9**) [24] by a comparison of their spectroscopic data with those reported in the literature. Selected spectra of these compounds are reported as Supplementary Materials. All these phenolic derivatives are reported from *A. garcinii* for the first time.

Compound **1** was isolated as a white solid with the molecular formula $C_{15}H_{22}O_5$, determined by high-resolution electrospray ionization mass spectrometry (HR-ESIMS) (*m/z* 281.1400 [M–H]$^-$; calculated for $C_{15}H_{21}O_5$, 281.1394), indicating five unsaturation degrees. The ^{1}H NMR spectrum of **1** showed the presence of a pair of sp^2 methylene protons (δ_H 5.90 and 5.36, each bs); two oxygenated methine protons at δ_H 3.58 (1H, d, *J* = 2.5 Hz) and 4.17 (1H, dd, *J* = 9.5, 11.0 Hz); three relatively deshielded methines at δ_H 2.00 (1H, brd, *J* = 11.0 Hz), 2.87 (overlapped), and 2.84 (overlapped); three methylene protons, and two methyl singlets at δ_H 0.95 and 1.10 (see Table 1). The ^{13}C NMR spectral data of **1**, which was analyzed with the help of the 2D NMR HSQC spectrum, disclosed the presence of one ester carbonyl at δ_C 170.8; one sp^2 methylene at δ_C 118.7, and an additional unprotonated sp^2 carbon at δ_C 139.8; two oxymethine carbons at δ_C 82.6 and 76.0 and two unprotonated oxygenated carbons at 79.6 and 76.6. The remaining carbon atoms were assigned as three sp^3 methylenes at δ_C 24.6, 31.6, and 40.3, three sp^3 methines at δ_C 40.5, 40.7, and 54.6, and two methyl carbon atoms at δ_C 21.7 and 22.0.

The guaianolide-type skeleton of compound **1** was assembled on the basis of the 2D NMR COSY and heteronuclear multiple bond coherence (HMBC) spectra. The COSY spectrum disclosed the single extended spin system (highlighted in red in Figure 2), which was arranged on the bicyclic system on the basis of the HMBC correlations from methyl singlets H$_3$-14 and H$_3$-15. The HMBC correlations from the methylene H-13 to C-12, the nuclear Overhauser enhancement spectroscopy (NOESY) correlations H-6/H$_3$-15, H-6/H$_3$-14, and H-9/H$_3$-14, and the remaining NOESY correlation of **1**, shown in Figure 2, indicated the relative configuration of compound **1**. Thus, using all the above-mentioned data, compound **1** was elucidated as 4α,9α,10α-trihydroxyguaia-11(13)-en-12,6α-olide.

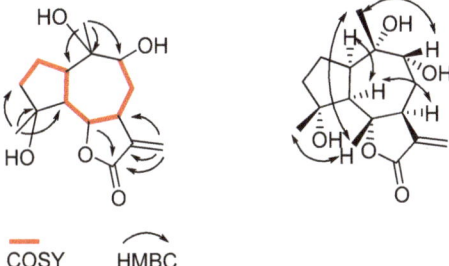

Figure 2. Some key two-dimensional (2D) NMR correlations of **1** (left, correlated spectroscopy (COSY) and heteronuclear multiple bond coherence (HMBC) and right, nuclear Overhauser enhancement spectroscopy (NOESY)).

Interestingly, the presence of **1** as a component of the sesquiterpenoid pool of *A. garcinii* was anticipated by us at the time of isolation of garcinamine E [13]. Indeed, garcinamine E, co-occurring in the *n*-butanol fraction of the leaves of *A. garcinii*, is the L-proline adduct at C-13 of **1**.

Table 1. ^{1}H (500 MHz) and ^{13}C (125 MHz) NMR data for compounds **1** and **2** in CD$_3$OD.

Pos.	1 δ_H (mult., *J* in Hz)	δ_C	2 δ_H (mult., *J* in Hz)	δ_C
1	2.80 (m)	40.5	5.56 (dd, 9.5, 11.5)	129.4
2α	1.64 (dddd, 1.5, 3.5, 7.5, 12.5)	24.6	2.61 (m)	23.5
2β	1.49 (tdd, 2.0, 6.5, 12.5)		2.22 (m)	
3	1.53 (m)	40.4	2.13 (m)	35.9
			1.22 (m)	
4	-	79.6	-	61.8
5	2.00 (t, 11.0)	54.6	2.79 (d, 9.0)	65.9
6	4.17 (dd, 9.5, 11.0)	82.6	4.04 (t, 9.0)	81.4
7	2.87 (ddd, 9.5, 3.5, 1.5)	40.7	2.11 (m)	48.2
8α	1.99 (ddd, 2.5, 3.5, 9.2)	31.6	2.09 (dd, 2.1, 9.2)	35.0
8β	1.53 (ddd, 1.0, 1.5, 9.2)	-	1.98 (bdd, 9.2, 7.5)	-
9	3.58 (dd, 2.5, 1.0)	76.0	4.37 (dd, 7.5, 2.1)	83.1
10	-	76.6	-	133.9
11	-	139.8	2.49 (dt, 2.5, 7.0)	41.7
12	-	170.8	-	178.7
13a	5.90 (brs)	118.7	1.27 (d, 7.0)	12.0
13b	5.36 (brs)	-		
14	0.95 (s)	21.8	1.76 (s)	10.0
15	1.10 (s)	22.0	1.36 (s)	16.3
1'			4.11 (d, 7.5)	98.7
2'			3.23 (t, 7.5)	73.5
3'			3.17 (m)	76.5
4'			3.29 (m)	70.3
5'			3.31 (m)	76.7
6'a			3.67 (m)	61.4
6'b			3.86 (m)	

Compound **2** was obtained as an optically active ($[\alpha]^{25}$ D = −55, *c* = 0.10, CH$_3$OH) yellow gummy solid with molecular formula C$_{21}$H$_{32}$O$_9$, as established by HR-ESIMS. The ^{13}C NMR spectrum, which was interpreted taking into account data from the 2D NMR HSQC and HMBC experiments, indicated the presence of one ester carbonyl (δ_C 178.7); two olefinic carbons (δ_C 129.4 and 133.9); one anomeric carbon (δ_C 98.7); seven additional oxygenated methines (δ_C 83.1, 81.4, 76.7, 76.5, 73.5, 70.3 and 65.9); one oxygenated unprotonated carbon (δ_C 61.8); one oxygenated methylene (δ_C 61.4); and eight additional sp^3 carbons, including two methines, three methylenes, and three methyls (Table 1). Accordingly, the ^{1}H NMR spectrum of **2** (Table 1) showed a *sp^2* methine signal at δ_H 5.56, a series of oxymethine and oxymethylene protons between δ_H 4.37 and 3.17, and three methyl signals, namely a deshielded singlet at δ_H 1.76, a singlet at δ_H 1.36, and a doublet at δ_H 1.27. These data were indicative of the sesquiterpene lactone glycoside nature for compound **2**, whose structure was assigned on the basis of a detailed inspection of the 2D NMR correlations and comparison with data of known compounds [12].

In particular, the COSY spectrum of **2** revealed the presence of three spin systems, namely (i) from the sp^2 methine H-1 to H$_2$-3, (ii) from H-5 to H-9 including the H-11/H$_3$-13 branching, and (iii) the sugar spin system (H-1' to H$_2$-6'). The sugar unit was assigned as a β-D-glucopyranoside on the basis of the coupling constant H-1'/H-2' (*J* = 7.5 Hz) and acid hydrolysis of **2**, which afforded the free sugar unit, identified as D-glucose through co-TLC and optical rotation sign.

The HMBC correlations of **2** were instrumental to join the above deduced fragments. In particular, ^3J cross-peaks of H$_3$-14 with C-1, C-9, and the unprotonated sp^2 C-10 and of H$_3$-15 with C-3, C-4, and C-5 indicated the presence of the ten-membered ring. Moreover, cross-peaks of both H-6 and H$_3$-13 with the ester carbonyl carbon C-12 indicated the presence of the lactone ring. The linkage of the D-glucopyranose moiety at position 9 was indicated by the ^3J HMBC correlation of H-1' (δ_H 4.10) with C-9 (δ_C 83.1). The presence of an epoxyde ring at C-4/C5, which accounted for the remaining unsaturation degree, was in perfect agreement with the NMR resonances of the involved carbons (C-4 = 61.8 ppm and C-5 = 65.9 ppm). The NOESY correlations were, then, used to deduce the relative configuration of compound **2**. In particular, NOESY cross-peak of H-1 with H$_3$-14 indicated the Z configuration of the endocyclic double bond. The relative configuration of the five consecutive stereogenic centers (C-4 to C-11) was deduced on the basis of the following NOESY correlations: H$_3$-15/H-6, H-5/H-7, H$_2$-3/H-5, and H-7/H$_3$-13. Finally, the NOESY cross-peak of H-7 with H-9 pointed to the α-orientation of both protons. Thus, compound **2** was identified as the new 1Z-9β-hydroxyparthenolide-9-O-β-D-glucopyranoside. The $\Delta^{1,10}$-E isomer of **2** has been recently isolated from *Asteriscus graveolens* [25] and, accordingly, its reported ^{13}C NMR resonances for C-1 and C-10 showed significant differences as compared with those of **2**. Both compounds **1** and **2** are close analogues of sesquiterpenoids previously isolated from the same species and we have assumed that they share the absolute configuration of their co-occurring analogues.

The isolated metabolites (**1–9**) were evaluated for their antimicrobial activity against pathogenic bacteria and fungi (Tables 2 and 3). Compounds **1–3** showed antifungal activities against human pathogenic fungi, with a growth inhibitory activity around 80% at 50 µg mL^{-1} against *Candida albicans* and *C. parapsilosis*, respectively. The respective minimum inhibitory concentrations (MIC) of **1–3** were 0.21, 0.26, and 0.38 µg mL^{-1} against *C. albicans* and 0.25, 0.31, and 0.34 against *C. parapsilosis*. This finding is in agreement with our previously reported results on antifungal activity of guaianolide sesquiterpenoids [26]. In addition, **1–3** also showed activity against Gram-positive and Gram-negative pathogenic bacteria with MIC ranging from 2.3 to 6.3 µg mL^{-1} (Table 3). Chlorogenic acid (**4**), a non-sesquiterpenoid, showed a significant inhibition against pathogenic fungi (Table 2) and strong antibacterial activity against the Gram-negative bacteria *E. xiangfangensis* and *E. fergusonii*. Ester derivatives **6** and **7** showed neither antifungal nor antibacterial activity at 25 µg mL^{-1}.

Table 2. Antifungal activity of compounds **1–9**.

Compound	Growth Inhibition (%, mean ± SD) *		MIC (µg mL^{-1})	
	C. albicans	*C. parapsilosis*	*C. albicans*	*C. parapsilosis*
1	83.4 ± 3.3	81.3 ± 2.6	0.21 ± 0.04	0.25 ± 0.05
2	79.8 ± 5.3	76.5 ± 4.5	0.26 ± 0.07	0.31 ± 0.02
3	85.0 ± 3.4	80.0 ± 2.7	0.38 ± 0.03	0.34 ± 0.06
4	61.2 ± 3.3	69.5 ± 2.4	0.89 ± 0.02	0.61 ± 0.08
5	23.6 ± 5.2	18.9 ± 3.7	0.68 ± 0.01	0.79 ± 0.03
6	19.5 ± 2.9	21.7 ± 3.4	0.73 ± 0.08	0.86 ± 0.07
7	15.8 ± 3.2	10.9 ± 4.7	0.97 ± 0.12	0.79 ± 0.06
8	42.7 ± 4.4	51.8 ± 2.5	0.74 ± 0.05	0.62 ± 0.03
9	45.3 ± 3.7	49.9 ± 4.8	0.68 ± 0.08	0.74 ± 0.02
Itraconazole	54.7 ± 2.6	51.5 ± 4.1	0.29 ± 0.06	0.33 ± 0.04

* Results expressed as mean ± standard deviation (SD).

Table 3. Antibacterial activity of compounds 1–9.

Compound	MIC (µg mL^{-1})				
	Staphilococcus aureus	Bacillus licheniformis	Escherichia xiangfangensis	Escherichia fergusonii	Pseudomonas aeruginosa
1	2.3	2.3	>25	5.7	>25
2	3.4	3.1	>25	6.3	>25
3	5.2	4.4	3.8	>25	>25
4	>25	>25	5.2	4.6	>25
5	>25	>25	>25	>25	>25
6	>25	>25	>25	>25	>25
7	>25	>25	>25	>25	>25
8	9.4	>25	>25	6.8	>25
9	>25	7.5	>25	8.4	>25
Amikacin	0.523	0.523	0.523	0.523	0.523

* Results expressed as mean ± standard deviation (SD).

3. Materials and Methods

3.1. General

Optical rotations were measured in analytical grade methanol using a JASCO P-2000 polarimeter (JASCO, 2967-5, Tokyo, Japan). The 1D and 2D NMR data were acquired using a Bruker AVANCE spectrometer (Bruker, Billerica, MA, USA) (500 MHz for ^{1}H and 125 MHz for ^{13}C). Chemical shifts (δ) in ppm, relative to tetramethylsilane, were calculated basing on the residual solvent signal, and *J* scalar coupling constants are reported in Hz (Hertz). The ESI-MS analyses were measured on an Triple Quadrupole 6410 QQQ LC/MS mass spectrometer (Agilent, Santa Clara, CA, USA) with ESI ion source (gas temperature was 350 °C, nebulizer pressure was 60 psi, and gas flow rate was 12 L/min), operating in the negative and positive scan modes of ionization through direct infusion method using CH$_3$OH\H$_2$O (4:6 *v/v*) at a flow rate of 0.5 mL/min. Column chromatography procedures were performed using silica gel 70–230 mesh, RP-18, Sephadex LH-20 (each from; E. Merck, Darmstadt, Germany). TLC analysis was performed using precoated silica gel 60 F$_{254}$ and RP-18 (Merck, Darmstadt, Germany) plates, and spots were visualized via exposure under UV light (254/365 nm) and by spraying with different spray reagent. Analytical grade solvents and reagents were purchased from Sigma-Aldrich (St. Louis, MO, USA). Deuterated methanol (CD$_3$OD-*d*) and dimethylsulfoxide (DMSO-d_6) were obtained from Cambridge Isotope Laboratories (Tewksbury, MA, USA).

3.2. Plant Material

The aerial parts of *A. garcinii* were collected in March 2018 in the area 17 km South West of Al-Kharj city and identified by taxonomist, Dr. M. Atiqur Rahman, College of Pharmacy, Medicinal, Aromatic and Poisonous Plants Research Center, King Saud University. A voucher specimen (PSAU-CPH-6-2018) is kept in the herbarium of College of Pharmacy, Prince Sattam Bin Abdulaziz University.

3.3. Extraction and Isolation

The shade dried powdered aerial parts of *A. garcinii* (0.5 kg) were extracted with methanol at room temperature (3 × 2.5 L). Total methanol extract was concentrated under reduced pressure using a rotary evaporator (Büchi Rotavapor RII, Flawil, Switzerland). The crude extract (50 g) was suspended in H$_2$O (0.5 L) and extracted successively with chloroform and *n*-butanol, and then the residual water fraction was lyophilized. The *n*-butanol soluble fraction (30 g) was subjected to a silica gel open column and eluted with a gradient of CH$_2$Cl$_2$:CH$_3$OH (9.5:0.5→1.0:9.0), to afford nine major fractions 1–9 based on their TLC image. Fraction 3 (0.8 g) was further subjected to RP C-18 column chromatography, eluted under medium pressure with a gradient of water/methanol (4.0:6.0→9.0:1.0), to obtain two subfractions which was further loaded on a RP C-18 column and eluted with a gradient mixture of water/methanol

(6.0:4.0→1.0:9.0), which yielded compounds **1** (10 mg) and **3** (8 mg). Fraction 5 (0.3 g) was applied to a RP C-18 column using water/methanol (8.0:2.0→1.0:1.0) to yield compound **2** (15 mg). Fraction 6 (0.6 g) was rechromatographed on a Sephadex LH-20 column with water/methanol (1:1–100:0) to afford two compounds **4** (10 mg) and **5** (12 mg). Fraction 7 (0.5 g) was separated on a Sephadex LH-20 column with a gradient mixture of water/methanol (9.0:1.0→7.0:3.0), and finally was divided on a silica gel column with $CHCl_3$/MeOH (8.5:1.5) to afford compounds **6** (6.0 mg) and **7** (11 mg). Subfraction 8 (0.2 g) was further purified by HPLC (flow rate 1 mL/min, wavelength 254 nm, and CH_3OH–0.01%HCOOH/H_2O, 4:6) to afford **8** (15 mg, Rt 25.5 min). Subfraction 9 (0.1 g) was purified by HPLC (flow rate 1.0 mL/min, wavelength 254 nm, CH_3OH–0.01%HCOOH/H_2O, 1:1) to afford compound **9** (12 mg, Rt 27.5 min).

4α,9α,10α-Trihydroxyguaia-11(13)en-12,6α-olide (**1**): Yellow gummy solid, $[\alpha]_D^{25}$ + 72 (c 0.10, MeOH); UV (MeOH), λ_{max} 223 nm (ε 4000); ^{1}H NMR (500 MHz, in CD_3OD) and ^{13}C NMR (125 MHz, in CD_3OD) see Table 1; negative ions ESIMS, m/z 281.1400 [M–H]$^-$, calculated for $C_{15}H_{21}O_5$, 281.1394.

1Z-9β-Hydroxyparthenolide-9-O-β-D-glucopyranoside (**2**): Yellow gummy solid, $[\alpha]_D^{25}$ + 55 (c 0.10, MeOH); UV (MeOH), λ_{max} 211 nm (ε 3200); ^{1}H NMR (500 MHz, in CD_3OD) and ^{13}C NMR (125 MHz, in CD_3OD) see Table 1; positive ions ESIMS, m/z 451.1948 [M+ Na]$^+$, calculated for $C_{21}H_{32}NaO_9$, 451.1944.

3.4. Acid Hydrolysis of 2

Compound **2** (3.0 mg) was dissolved in 0.6 mL of a solution of 1N HCl–methanol (1:1). The mixture was heated at 65 °C for 60 min and concentrated in vacuo, water was added and the whole was extracted with ethyl acetate. The aqueous portion was filtered, the filtrate was evaporated, and D-glucose (0.9 mg, 71%) was identified from the sign of its optical rotation ($[\alpha]^{25}_D$ + 52.0) and co-TLC (n-butanol/water/acetic acid, 8:2:10, Rf 0.17) with an authentic sample of D-glucose (Merck) using anisaldehyde as spray reagent for visualization.

3.5. Antibacterial Bioassay

The antibacterial activity was determined according the reported method [27]. Muller Hinton agar plate contained microorganisms after suspension in a nutrient broth for 24 h wells were created in the plate and loaded with 10 μL of the sample solution obtained using DMSO as solvent. Amikacin was used as standard antibiotic for five different pathogenic bacteria two were Gram-positive, i.e., *Staphylococcus aureus* (CP011526.1) and *Bacillus licheniformis* (KX785171.1) and three were Gram-negative, i.e., *Enterobacter xiangfangensis* (CP017183.1), *Escherichia fergusonii* (CU928158.2), and *Pseudomonas aeruginosa* (NR-117678.1).

The clear area which was free of microbial growth was measured three times to detect the diameter of the zone of inhibition and the mean were recorded. The minimal inhibitory concentration (MIC, μg mL^{-1}) of the tested isolated compounds that inhibited the visible bacterial growth was calculated using varying concentrations of the tested compounds following the broth microdilution method [27,28].

3.6. Antifungal Assay

Well diffusion and broth microdilution techniques were used in this study to detect the antifungal activity of the isolated compounds. According to Gong and Guo [29], in SDA plate the sample solutions (100 μL), approximately 3 × 10^6 colony-forming units (CFU) mL^{-1} was smeared of two pathogenic fungi, *Candida albicans* and *Candida parapsilosis*. Wells were created in SDA plates and loaded with the 10 μg of the tested compounds dissolved in DMSO and incubated at 37 °C for 1 day. Itraconazole was used as a standard antifungal and the diameters (in mm) of zone of inhibition were measured. The rates of growth inhibition were obtained according to the following formula taking into consideration ± SD as means:

$$\% \text{ Growth inhibition rate} = (d_c - d_s) / (d_c - d_0) \times 100$$

where d_c is the diameter of the untreated control fungus, d_s is the diameter of the sample-treated fungus, and d_0 is the diameter of the fungus cut.

The minimal inhibitory concentration (MIC) of the isolated compounds **1–9** against *Candida albicans* and *C. parapsilosis* was determined by using varying concentrations of the tested compounds following the broth microdilution method following the instructions of the Clinical and Laboratory Standards Institute. Serial dilution of the isolated compounds was prepared into two-fold using sterile Roswell Park Memorial Institute (RPMI) 1640 medium with MOPS (0.165 mol L-1) and presence of glucose (2%). The 96-well microplates were performed and incubated at 37 °C for 24 h.

3.7. Statistical Analysis

Data analysis was expressed as mean ± standard deviation (SD) of three replicates. Where applicable, the data were subjected to one-way analysis of variance (ANOVA). According to a Microsoft Excel 2010 statistical package analyses, the significant differences were considered statistically significant P values < 0.05.

4. Conclusions

This investigation on the Saudi Arabia plant *A. garcinii* yielded two additional members of the sesquiterpene lactone class, a new guaianolide, anticipated as precursor of garcinamine E, and a new parthenolide glycoside. Both of these compounds have been evidenced to have a significant antifungal activity, complementing that which had already been revealed for previously isolated congeners of the same family. Therefore, this study clearly evidences the potential of even a single plant to provide a countless list of bioactive phytochemicals and, more in general, of the Saudi Arabian flora to enrich the global phytochemical effort. Although less diverse than others, Saudi Arabian flora is well worth of being studied in detail, also to provide scientific basis to the traditional use of medicinal plants in this area.

Supplementary Materials: The following are available online at http://www.mdpi.com/1420-3049/25/7/1730/s1. Figures S1 and S2: ^{1}H and ^{13}C NMR spectra of compound **1**. Figures S3 and S4: DEPT-90 and DEPT-135 of compound **1**. Figures S5 and S6: 2D NMR COSY and HSQC spectra of compound **1**. Figure S7: negative ESIMS spectrum of compound **1**. Figures S8 and S9: ^{1}H and ^{13}C NMR spectra of compound **2**. Figures S10 and S11: DEPT-135 and DEPT-90 of compound **2**. Figures S12 and S13: 2D NMR COSY and HSQC spectra of compound **2**. Figure S14: positive ESIMS spectrum of compound **2**. Figures S15 and S16: ^{1}H and ^{13}C NMR spectra of compound **3**. Figures S17 and S18: ^{1}H and ^{13}C NMR spectra of compound **4**. Figure S19: DEPT-90 of compound **4**. Figures S20 and S21: ^{1}H and ^{13}C NMR spectra of compound **5**. Figures S22 and S23: ^{1}H and 2D HSQC spectra of compound **6**.

Author Contributions: Investigation, J.A., R.O., H.Y.A., A.M.A.-T., T.A.I., A.K., H.S.Y., M.S.A.-K.; writing—original draft preparation, S.P. and O.T.S.; writing—review and editing, S.P. and O.T.S.; funding acquisition, S.P. and O.T.-S. All authors have read and agreed to the published version of the manuscript.

Funding: The authors would like to extend their sincere appreciation to the Deanship of Scientific Research at King through the "Research Group Project no RGP-221". J. Alqahtani thanks the supporting of EJSP for her PhD program at the University of Naples Federico II.

Conflicts of Interest: The authors declare no conflict of interest.

References

1. Aati, H.; El-Gamal, A.; Shaheen, H.; Kayser, O. Traditional use of ethnomedicinal native plants in the Kingdom of Saudi Arabia. *J. Ethnobiol. Ethnomed.* **2019**, *15*, 2. [CrossRef] [PubMed]
2. Bitsindou, M.; Lejoly, J. Plants used in hepatoprotective remedies in traditional African medicine. In Proceedings of the WOCMAP I-Medicinal and Aromatic Plants Conference, Maastrcht, The Netherland, 19 July 1992; part 2 of 4 332. pp. 73–80.
3. Oshkondali, S.T.; Elshili, M.M.; Almunir, N.; Rashed, A.; Kushlaf, N.; EL-mahmoudy, A.M.; Shaeroun, A.; Alqamoudy, H.; Ahmed, B.A.; Mohamed, K.S. Therapeutic potentials of bioactive compounds in some species (*Amberboa Tubiflore*, *Anacyclus Clavatus* and *Anvillea Garcinii*) in the family Asteraceae. *Sch. Acad. J. Pharm.* **2019**, *8*, 456–460. [CrossRef]

4. El Hassany, B.; El Hanbali, F.; Akssira, M.; Mellouki, F.; Haidour, A.; Barrero, A.F. Germacranolides from *Anvillea radiata*. *Fitoterapia* **2004**, *75*, 573–576. [CrossRef] [PubMed]
5. Tyson, R.L.; Chang, C.J.; McLaughlin, J.L.; Cassady, J.M. A novel sesquiterpene lactone from *Anvillea garcinii* (Burm.). *J. Nat. Prod.* **1979**, *42*, 680–681.
6. Tyson, R.L.; Chang, C.J.; McLaughlin, J.L.; Aynehchi, Y.; Cassady, J.M. 9-α-hydroxyparthenolide, a novel antitumor sesquiterpene lactone from *Anvillea garcinii* (Burm.) DC. *Experientia* **1981**, *37*, 441–442. [CrossRef]
7. Rustaiyan, A.; Dabiri, M.; Jakupovic, J. Germacranolides from *Anvillea garcinii*. *Phytochemistry* **1986**, *25*, 1229–1230. [CrossRef]
8. Khan, M.; Saeed Abdullah, M.M.; Mousa, A.A.; Alkhathlan, H.Z. Chemical composition of vegetative parts and flowers essential oils of wild *Anvillea garcinii* grown in Saudi Arabia. *Rec. Nat. Prod.* **2016**, *10*, 251–256.
9. Sattar, E.A.; Galal, A.M.; Mossa, G.S. Antitumor germacranolides from *Anvillea garcinii*. *J. Nat. Prod.* **1996**, *59*, 403–405. [CrossRef]
10. Ulubelen, A.; Mabry, T.J.; Aynehchi, Y. Flavonoids of *Anvillea garcinii*. *J. Nat. Prod.* **1980**, *42*, 624–626. [CrossRef]
11. Perveen, S.; Al-Taweel, A.M.; Yusufoglu, H.S.; Fawzy, G.A.; Foudah, A.; Abdel-Kader, M.S. Hepatoprotective and cytotoxic activities of *Anvillea garcinii* and isolation of four new secondary metabolites. *J. Nat. Med.* **2018**, *72*, 106–117. [CrossRef]
12. Perveen, S.; Fawzi, G.A.; Al-Taweel, A.M.; Orfali, R.S.; Yusufoglu, H.S.; Abdel-Kader, M.S.; Al-Sabbagh, R.M. Antiulcer activity of different extract of *Anvillea garcinii* and isolation of two new secondary metabolites. *Open Chem.* **2018**, *16*, 437–445. [CrossRef]
13. Perveen, S.; Alqahtani, J.; Orfali, R.; Al-Taweel, A.M.; Yusufoglu, H.S.; Abdel-Kader, M.S.; Taglialatela-Scafati, O. Antimicrobial guaianolide sesquiterpenoids from leaves of the Saudi Arabian plant *Anvillea garcinii*. *Fitoterapia* **2019**, *134*, 129–134. [CrossRef]
14. Chae, Y.K.; Bobin, K.; Jungil, H.; Hyeon-Son, C. Parthenolide inhibits lipid accumulation via activation of Nrf2/ Keap1 signaling during adipocyte differentiation. *Food Sci. Biotechnol.* **2020**, *29*, 431–440.
15. Abdel-Sattar, E.; McPhail, A.T. Cis-Parthenolid-9-one from *Anvillea garcinia*. *J. Nat. Prod.* **2000**, *63*, 1587–1589. [CrossRef]
16. Drew, D.P.; Krichau, N.; Reichwald, K.; Simonsen, H.T. Guaianolides in Apiaceae: Perspectives on pharmacology and biosynthesis. *Phytochem. Rev.* **2009**, *8*, 581–599. [CrossRef]
17. Galal, A.M. Minor guaianolides from *Anvillea garcinia*. *Al Azhar J. Pharm. Sci.* **1997**, *19*, 30–33.
18. Tan, R.X.; Tang, H.Q.; Hu, J.; Shuai, B. Lignans and sesquiterpene lactones from *Artemisia sieversiana* and *Inula racemosa*. *Phytochemistry* **1998**, *49*, 157–161. [CrossRef]
19. Tosovic, J.; Markovic, S. Structural and antioxidative features of chlorogenic acid. *Croat. Chem. Acta* **2016**, *89*, 535–541. [CrossRef]
20. Erel, S.B.; Karaalp, C.; Bedir, E.; Kaehlig, H.; Glasl, S.; Khan, S.; Krenn, L. Secondary metabolites of *Centaurea calolepis* and evaluation of cnicin for anti-inflammatory, antioxidant, and cytotoxic activities. *Pharm. Biol.* **2011**, *49*, 840–849. [CrossRef]
21. Azam, F.; Chaudhry, B.A.; Ijaz, H.; Qadir, M.I. Caffeoyl-β-D-glucopyranoside and 1,3-dihydroxy-2-tetracosanoylamino-4-(E)-nonadecene isolated from *Ranunculus muricatus* exhibit antioxidant activity. *Sci. Rep.* **2019**, *9*, 15613. [CrossRef]
22. Delazar, A.; Nazemiyeh, H.; Afshar, F.H.; Barghi, N.; Esnaashari, S.; Asgharian, P. Chemical compositions and biological activities of *Scutellaria pinnatifida* A. Hamilt aerial parts. *Res. Pharm. Sci.* **2017**, *12*, 187–195.
23. Aisah, L.S.; yun, Y.F.; Herlina, T.; Julaeha, E.; Zainuddin, A.; Nurfarida, I.; Hidayat, A.T.; Supratman, U.; Shiono, Y. Flavonoid compounds from the leaves of *Kalanchoe prolifera* and their cytotoxic activity against P-388 murine leukemia cells. *Nat. Prod. Sci.* **2017**, *23*, 139–145. [CrossRef]
24. Lee, S.B.; Shin, J.S.; Han, H.S.; Lee, H.H.; Park, J.C.; Lee, K.T. Kaempferol 7-O-β-D-glucoside isolated from the leaves of *Cudrania tricuspidata* inhibits LPS-induced expression of pro-inflammatory mediators through inactivation of NF-κB, AP-1, and JAK-STAT in RAW 264.7 macrophages. *Chem. Biol. Interact.* **2018**, *284*, 101–111. [CrossRef]
25. Achoub, H.; Mencherini, T.; Esposito, T.; Rastrelli, L.; Aquino, R.; Gazzerro, P.; Zaiter, L.; Benayache, F.; Benayache, S. New sesquiterpenes from *Asteriscus graveolens*. *Nat. Prod. Res.* **2019**, in press. [CrossRef]
26. Meng, J.C.; Hu, Y.F.; Chen, J.H.; Tan, R.X. Antifungal highly oxygenated guaianolides and other constituents from *Ajania fruticulosa*. *Phytochemistry* **2002**, *58*, 1141–1145. [CrossRef]

27. Ebrahim, W.; El-Neketi, M.; Lewald, L.; Orfali, R.; Lin, W.; Rehberg, N.; Kalscheuer, R.; Daletos, G.; Proksch, P. Metabolites from the fungal endophyte *Aspergillus austroafricanus* in axenic culture and in fungal–bacterial mixed cultures. *J. Nat. Prod.* **2016**, *79*, 914–922. [CrossRef]
28. Berghe, V.; Vlietinck, A. Screening methods for antibacterial and antiviral agents from higher plants. *Methods Plant Biochem.* **1991**, *6*, 47–68.
29. Gong, L.; Guo, S. Endophytic fungi from *Dracaena cambodiana* and *Aquilaria sinensis* and their antimicrobial activity. *Afr. J. Biotechnol.* **2009**, *8*, 731.

Sample Availability: Samples of the compounds are available from the authors.

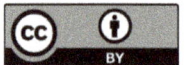

© 2020 by the authors. Licensee MDPI, Basel, Switzerland. This article is an open access article distributed under the terms and conditions of the Creative Commons Attribution (CC BY) license (http://creativecommons.org/licenses/by/4.0/).

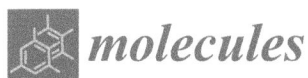

Article

Phytochemical and Safety Evaluations of Volatile Terpenoids from *Zingiber cassumunar* Roxb. on Mature Carp Peripheral Blood Mononuclear Cells and Embryonic Zebrafish

Raktham Mektrirat [1,2], Terdsak Yano [3], Siriporn Okonogi [2,4], Wasan Katip [5] and Surachai Pikulkaew [2,3,*]

[1] Department of Veterinary Biosciences and Public Health, Faculty of Veterinary Medicine, Chiang Mai University, Chiang Mai 50100, Thailand; raktham.m@cmu.ac.th
[2] Research Center for Pharmaceutical Nanotechnology, Chiang Mai University, Chiang Mai 50200, Thailand; okng2000@gmail.com
[3] Department of Food Animal Clinic, Faculty of Veterinary Medicine, Chiang Mai University, Chiang Mai 50100, Thailand; vetjek@gmail.com
[4] Department of Pharmaceutical Sciences, Faculty of Pharmacy, Chiang Mai University, Chiang Mai 50200, Thailand
[5] Department of Pharmaceutical Care, Faculty of Pharmacy, Chiang Mai University, Chiang Mai 50200, Thailand; wasankatip@gmail.com
* Correspondence: surapikulkaew@gmail.com; Tel.: +66-(53)-948-023; Fax: +66-(53)-274-710

Received: 30 December 2019; Accepted: 28 January 2020; Published: 30 January 2020

Abstract: Pharmaceutical products of essential oil from *Zingiber cassumunar* Roxb. are extensively being developed, while the research on their safety is seldom documented. The aim of the present study was to evaluate the phytochemical profile and the effect of cassumunar ginger oil on cell-based assay and the zebrafish model. The essential oil was isolated from fresh rhizomes of *Z. cassumunar* using simultaneous steam-distillation. Chemical composition was analyzed using gas chromatograph coupled to a mass spectrometer (GC-MS). Effect of cassumunar ginger oil on adult carp fish peripheral blood mononuclear cells (PBMCs) was investigated using MTT assay. The embryotoxic and teratogenic effects of cassumunar ginger oil were studied in zebrafish embryos. GC-MS results showed that the essential oil was composed of sabinene (43.54%) and terpinen-4-ol (29.52%) as the major phytoconstituents. No fish PBMC cytotoxic effect was observed with the concentration less than 50 µg/mL of cassumunar ginger oil. Our results showed for the first time the embryotoxic and teratogenic effects of cassumunar ginger oil in zebrafish embryos. The result indicated that the cassumunar ginger oil induced zebrafish embryotoxicity in a concentration-dependent manner. At 500 µg/mL of cassumunar ginger oil demonstrated significantly moderated embryotoxicity within 24 h ($p < 0.05$). The survival rate of 100 µg/mL of cassumunar ginger group was markedly declined to zero at 96-h post-fertilization (log-rank test, $p = 0.001$). However, survival rates of zebrafish embryo in the 1 and 10 µg/mL cassumunar ginger groups were more than 90% throughout the trial period. Moreover, very low teratogenicity to the zebrafish embryo was also observed in 1 and 10 µg/mL of cassumunar ginger groups. Our findings suggest that there is hardly any cytotoxicity, embryotoxicity and teratogenicity at concentrations less than 10 µg/mL of cassumunar ginger oil. However, the toxicity assessment of its pharmaceutical product should prove for further consumer protection.

Keywords: Zingiberaceae; essential oil; terpene; cytotoxicity; embryotoxicity; zebrafish

1. Introduction

The perennial angiosperm plants of family Zingiberaceae is distributed widely the tropical climatic areas including Asia, Africa and America [1]. This plant family is a significant bioresource provided various utilizations including food ingredients and spices, medicinal herbs, aromatherapy agents and textile dyes [2]. In the last decades, the phytotherapies of the plant extracts is worldwide exceeding in both human and veterinary medicines [3]. As a consequence, the rhizome of Zingiberaceous plants are a valuable source of terpenes and terpenoids, which exhibits a broad spectrum of biological effects. Plants of the Zingiber genera particularly represent useful herbal remedies under Zingiberaceous plants including Z. cassumunar Roxb., Z. corallinum Hance., Z. nimmonii Dalzell., Z. officinale Rosc., Z. wrayi C.K. Lim. and Z. zerumbet (L.) Smith. [1]. Increasingly, Z. cassumunar (cassumunar ginger) is commonly used as a traditional medicinal plant with treatment of a variety of illnesses in Thailand and many Asian countries [4]. The essential oils of the cassumunar ginger have previously identified the major terpenic compounds containing sabinene and terpinen-4-ol [5,6]. The modern pharmaceutical products of the functional terpenoids from cassumunar ginger have recently been developed because of its pharmacological properties including anti-inflammatory, antifungal and antibacterial efficacies [1,4,7]. The pharmacological efficacy is hindered by the low hydrophilicity of the terpene derivatives; therefore, some thermodynamically stable dosage forms are prepared for overcoming this problem [6]. Therefore, the toxicity assessments of the cassumunar ginger oils are essential to ensure the safety of phytopharmaceuticals, although the acute and the chronic oral toxicity of Z. cassumunar extracts using Organization of Economic Cooperation and Development (OECD) and World Health Organization (WHO) guidelines has been previously reported [8]. Geographical origin is one of the most important aspects that influence the chemical composition of plants. Unfortunately, a review of the literature revealed that there is no documented in the considering embryotoxic and teratogenic assessments of essential oil from Z. cassumunar from Thailand. Therefore, the present research planned to fill this gap.

In recent year, the zebrafish (Danio rerio) has been widely used as animal model in scientific research areas such as genetic model, cancer research and biology development [9]. The zebrafish embryo is a useful small model for investigating vertebrate development because of its rapid development, high fecundity and easy observation of transparent embryos [10]. Interestingly, the processes of development in zebrafish embryo are similar to embryogenesis of other higher vertebrates, including humans [11]. Moreover, the usage of the zebrafish model unforgettably tapers the toxicity studies using the higher vertebrate models. From these benefits, the zebrafish embryo has been considered as an alternative model for vertebrate model for toxicological assessment [9,10], as well as for new drug discovery of herb [12,13]. Recent studies on embryotoxic and developmental toxicity assessments of Curcuma longa Linn. extract using a zebrafish model are reported. [14]. Thus, the current investigation was used the zebrafish embryo model to assessment the embryotoxicity and teratogenicity of essential oil from Z. cassumunar. However, the cell-based toxicity assay should be performed for prognosticating toxicity prior to study in the whole organisms. The ability of the phytoconstituents in inhibiting the cell viability of peripheral blood mononuclear cells (PBMC) is ascertained as an indication of its systemic toxicity. Consequently, the aim of the present study was to identify chemical composition of the cassumunar ginger oil and evaluate its toxicity on in vitro adult carp PBMCs and in vivo zebrafish embryos.

2. Results

2.1. Chemical Compositions of Essential Oil

The ginger cassumunar oil appeared as a clear pale yellowish liquid. The phytoconstituents were characterized by GC-MS method with a running time of 50 min. A list of the constituents identified in the ginger cassumunar oil and their percentage composition is shown in Table 1. The composition of essential oil was identified by terpenoids (87.97%), which consisted mainly of monocyclic monoterpenoids (87.47%) and small amounts of sesquiterpenes (0.52%). The monoterpenoids were divided into the monoterpene hydrocarbons (58.45%) and the oxygen-containing compounds (29.25%). Interestingly, an indolizidine alkaloid was present in little amounts (11.10%). The chromatogram demonstrated the presence of predominated identifiable spectra (Figure 1). The most abundant compounds were sabinene, accounting for about 43.54% of the total peak area, followed by terpinen-4-ol (29.52%), 1,2-dimethyl-6-nitroindolizine (11.10%), and γ-Terpinene (7.38%).

Table 1. Chemical composition of essential oil from *Z. cassumunar* Roxb. obtained by GC-MS analysis. The cassumunar ginger oil was extracted from the rhizomes of *Z. cassumunar* by simultaneous steam-distillation and analyzed by GC-MS. RT: Retention time; MW: Molecular weight.

Peak	RT (min)	Component	Formula	MW (g/mol)	Amount (%)
1	5.64	α-Thujene	$C_{10}H_{16}$	136.23	0.60
2	5.83	α-Pinene	$C_{10}H_{16}$	136.23	1.58
3	7.16	Sabinene	$C_{10}H_{16}$	136.23	43.54
4	7.84	Myrcene	$C_{10}H_{16}$	136.23	1.17
5	8.74	α-Terpinene	$C_{10}H_{16}$	136.23	2.82
6	9.09	Benzene	C_6H_6	78.11	0.94
7	10.46	γ-Terpinene	$C_{10}H_{16}$	136.23	7.38
8	11.69	α-Terpinolene	$C_{10}H_{16}$	136.23	0.84
9	15.68	Terpinen-4-ol	$C_{10}H_{18}O$	154.25	29.52
10	30.24	β-Sesquiphellandrene	$C_{15}H_{24}$	204.35	0.52
11	34.63	1,2-Dimethyl-6-nitroindolizine	$C_{10}H_{10}O_2N_2$	190.20	11.10

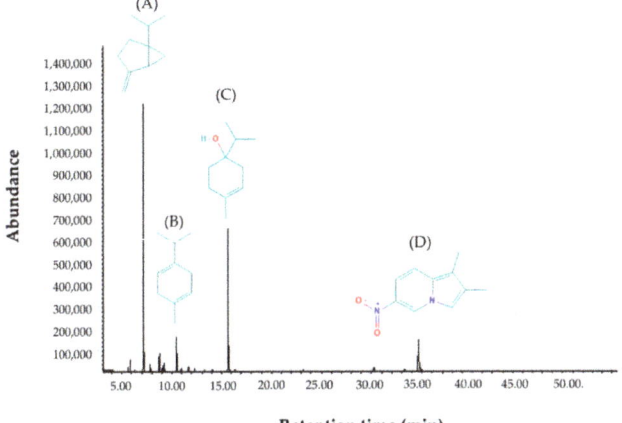

Figure 1. GC-MS chromatograph for essential oil isolated from *Zingiber cassumunar* Roxb. The phytoconstituents were characterized by a GC-MS method with a running time of 50 min. Chemical structures of the four major constituents identified from the cassumunar ginger oil including (**A**) Sabinene, (**B**) γ-Terpinene, (**C**) 4-Terpineol and (**D**) 1,2-Dimethyl-6-nitroindolizine.

2.2. Cytotoxicity on Adult Fish PBMCS

To examine the essential oil from *Z. cassumunar* induced cytotoxicity, cell viability for PBMCs of adult carp fish was determined using MTT reduction assay. The cell viability was represented by the detection of enzyme mitochondrial dehydrogenase activity. The cytotoxic effect of the cassumunar ginger oil on PBMCs for 24 h was shown in Figure 2. The results summarized that the cassumunar ginger oil induced PBMCs cytotoxicity in a concentration-dependent manner. The viability rate of the PBMCs from the control group was 100%, while that of the PBMCs treated with 5, 10, 50, 100 and 500 µg/mL of the cassumunar ginger oils was 89.75 ± 3.04%, 82.32 ± 6.12%, 71.08 ± 1.92, 62.94 ± 4.73 and 59.25 ± 5.73%, respectively. The essential oil concentrations of 100 and 500 µg/mL exhibited significantly higher cytotoxicity than that of the concentration range at 5 and 10 µg/mL ($p < 0.05$).

On the other hand, the cassumunar ginger oils at the concentration less than 50 µg/mL were not significantly toxic to the PBMCs by this assay.

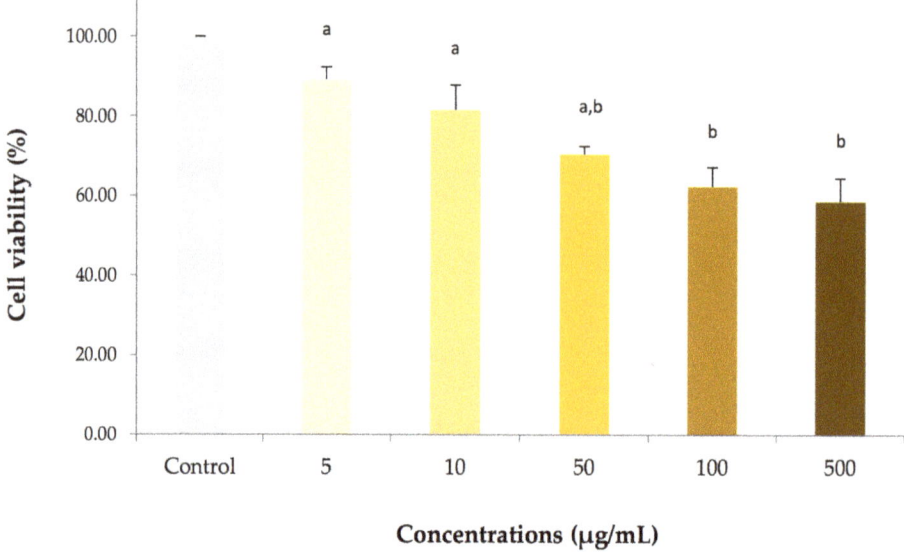

Figure 2. The cytotoxic effect of essential oil from *Zingiber cassumunar* Roxb. on adult carp fish PBMCs. The cells were treated with a series of concentrations in the range 5–500 µg/mL for 24 h. Percentages of cell viability were calculated from the PBMCs exposed to 0.1% DMSO (control), and 5, 10, 50, 100 and 500 µg/mL essential oils. Data represent the mean (±standard deviation, SD) of four independent experiments. Experiments were analyzed using two-way ANOVA and Tukey's multiple comparison test. Bars not sharing a common letter are significantly different ($p < 0.05$).

2.3. Dose-response Embryotoxicity in Zebrafish

The embryotoxicity was determined at multiple concentrations of the cassumunar ginger oils (5, 10, 50, 100 and 500 µg/mL) prior to evaluating its killing-kinetic effect. Absence of larvae heartbeat and coagulation of embryo were used as criteria to differentiate viable from non-viable zebrafish embryo (Figure 5B). Our results revealed that the toxic effect of cassumunar ginger oils were found to be dependent on dose. The mean mortality of zebrafish embryo at 24 h was obtained as shown in Figure 3. The results summarized that no mortality was observed in embryos exposed to 0.1% DMSO (control) and 5 µg/mL of the cassumunar ginger oils. A few mortality rates of embryos exposed treated with 10, 50, 100 µg/mL of the cassumunar ginger oils was 2.50 ± 5.00%, 2.50 ± 5.00%, and 15.00 ± 5.77%, respectively. Significantly increasing mortality rates ($p < 0.05$) were demonstrated in treatment at 500 µg/mL when compared with the low concentration of cassumunar ginger oils (≤100 µg/mL).

2.4. Time-kill Analysis in Zebrafish Embryos

The study of dose-response embryotoxicity suggested that a value corresponding to the maximum safety concentration on zebrafish embryos are given at 100 µg/mL of the cassumunar ginger oils. Therefore, the time-kill analysis of three different concentrations of cassumunar ginger oils (1, 10 and 100 µg/mL) was performed to evaluate the kinetic killing of zebrafish embryos at 24, 48, 72 and 96 h. The Kaplan–Meier curve is used to demonstrate the survival time from a certain date to time of zebrafish embryo death (Figure 4). The result showed that the killing ability of cassumunar ginger oil was performed in a time dependent manner. However, survival rates of embryo in the control, 1 and

10 µg/mL of cassumunar ginger groups were more than 90% throughout the trial period. Whereas, the survival rate of 100 µg/mL of cassumunar ginger groups was markedly declined to zero at 96 h post-exposure observation time (log-rank test, $p = 0.001$).

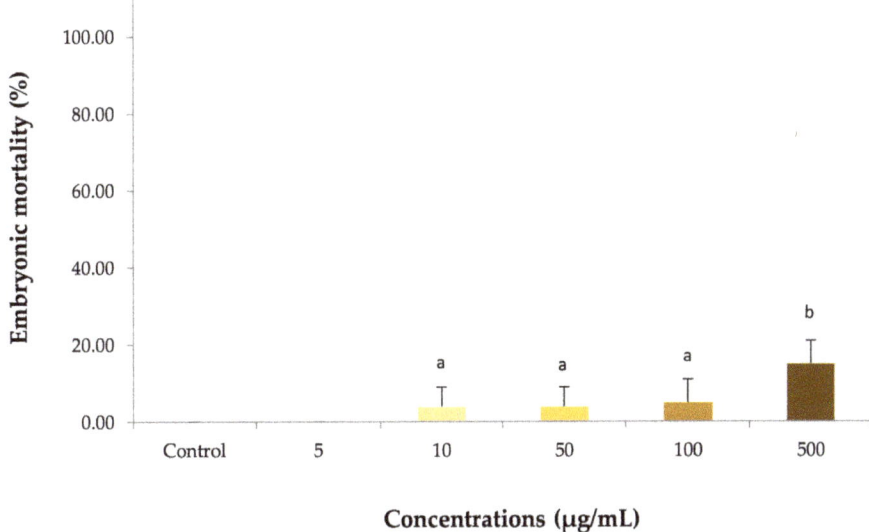

Figure 3. The embryotoxic effect of various concentrations of essential oil from *Zingiber cassumunar* Roxb. in embryonic zebrafish. The zebrafish embryos were treated with a series of concentrations in the range 5–500 µg/mL Percentages of embryonic mortality were calculated from zebrafish embryos exposed to 0.1% DMSO (control), and 5, 10, 50, 100 and 500 µg/mL of the cassumunar ginger oils. Data represent the mean ± SD of four independent experiments ($n = 40$ per group). Experiments were analyzed using two-way ANOVA and Tukey's multiple comparison test. Bars not sharing a common letter are significantly different ($p < 0.05$).

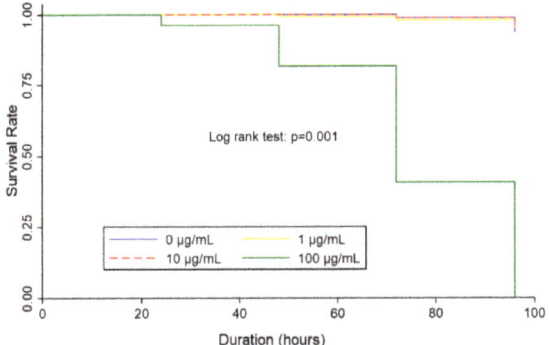

Figure 4. The embryotoxic effect of essential oil from *Zingiber cassumunar* Roxb. on time-killing in embryonic zebrafish. The zebrafish embryos were exposed to 0.1% DMSO (control), and 1, 10 and 100 µg/mL of the cassumunar ginger oils. Kaplan–Meier plot represents survival rate in four different groups of four independent experiments (n = 40 per group). The Log Rank test was used for statistical analysis ($p < 0.01$).

2.5. Teratogenicity in Zebrafish

To examine the essential oil from *Z. cassumunar* induced teratogenicity, the zebrafish embryos were determined at multiple concentrations of the cassumunar ginger oils (1, 10 and 100 µg/mL) during range of exposure time 24–96 h. The teratogenic effect of the cassumunar ginger oil in zebrafish embryos was shown in Table 2. The result illustrated that the malformation rate of embryonic zebrafish exposed to 10 and 100 µg/mL of cassumunar ginger oils for 24 h was 1 ± 0.8% and 24.5 ± 6.6%, respectively. The embryonic morphology was observed including the malformation of yolk sac and the malformation of head and tail development (Figure 5D). Surprisingly, accumulative abnormality to the zebrafish embryo was not found in all experiment groups at 48 h. However, some remaining embryos that were exposed to 100 µg/mL showed pericardial sac edema, the abnormality of the spinal column and the poor reabsorption of yolk sac (Figure 5F,H) with 10.5 ± 1.9% at 72 h. Mortality rate of 100% was observed at 96 h after exposure to 100 µg/mL of cassumunar ginger oils and all embryos were defined as coagulation of embryo (Figure 5B). Interestingly, no teratogenic abnormality of the zebrafish embryo was found in control and 1 µg/mL groups throughout the trial period. (Figure 5A,E).

Table 2. Teratogenic effects of essential oil from *Zingiber cassumunar* Roxb. on early development of zebrafish. The zebrafish embryos were treated to 0.1% DMSO (control), and 1, 10 and 100 µg/mL of the cassumunar ginger oils at different times of exposure (24, 48, 72 and 96 h). Descriptive data represent the mean ± SD of teratogenic embryo percentage of four independent experiments (*n* = 40 per group). NE = no surviving embryo.

Concentrations (µg/mL)	Times of Exposure (h)			
	24	48	72	96
0	0	0	0	0
1	0	0	0	0
10	1.0 ± 0.8	0	0	0
100	24.5 ± 6.6	0	10.5 ± 1.9	NE

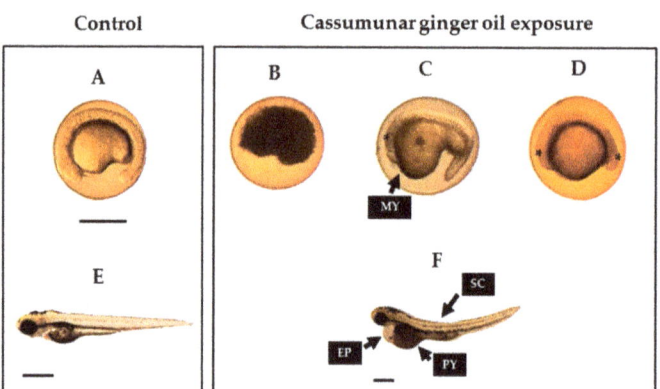

Figure 5. Effect of essential oil from *Zingiber cassumunar* Roxb. on typical malformations in zebrafish embryos. The zebrafish embryos were exposed to 0.1% DMSO (control), and 1, 10 and 100 of the cassumunar ginger oils. The normal morphology of zebrafish embryo and larvae exposure to filtered water and to 0.1% DMSO (control) at 24 h (**A**) and 72 h (**E**). Typical malformations caused by 100 µg/mL of cassumunar ginger oils on zebrafish embryonic development at 24 h (**B,C,D**) and 72 h (**F**). Description: coagulation (**B**) and embryo with teratogenic effect (**C,D,F**). Abbreviations: MY, malformation of yolk sac; PY, poor reabsorption of yolk sac; and SC, spinal column curving. (Scale bars = 1 µm).

3. Discussion

Terpenes and their derivatives are worldwide exceeding in both human and veterinary medicine. Fortunately, the essential oil from Z. cassumunar Roxb. was previously characterized as the natural terpenic compounds. The major component including sabinene (53.50%) and terpinen-4-ol (29.96%), γ-Terpinene (7.25%), and (E)-1-(3,4-dimethoxyphenyl) butadiene (16.16%) had found in essential oil isolated from a native Thai species of Z. cassumunar [5]. The phytochemical composition of essential oil from Z. montanum Koenig Link ex A. Dietr were also sabinene (56.34%), terpinen-4-ol (10.17%) and (E)-1-(3,4-dimethoxyphenyl) butadiene (14.7%) [15]. These findings are in agreement with our results on cassumunar ginger oil which the major constituents were sabinene (43.54%), terpinen-4-ol (29.52%) and γ-Terpinene (7.38%), respectively. Our results demonstrated differences in their constituents from an indolizidine alkaloid of 1,2-dimethyl-6-nitroindolizine (11.10%). On the other hand, the essential oil from Z. cassumunar cultivated in Malaysia showed the distinctive compounds including 6,9,9-tetramethyl-2,6,10-cycloundecatrien-1-one (60.77%) and α-caryophyllene (23.92%) [16]. The amount and phytochemicals of essential oils are decided by the plant ontogenesis; therefore, the growing season and the harvesting time are the exogenous factors affecting quality and quantity [15,17]. The extraction techniques of the distillations and the solvent extractions are also influencing both yield and quality of essential oils [18]. Moreover, the different cultivation areas affecting the phytochemical constituents of Z. montanum have previously been published [15].

The major component of the cassumunar ginger oil consists of monocyclic monoterpenoid with sabinene and terpinen-4-ol were well documented. Moreover, both sabinene and terpinen-4-ol exhibit a broad spectrum of biological effects [19,20]. Therefore, many efforts are development of cassumunar ginger oil as a value-added material that is useful as a pharmaceutical excipient for pharmaceutical, cosmetic and food industries [1,21]. In the most interest of the anti-inflammatory activity, attempts have recently been made to derive this cassumunar ginger oil to formulate the tropical preparations for local and systemic administrations. The topical and the transdermal deliveries of cassumunar ginger oil have been successfully developed by microemulsion, gels and patches [6,22–24]. Development of pharmaceutical products from cassumunar ginger oil are extensively growing, while the research on their toxicity is still limited. The acute and chronic oral toxicity of Z. cassumunar extract granules in Sprague–Dawley rats using OECD and WHO guidelines have been previously reported [8]. Their results demonstrated that the animals treated with the granules of Z. cassumunar extract were not showing the clinical signs related to toxicity in both single and chronic administration. Therefore, the oral no-observed-adverse-effect level (NOAEL) in rats was documented at 1,125 mg/kg body weight/day. Unfortunately, there is no documentation considering embryotoxic and teratogenic assessments of essential oil from Z. cassumunar.

The cell-based toxicity assay on adult fish PBMCs was performed for prognosticating toxicity of cassumunar ginger oil prior to study in the whole organism of zebrafish. The cytotoxicity result of the essential oil on adult fish PBMCs was in dose-dependent manner. The concentration at 5, 10 and 50 μg/mL of the essential oils showed low effect to adult fish PBMCs; whereas, the essential oil concentrations of 100 and 500 μg/mL exhibited significantly higher cytotoxicity than that of the low concentration (≤50 μg/mL). The mechanisms of cassumunar ginger oil-mediated cell death are difficult to delineate under this methodologic study. In the reaction mixture, MTT is reduced by mitochondrial enzymes of metabolically active cells and the amount of MTT formazan generated is directly proportional to the viable cell number [25]. Therefore, the MTT assay is used for measuring the screening results of cytotoxicity or proliferative effect of the medicinal substances. However, the percentage of cytotoxicity at highest concentration of the essential oils (500 μg/mL) is lower the inhibitory concentration 50% (IC_{50}) in this study. Moreover, a previous study demonstrated that cytotoxicity of purified compounds from crude extract of Z. cassumunar has weak toxic activity with IC_{50} values of L929 cell line (1263.42 to 2857.83 μg/mL) and Vero cell line (1537.83 to 2698.45 μg/mL) [26]. These results suggest that cassumunar ginger oil has strong safety on the animal cells exposed directly.

The effects of cassumunar ginger oil on in vivo embryotoxicity or teratogenicity in zebrafish embryos were investigated. No embryonic mortality or malformation were observed in the low concentration of cassumunar ginger oil (≤10 µg/mL). At the concentration of 100 ug/mL, an increase in embryotoxicity by a time-dependent manner was observed. This corresponds to the previous finding on *Curcuma longa* Linn. extract which exhibited embryotoxicity at high concentrations (125 µg/mL) on developing zebrafish [14]. The zebrafish fed with the essential oil from *Pistacia lentiscus* Var. *chia* with high concentrations of 100 and 200 ppm also demonstrated in increased larvae mortality [27]. It is already known from many research reports that both *Z. cassumunar* and *C. longa* plants of family Zingiberaceae represent terpenic and phenolic structures. It can readily pass through the cytoplasmic membrane of zebrafish embryos. Effective permeability of terpenic compounds depends on its chemical structure including hydrophobicity, small size, energy of vaporization and degree of unsaturation [28]. Moreover, it is notable that outer membrane enclosing the embryo was uninterruptedly altered with advancing age of embryo development. This alteration of the protective layer has caused in opening and widening of the chorion pore channel; therefore, the increased uptake of external solutes occurred [29].

Current evidence suggests that the essential oil from *Z. cassumunar* possess certain toxic effects on embryos and development of larvae at high dosage. It should be noted that the toxicity of *Z. cassumunar* are on the basis of their isolated active phytochemical compounds. The pharmaceutical necessities use in pharmaceutical products may also cause toxicity and other disadvantage to the formulation. Therefore, the toxicity assessment of the pharmaceutical product of *Z. cassumunar* should be studied further. Among the 808 articles of the clinical efficacy and safety on *Z. cassumunar* previously was identified by a systematic review [30]. Moreover, the pharmacokinetics of the major bioactive components from *Z. cassumunar* following oral and topical administrations in rats were previously evaluated [31–33]. In drug development, is critical to ensure that the preclinical study properly supports the patient safety and quality of health care. Our results contribute to understanding the developmental toxicity of essential oil which has a predictive value with regard to its safety.

4. Materials and Methods

4.1. Plant Materials

The fresh rhizomes of cassumunar ginger were purchased from the local market in Chiang Mai, Thailand (Lat 18° 47' 46.1148'' N and Long 98° 58' 45.3468'' E). The voucher specimens were deposited at the Herbarium of the Faculty of Pharmacy, Chiang Mai University, Thailand. The rhizomes were cleaned with water and chopped into pieces. The sample was shade dried and powdered using a dry grinder. The powdered material was stored in light-resistant container until used in the extraction studies.

4.2. Distillation of Essential Oil and Chemical Characterization

The essential oil was isolated by the simultaneous steam-distillation using a Clevenger apparatus for 3 h. The essential oil obtained was dried and stored in an airtight dark bottle at −20 °C until use. Chemical characterizations of the obtained essential oil were analyzed using a gas chromatography-mass spectrometry (GC-MS) method. The GC-MS analysis was performed using a model 6890 gas chromatograph equipped with a 5973 mass-selective detector using HP-5MS column (30 m × 250 µm i.d. × 0.25 µm film thickness). The identification of each compound was based on their retention times relative to those of authentic samples and matching spectral peaks available in Wiley, NIST, and NBS mass spectral libraries. The percentage of each component was calculated based on the total area of all peaks obtained from the oil.

4.3. Animal and Ethic Statement

Koi carp (*Cyprinus carpio* Koi) and Zebrafish (*Danio rerio*) were obtained from the stock of the Faculty of Veterinary Medicine, Chiang Mai University. Adult fish were kept in the glass tanks using filtered tap water (pH 7.4–7.6) and held in natural light conditions. Water parameters including temperature and pH were monitored daily. The fish were fed twice daily with frozen brine shrimp in the morning and with commercial dry feed in the afternoon. Feces were siphoned out of the tanks every day. The experiment was conducted in accordance with the protocols approved by the Animal Ethics Committee, Faculty of Veterinary Medicine, Chiang Mai University (Ethic Permit No. S5/2562).

4.4. Fish Blood Collection and PBMC Isolation

The pooled blood samples were collected from twelve anesthetized carp fish. Each of four fish in three independent experiments were recruited into the study. About three ml of whole blood was collected by caudal venipuncture into a coagulation tubes containing a buffered sodium citrate solution. The PBMCs were isolated by Ficoll gradient centrifugation according to the manufacturer's instructions. Briefly, a stratified sample between 6 mL of Ficoll–Hypaque and 12 mL of peripheral blood was prepared and centrifuged at $400 \times g$ for 20 min. the PBMCs were carefully aspirated from the Ficoll-plasma interface and washed three times with sterile phosphate-buffered saline (PBS). The cell viability was assessed by trypan blue exclusion under the light microscope.

4.5. In Vitro MTT Reduction Assay

Isolated PBMCs of carp fish were adjusted to 5×10^5 cells/mL in RPMI 1640 supplemented with 1% heat-inactivated fetal bovine serum. The fish PBMCs were treated with various concentration of 0, 5, 10, 50, 100 and 500 µg/mL cassumunar ginger oil and incubated in 5% CO_2 incubator under humidified conditions at 37 °C. Briefly, the solutions were freshly prepared by mixing the appropriate amount of oil and pure solvent DMSO in a sterile tube and subsequently mixing under moderate agitation using a vortex mixer until homogenous. The cytotoxicity was measured by MTT (3-(4,5-dimethylthiazol-2-yl)-2,5-diphenyl tetrazolium bromide) reduction assay at 24 h after exposure of cassumunar ginger oil. The volume of 10 µL of 5 mg/mL MTT was added into 200 µL of cell suspension and incubated for 4 h. The volume of 100 µl 0.1 M HCl in absolute isopropanol was added after incubation. The colorimetric determination of formazan product was spectrophotometrically measured at 570 nm. Cell viability was expressed as a percentage of the control culture with 0.1% DMSO.

4.6. Zebrafish Breeding and Embryo Acquisition

One male and two female adult zebrafishes were kept during the breeding period. Zebrafish embryos were spawned by natural mating. The fertilized eggs collected and were rinsed with sea salt egg water (60 mg/L sea salt and 2 mg/L methylene blue). Selections of fertilized egg in a stage 3–4 h postfertilization (hpf) were performed under a stereomicroscope (Nikon, Tokyo, Japan). Qualified embryos were maintained at 28.5 °C in clean petri dishes with previously egg water until analysis.

4.7. Zebrafish Embryonic Toxicity Test

4.7.1. Dose-response Embryotoxicity

Sample embryotoxicity was determined by means of mortality rate in the zebrafish embryos. Briefly, the zebrafish embryos ($n = 10$) were transferred to individual wells of 24-well plates. The embryos were exposed to various concentrations of essential oil from *Z. cassumunar* in DMSO (100 mg/mL) to make 0, 5, 10, 50, 100 and 500 µg/mL of final concentration. The embryos were observed under a stereomicroscope at 24 h post-fertilization (hpf). The identification of death embryo was defined with coagulation of embryo or no visual heartbeat of larvae. The number of dead embryos were recorded, and the mortality rate was calculated.

4.7.2. Time-killed Analysis

The killing kinetic of essential oil from *Z. cassumunar* was performed to determine the time killing rates of Zebrafish embryos. Briefly, ten fertilized eggs ($n = 10$) for each concentration of treatment essential oil from Z. *cassumunar* were studied. The experiment was performed in four independent replicates in a 24-well plate containing 2 mL of embryo media with 0.1% DMSO containing 100 μg of essential oil from Z. *cassumunar*. It was serially diluted via 10-fold serial dilution to produce 3 different concentrations of essential oil from Z. *cassumunar*. The death embryos were identified under a stereomicroscope and the time-killed analysis was studied at 24, 48, 72 and 96 h. The data was recorded, and the Kaplan–Meier curve was generated.

4.8. Zebrafish Teratogenicity Test

Sample teratogenicity was determined by morphological appearance and development of the zebrafish embryos. Briefly, the zebrafish embryos ($n = 10$) were transferred to individual wells of 24-well plates containing the essential oil from Z. *cassumunar* (0, 5, 10, 50, 100 and 500 μg/mL of final concentration). After incubation, the morphological defects of the exposed embryos were evaluated every 24 h under a stereomicroscope. Embryonic morphology was determined according to OECD test guidelines [34] and normal development of embryo was compared with previous described by Kimmel et al. [11]. The teratogenicity was assessed by descriptive determining the percentage of embryos or larvae with abnormality over remaining embryos.

4.9. Statistical Analysis

The experiments were done with four independent replications of each treatment and each killing time of study. The PBMC viability and the mortality of zebrafish embryos were compared by means of two-way analysis of variance (ANOVA) and Tukey's multiple comparison test using R analysis program. All data are presented as mean ± standard deviation of the mean (SD), and the probabilities less than 0.05 were considered significant. Statistical analysis of killing time was performed using Stata software, version 14 (Stata-Corp, College Station, TX). Differences between the four groups in rates of time to outcome, was compared using the Kaplan–Meier curve and the log-rank test for significance.

5. Conclusions

This present research has indicated that the phytochemical characterization of cassumunar ginger oil has demonstrated sabinene and 4-terpineol as the major composition, along with other volatile compounds to sum a total of 11 identified phytoconstituents. Our results highlighted for the first study of embryotoxicity and teratogenicity of essential oil isolated from Z. *cassumunar* Roxb. This study provides safety information of cassumunar ginger oil in the cell-based toxicity assay and the zebrafish model. The cassumunar ginger oil at the concentration less than 50 μg/mL was not toxic to the adult fish PMMCs by MTT reduction test, whereas, no embryotoxicity and teratogenicity since 10.8% teratogenic effect is not significant. However, the toxicity assessment of its pharmaceutical product should prove for further consumer protection.

Author Contributions: Project administration and conceptualization, R.M., S.P. and S.O.; methodology, investigation and validation, R.M. and S.P.; data curation, formal analysis and visualization, R.M., S.P., T.Y., and W.K.; original draft preparation, R.M. and S.P.; review, editing and approval of final draft, R.M. and S.P. All authors have read and agreed to the published version of the manuscript.

Funding: The authors are grateful for the financial support received from the National Research Council of Thailand (NRCT).

Acknowledgments: This research work was partially supported by Chiang Mai University. The authors are thankful for the Research Center of Pharmaceutical Nanotechnology and the Research Center of Producing and Development of Products and Innovations for Animal Health and Production, Chiang Mai University for the facility and instrument support.

Conflicts of Interest: The authors declare no conflict of interest.

References

1. Sharifi-Rad, M.; Varoni, E.M.; Salehi, B.; Sharifi-Rad, J.; Matthews, K.R.; Ayatollahi, S.A.; Kobarfard, F.; Ibrahim, S.A.; Mnayer, D.; Zakaria, Z.A.; et al. Plants of the Genus *Zingiber* as a Source of Bioactive Phytochemicals: From Tradition to Pharmacy. *Molecules* **2017**, *22*, 2145. [CrossRef] [PubMed]
2. Sharifi-Rad, J.; Sureda, A.; Tenore, G.C.; Daglia, M.; Sharifi-Rad, M.; Valussi, M.; Tundis, R.; Sharifi-Rad, M.; Loizzo, M.R.; Ademiluyi, A.O.; et al. Biological Activities of Essential Oils: From Plant Chemoecology to Traditional Healing Systems. *Molecules* **2017**, *22*, 70. [CrossRef] [PubMed]
3. Ghosh, S.; Majumder, P.B.; Mandi, S.S. Species-specific AFLP markers for identification of *Zingiber officinale*, *Z. montanum* and, *Z. zerumbet* (Zingiberaceae). *Genet. Mol. Res.* **2011**, *10*, 218–229. [CrossRef] [PubMed]
4. Singh, C.B.; Manglembi, N.; Swapana, N.; Chanu, S.B. Ethnobotany, Phytochemistry and Pharmacology of *Zingiber cassumunar* Roxb. (Zingiberaceae). *J Pharmacogn. Phytochem.* **2015**, *4*, 1–6.
5. Sukatta, U.; Rugthaworn, P.; Punjee, P.; Chidchenchey, S.; Keeratinijakal, V. Chemical composition and physical properties of oil from Plai (*Zingiber cassumunar* Roxb.) obtained by hydrodistillation and hexane extraction. *Kasetsart J. (Nat. Sci.)* **2009**, *43*, 212–217.
6. Chaiyana, W.; Anuchapreeda, S.; Leelapornpisid, P.; Phongpradist, R.; Viernstein, H.; Mueller, M. Development of microemulsion delivery system of essential oil from *Zingiber cassumunar* Roxb. rhizome for improvement of stability and anti-inflammatory activity. *AAPS PharmSciTech* **2017**, *18*, 1332–1342. [CrossRef]
7. Boonyanugomol, W.; Kraisriwattana, K.; Rukseree, K.; Boonsam, K.; Narachai, P. In vitro synergistic antibacterial activity of the essential oil from *Zingiber cassumunar* Roxb against extensively drug-resistant *Acinetobacter baumannii* strains. *J. Infect. Public Health* **2017**, *10*, 586–592. [CrossRef]
8. Koontongkaew, S.; Poachanukoon, O.; Sireeratawong, S.; Decatiwongse Na Ayudhya, T.; Khonsung, P.; Jaijoy, K.; Soawakontha, R.; Chanchai, M. Safety evaluation of *Zingiber cassumunar* roxb rhizome extract: Acute and chronic toxicity studies in rats. *Int. Sch. Res. Not.* **2014**, *16*, 1–14.
9. Nishima, Y.; Inoue, A.; Sasagawa, S.; Koiwa, J.; Kawaguchi, K.; Kawase, R.; Maruyama, T.; Kim, S.; Tanaka, T. Using zebrafish in systems toxicology for developmental toxicity testing. *Congenit. Anom. (Kyoto)* **2016**, *56*, 18–27. [CrossRef]
10. Tran, S.; Facciol, A.; Gerlai, R. The Zebrafish, a Novel Model Organism for Screening Compounds Affecting Acute and Chronic Ethanol-Induced Effects. *Int. Rev. Neurobiol.* **2016**, *126*, 467–484.
11. Kimmel, C.B.; Ballard, W.W.; Kimmell, S.R.; Ullmann, B.; Schilling, T.F. Stages of embryonic development of the zebrafish. *Dev. Dyn.* **1995**, *203*, 253–310. [CrossRef] [PubMed]
12. Falcão, M.A.P.; de Souza, L.S.; Dolabella, S.S.; Guimarães, A.G.; Walker, C.I.B. Zebrafish as an alternative method for determining the embryo toxicity of plant products: a systematic review. *Environ. Sci. Pollut. Res. Int.* **2018**, *25*, 35015–35026. [CrossRef] [PubMed]
13. Yang, J.B.; Li, W.F.; Liu, Y.; Wang, Q.; Chen, X.L.; Wang, A.G.; Jin, H.T.; Ma, S.C. Acute toxicity screening of different extractions, components and constituents of *Polygonum multiflorum* Thunb. on zebrafish (*Danio rerio*) embryos in vivo. *Biomed. Pharmacother.* **2018**, *99*, 205–213. [CrossRef] [PubMed]
14. Alafiatayo, A.A.; Lai, K.S.; Syahida, A.; Mahmood, M.; Shaharuddin, N.A. Phytochemical evaluation, embryotoxicity, and teratogenic effects of *Curcuma longa* extract on zebrafish (*Danio rerio*). *Evid. Based Complement Alternat. Med.* **2019**, *10*, 3807207. [CrossRef] [PubMed]
15. Manochai, B.; Paisooksantivatana, Y.; Choi, H.; Hong, J.H. Variation in DPPH scavenging activity and major volatile oil components of cassumunar ginger, *Zingiber montanum* (Koenig), in response to water deficit and light intensity. *Sci. Hortic.* **2010**, *126*, 462–466. [CrossRef]
16. Kamazeri, T.S.A.T.; Samah, O.A.; Taher, M.; Susanti, D.; Qaralleh, H. Antimicrobial activity and essential oils of *Curcuma aeruginosa*, *Curcuma mangga*, and *Zingiber cassumunar* from Malaysia. *Asian Pac. J. Trop. Med.* **2012**, *5*, 202–209. [CrossRef]
17. Younis, A.; Riaz, A.; Khan, M.A.; Khan, A.A. Effect of Time of Growing Season and Time of Day for Flower Harvest on Flower Yield and Essential Oil Quality and Quantity of Four Rosa Cultivars. *Floric. Ornam. Biotech.* **2009**, *3*, 98–103.
18. Akram, A.; Younis, A.; Akhtar, G.; Ameer, K.; Farooq, A.; Hanif, M.A.; Saeed, M.; Lim, K. Comparative Efficacy of Various Essential Oil Extraction Techniques on Oil Yield and Quality of *Jasminum sambac* L. *Sci. Int.* **2017**, *5*, 84–95. [CrossRef]

19. Sharma, S.; Gupta, J.; Prabhakar, P.K.; Gupta, P.; Solanki, P.; Rajput, A. Phytochemical Repurposing of Natural Molecule: Sabinene for Identification of Novel Therapeutic Benefits Using In Silico and In Vitro Approaches. *Assay Drug Dev. Technol.* **2019**, *17*, 339–351. [CrossRef]
20. Pazyar, N.; Yaghoobi, R.; Bagherani, N.; Kazerouni, A. A review of applications of tea tree oil in dermatology. *Int. J. Dermatol.* **2013**, *52*, 784–790. [CrossRef]
21. Li, M.X.; Bai, X.; Ma, Y.P.; Zhang, H.X.; Nama, N.; Pei, S.J.; Du, Z.Z. Cosmetic potentials of extracts and compounds from *Zingiber cassumunar* Roxb. rhizome. *Ind. Crop Prod.* **2019**, *141*, 111764. [CrossRef]
22. Suksaeree, J.; Charoenchai, L.; Madaka, F. *Zingiber cassumunar* blended patches for skin application: formulation, physicochemical properties, and in vitro studies. *Asian J. Pharm. Sci.* **2015**, *10*, 341–349. [CrossRef]
23. Priprem, A.; Janpim, K.; Nualkaew, S.; Mhakunakorn, P. Topical niosome gel of Zingiber cassumunar Roxb. extract for anti-inflammatory activity enhanced skin permeation and stability of compound D. *AAPS Pharm. Sci. Tech.* **2016**, *173*, 631–639. [CrossRef] [PubMed]
24. Thaweboon, S.; Thaweboon, B.; Kaypetch, R. Antifungal, Anti-Inflammatory and Cytotoxic Effects of *Zingiber cassumunar* Gel. *Key Eng. Mater.* **2018**, *773*, 360–364. [CrossRef]
25. Van Meerloo, J.; Kaspers, G.J.; Cloos, J. Cell sensitivity assays: the MTT assay. *Methods Mol. Biol.* **2011**, *731*, 237–245.
26. Taechowisan, T.; Suttichokthanakorn, S.; Phutdhawong, W.S. Antibacterial and cytotoxicity activities of phenylbutanoids from *Zingiber cassumunar* Roxb. *J. App. Pharm. Sci.* **2018**, *8*, 122–128.
27. Serifi, I.; Tzima, E.; Bardouki, H.; Lampri, E.; Papamarcaki, T. Effects of the Essential Oil from *Pistacia lentiscus* Var. chia on the Lateral Line System and the Gene Expression Profile of Zebrafish (*Danio rerio*). *Molecules* **2019**, *24*, 3919. [CrossRef]
28. Aqil, M.; Ahad, A.; Sultana, Y.; Ali, A. Status of terpenes as skin penetration enhancers. *Drug Discov. Today* **2007**, *12*, 1061–1067. [CrossRef]
29. Ali, M.K.; Saber, S.P.; Taite, D.R.; Emadi, S.; Irving, R. The protective layer of zebrafish embryo changes continuously with advancing age of embryo development (AGED). *J. Toxicol. Pharmacol.* **2017**, *1*, 9.
30. Chongmelaxme, B.; Sruamsiri, R.; Dilokthornsakul, P.; Dhippayam, T.; Kongkaew, C.; Saokaew, S.; Chuthapultti, A.; Chaiyakunapruk, N. Clinical effects of Zingiber cassumunar (Plai): A systematic review. *Complement. Ther. Med.* **2017**, *35*, 70–77. [CrossRef]
31. Chooluck, K.; Singh, R.P.; Sathirakul, K.; Derendorf, H. Dermal Pharmacokinetics of Terpinen-4-ol Following Topical Administration of *Zingiber cassumunar* (plai) Oil. *Planta Med.* **2012**, *78*, 1761–1766. [CrossRef] [PubMed]
32. Chooluck, K.; Singh, R.P.; Sathirakul, K.; Derendorf, H. Plasma and dermal pharmacokinetics of terpinen-4-ol in rats following intravenous administration. *Die Pharmazie* **2013**, *68*, 135–140. [PubMed]
33. Khemawoot, P.; Hunsakunachai, N.; Anukunwithaya, T.; Bangphumi, K.; Ongpipattanakul, B.; Jiratchariyakul, W. Pharmacokinetics of compound D, the major bioactive component of *Zingiber cassumunar*, in rats. *Planta Med.* **2016**, *82*, 1186–1191. [CrossRef] [PubMed]
34. OECD. *Guidelines for the Testing of Chemicals. Section 2-Effects on Biotic Systems Test (No 236 Fish Embryo Acute Toxicity (FET) Test)*; Organization for Economic Cooperation and Development: Paris, France, 2013.

Sample Availability: Samples of the compounds are not available from the authors.

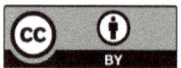

© 2020 by the authors. Licensee MDPI, Basel, Switzerland. This article is an open access article distributed under the terms and conditions of the Creative Commons Attribution (CC BY) license (http://creativecommons.org/licenses/by/4.0/).

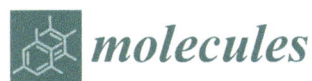

Article

Cytotoxic and Anti-Inflammatory Effects of *Ent*-Kaurane Derivatives Isolated from the Alpine Plant *Sideritis hyssopifolia*

Axelle Aimond [1,2,†], Kevin Calabro [3,†], Coralie Audoin [2], Elodie Olivier [1], Mélody Dutot [1], Pauline Buron [1], Patrice Rat [1], Olivier Laprévote [1], Soizic Prado [4], Emmanuel Roulland [4], Olivier P. Thomas [3,*] and Grégory Genta-Jouve [1,5,*]

1. Laboratoire de Chimie-Toxicologie Analytique et Cellulaire (C-TAC) UMR CNRS 8038 CiTCoM Université Paris-Descartes, 4, Avenue de l'Observatoire, 75006 Paris, France; axelle.aimond@clarins.com (A.A.); elodie.eolivier@gmail.com (E.O.); melodydutot@gmail.com (M.D.); pauline.buron92@gmail.com (P.B.); patrice.rat@parisdescartes.fr (P.R.); olivier.laprevote@parisdescartes.fr (O.L.)
2. Laboratoires Clarins, 5 Rue Ampère, 95300 Pontoise, France; coralie.audoin@clarins.com
3. Marine Biodiscovery, School of Chemistry and Ryan Institute, National University of Ireland Galway (NUI Galway), University Road, H91 TK33 Galway, Ireland; kevin.calabro@nuigalway.ie
4. Muséum National d'Histoire Naturelle, Unité Molécules de Communication et Adaptation des Micro-Organismes, UMR 7245, CP 54, 57 rue Cuvier, 75005 Paris, France; sprado@mnhn.fr (S.P.); emmanuel.roulland@parisdescartes.fr (E.R.)
5. Laboratoire Ecologie, Evolution, Interactions des Systèmes Amazoniens (LEEISA), USR 3456, Université De Guyane, CNRS Guyane, 275 Route de Montabo, 97334 Cayenne, French Guiana
* Correspondence: olivier.thomas@nuigalway.ie (O.P.T.); gregory.genta-jouve@parisdescartes.fr (G.G.-J.); Tel.: +353-9149-3563 (O.P.T.); +33-153-731-585 (G.G.-J.)
† These authors contributed equally to this work.

Received: 13 December 2019; Accepted: 26 January 2020; Published: 29 January 2020

Abstract: This paper reports the isolation and structural characterization of four new *ent*-kaurane derivatives from the Lamiaceae plant *Sideritis hyssopifolia*. Planar structures and relative configurations were determined using both mass spectrometry and nuclear magnetic resonance (1D and 2D). Absolute configurations were determined by comparing experimental and theoretical electronic circular dichroism spectra. The cytotoxic and microbial activities of all new compounds were tested. Compounds that were non-cytotoxic were further evaluated for anti-inflammatory activity.

Keywords: *Sideritis hyssopifolia*; *ent*-kaurane; anti-inflammatory; NMR

1. Introduction

The cosmetics sector represents a huge potential for growth in today's society. The quest for wellness and beauty has led to an intensive search for new products that can improve both the appearance and hygiene of an aging population. In this context, an increasing number of cosmetic companies are using nature as a unique source for their formulations. To discover new compounds of interest, the French company Laboratoires Clarins has been conducting an in-depth investigation of plants in their unique outdoor fields situated in the French Alps. *Sideritis*, containing around 190 species, is a widespread genus of the family Lamiaceae, which is commonly found in the Northern Hemisphere [1]. Around 250 natural products have been reported from the genus *Sideritis*, of which 160 are in the diterpene class, specifically in the kaurane group [2,3]. These kauranes and their enantiomers, *ent*-kauranes, exhibit a wide range of bioactivities, with antioxidant, anti-tyrosinase, anti-cholinesterase, and anti-inflammatory properties reported [4–6]. The focus of this study was the species *Sideritis hyssopifolia* grown in the French Alps. The phytochemical composition of this species is poorly described, with only two publications reporting the isolation and characterization of its flavonoids and its essential oil composition [7,8]. Except for siderol [9], diterpenoids have yet to be reported in *S. hyssopifolia* [10]. Because these compounds are commonly found throughout the *Sideritis* genus, we re-investigated the phytochemical composition of *S. hyssopifolia* and, as a result, isolated 12 compounds, eight of which are reported in this species for the first time, namely, siderol [9], sideridiol [9], siderone [11], *ent*-kaurene I [12], sideritriol [13], *ent*-15β,16β-epoxykauran-18-ol [14], *epi*-candicandiol [12], and *ent*-3β-7α-dihydroxykaur-16-ene [15]. Additionally, four new *ent*-kauranes were fully characterized (Figure 1) using 1D and 2D NMR, MS, and ECD. The four novel compounds were evaluated for their cytotoxic, antimicrobial, and anti-inflammatory activities.

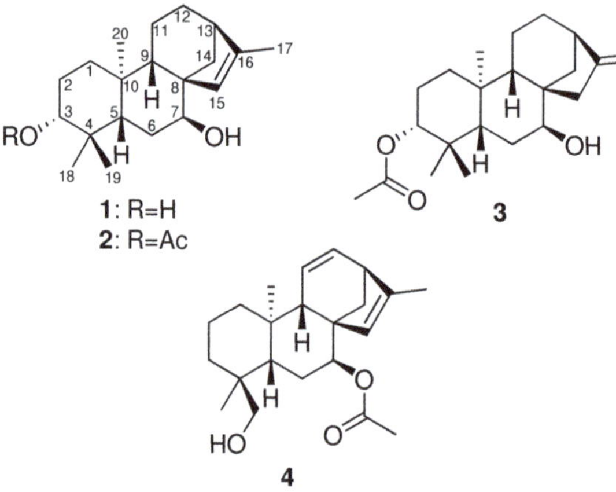

Figure 1. Structure of the new *ent*-kauranes compounds **1–4**.

2. Results and Discussion

Compound **1** was isolated as a light yellow oil. Its molecular formula was determined from the [M+H]$^+$ observed at *m/z* 305.2481 (calculated for $C_{20}H_{33}O_2$, 305.2475, δ 1.9 ppm) in the HRESIMS spectrum acquired in positive ionization mode; the formula required five degrees of unsaturation in the molecule. The ^{1}H NMR spectrum exhibited four methyl singlets at δ 0.76 (s, 3H, H$_3$-18), 0.95 (s, 3H, H$_3$-19), 1.07 (s, 3H, H$_3$-20), and 1.71 (s, 3H, H$_3$-17) ppm (Tables 1 and 2). A signal corresponding to a trisubstituted double bond at δ 5.52 (s, 1H, H-15) was also observed, together with two hydroxylated methines at δ 3.17 (dd, *J* = 11.6, 4.5 Hz, 1H, H-3) and 3.54 (br s, 1H, H-7). Inspection of the ^{1}H–^{1}H COSY spectrum led to the identification of three spin systems. The first one started with a clear correlation of H-3 with H-2a δ 1.67 (m, 1H) and H-2b δ 1.60 (m, 1H), which, in turn, correlated with the methylene protons H-1 at δ 1.84 (1H, m) and 0.95 (1H, m). A second spin system was observed between H-7 and H-6 δ 1.66 (m, 1H) and 1.62 (m, 1H), and the last correlation was observed between H6b and H-5 at δ 1.40 (d, *J* = 12.0 Hz, 1H). A last spin system comprising H-9/H-11/H-12/H-13/H-14 was identified, with correlations between δ 1.28 (d, *J* = 4.7 Hz, 1H, H-9), 1.54 (m, 2H, H$_2$-11), 1.51 (m, 2H, H$_2$-12), 2.33 (br s, 1H, H-13), and 1.96 (d, *J* = 9.9 Hz, 1H, H-14a). A ^4J cross-peak between H-15 and H-17 was also observed. Analysis of the HMBC spectrum revealed a connection between the three spin systems. The correlations of H-20 with C-1/C-5/C-9 and H-18/H-19 with C-3/C-5 indicated the presence of the first decalin ring. Two other cycles were identified using intense ^2J correlations between H-7/H-9/H-14/H-15 and C-8. The last cycle was confirmed by the cross-peak between H-13 and C-16. The full three-dimensional structure was determined using the coupling constant values of the ^{1}H NMR spectra and the NOESY correlations (see Figure 2).

Table 1. ^{1}H NMR data of compounds **1–4** (^{1}H 500 MHz).

No.	1 [a] δ_H (m, J in Hz)	2 [b] δ_H (m, J in Hz)	3 [b] δ_H (m, J in Hz)	4 [b] δ_H (m, J in Hz)
1a	1.84 (dt, 13.0, 3.5)	1.82 (dt, 13.2, 3.5)	1.84 (m)	1.84 (m)
1b	0.95 (m)	1.03 (m)	1.05 (td, 13.0, 4.0)	1.07 (dd, 12.5, 3.6)
2a	1.67 (m)	1.70 (m)	1.69 (m)	1.65 (m)
2b	1.60 (m)	1.62 (m)	1.64 (m)	1.52 (m)
3a	3.17 (dd, 11.6, 4.5)	4.52 (dd, 11.6, 5.1)	4.53 (dd, 11.6, 5.0)	1.55 (m)
3b	-	-	-	1.27 (dd, 14.3, 5.5)
4	-	-	-	-
5	1.40 (d, 12.0)	1.49 (m)	1.55 (m)	1.86 (m)
6a	1.66 (m)	1.65 (m)	1.68 (m)	1.74 (dd, 14.4, 3.8)
6b	1.62 (m)			1.56 (m)
7	3.54 (bs)	3.63 (t, 2.9)	3.62 (t, 3.1)	4.82 (t, 3.0)
8	-	-	-	-
9	1.28 (d, 4.7)	1.30 (d, 7.5)	1.42 (d, 6.6)	1.86 (m)
10	-	-	-	-
11	1.54 (m)	1.49 (m)	1.56 (m)	5.36 (dd, 9.7, 3.5)
12a	1.51 (m)	1.49 (m)	1.70 (m)	6.25 (dd, 9.6, 6.5)
12b			1.49 (m)	-
13	2.33 (bs)	2.37 (bs)	2.68 (m)	2.56 (m)
14a	1.96 (d, 9.9)	1.89 d (10.1)	1.82 (m)	2.01 (d, 9.4)
14b	1.35 (dd, 10.1, 5.3)	1.36 (d, 10.2, 5.2)	1.17 (dd, 11.4, 5.0)	1.50 (m)
15	5.52 (s)	5.47 (s)	2.25 (bs)	5.09 (s)
16	-	-	-	-
17a	1.71 (s)	1.72 (bs)	4.83 (bs)	1.77 (d, 1.1)
17b	-	-	4.80 (bs)	-
18	0.96 (s)	0.84 (s)	0.88 (s)	0.72 (s)
19a	0.76 (s)	0.85 (s)	0.86 (s)	3.36 (d, 10.8)
19b	-	-	-	3.04 (d, 10.8)
20	1.07 (s)	1.05 (s)	1.05 (s)	1.04 (s)
21	-	-	-	-
22	-	2.04 (s)	2.04 (s)	2.09 (s)

[a] CD$_3$OD, [b] CDCl$_3$.

The multiplicity of the signal at δ 3.17 (dd, J = 11.6, 4.5 Hz, 1H, H-3) indicated an axial orientation for H-3. The NOESY correlations between H-5/H-3 and H-5/H-9 confirmed the relative configuration of C-5 and the trans ring junction. The position of the trisubstituted double bond was supported by the NOESY correlation between H-15/H-9 and the correlation between H-14/H-20. Finally, the broad singlet signal for H-7 indicated a α orientation at C-7. This was further confirmed by the correlation between H-7/H-14b.

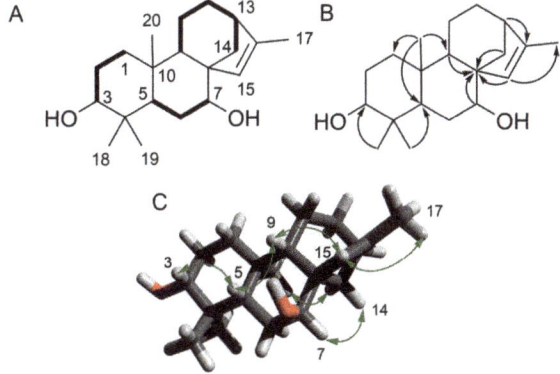

Figure 2. (**A**) COSY correlations; (**B**) HMBC key correlations; and (**C**) NOESY correlations.

The absolute configuration was determined by comparing experimental and theoretical electronic circular dichroism (ECD) spectra. As expected, the spectrum (Figure 3) revealed only one Cotton Effect (CE), which was due to the $\pi \rightarrow \pi^*$ transition. The sign of the CE agreed with compound **1** belonging to the *ent*-kaurane series. This compound was named hyssopifoliol A.

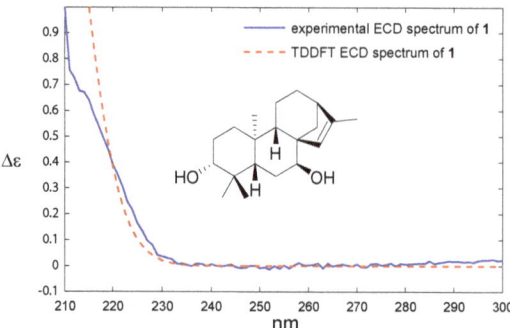

Figure 3. Comparison between experimental and theoretical ECD spectra of compound **1**.

Compound **2** was isolated as a light yellow oil. Its molecular formula was determined from the [M-AcOH+H]$^+$ observed at m/z 287.2361 (calculated for $C_{20}H_{31}O$, 287.2369, Δ -2.8 ppm) in the HRESIMS spectrum acquired in positive ionization mode. Inspection of the ^{1}H NMR spectrum suggested that compound **2** was very similar to compound **1** since only one additional signal, which was easily assigned to an acetyl moiety, was found at δ 2.04 (s, 3H, H$_3$-22) ppm. This was confirmed by the deshielding of the H-3 signal at δ 4.52 (dd, J = 11.6, 4.6 Hz, 1H, H-3) and the HMBC correlation between H-3 and C-21. The three-dimensional structure appeared to be similar to that determined for compound **1** because the coupling constants observed for the critical signals did not change. The multiplicities were similar with a doublet of doublets at δ 4.52 (dd, J = 11.6, 4.5 Hz) and 3.63 (J = 2.9 Hz) ppm for H-3 and H-7, respectively. The relative configurations at C-5, C-8, and C-9 were established using the correlations in the NOESY spectrum (see Supporting Information). The absolute configuration of compound **2** was determined by comparing the sign of the unique CE on the ECD spectrum. As for compound **1**, the positive band at ca. 215 nm led to the conclusion that compound **2** was an *ent*-kaurane and was named hyssopifoliol B.

Compound **3** was isolated as a light yellow oil. Its molecular formula was determined from the [M+H]$^+$ observed at m/z 347.2786 (calculated for $C_{22}H_{34}O_3Na$, 347.2780, δ +1.7 ppm) in the HRESIMS spectrum acquired in positive ionization mode; the formula required 6 degrees of unsaturation in the molecule. The ^{1}H NMR spectrum exhibited four methyl singlets at δ 0.86 (s, H$_3$-18), 0.86 (s, H$_3$-19), 1.05 (s, 3H, H$_3$-20), and 2.04 (s, 3H, H$_3$-22) ppm. The signal at 4.49 (dd, J = 11.4, 5.2 Hz) is typical of an axial acetylated methine at H-3, and a broad singlet assigned to a hydroxylated methine at H-7 was observed at δ 3.62 (t, J = 3.1 Hz, 1H, H-7). A major difference was observed between compounds **2** and **3**: two broad one-proton singlets at δ 4.76 and 4.80 ppm were observed in the ^{1}H NMR spectrum, while the singlet at δ 1.71 was absent. This difference was attributed to the isomerization of the double bond to obtain an *exo*-methylene group (H$_2$-17). The relative configuration was conserved between compounds **2** and **3**, and the multiplicities of the key stereogenic centers were very similar for both compounds (see Table 1). The relative configuration of **3** was confirmed by saponification (K$_2$CO$_3$/MeOH). The ^{1}H NMR spectrum of the resulting diol compound was compared with the published spectrum of *ent*-3β-7α-dihydroxykaur-16-ene [15], and a perfect match was obtained, thus confirming the relative configuration of compound **3**. According to the sign of the CE on ECD spectrum, the same absolute configuration was attributed to compound **3**. Compound **3** was thus named 3-acetoxy-*ent*-3β-7α-dihydroxykaur-16-ene.

Table 2. ^{13}C NMR data of compounds 1–4 (^{13}C 125 MHz).

No.	1 [a] δ_C	2 [b] δ_C	3 [b] δ_C	4 [b] δ_C
1	40.1	38.4	38.4	39.2
2	28.1	23.6	23.8	17.9
3	79.8	80.8	81.0	35.1
4	39.4	37.2	37.4	37.1
5	46.1	45.1	45.6	38.8
6	27.7	26.7	27.4	23.9
7	76.2	75.0	77.2	78.0
8	54.5	53.3	48.3	50.5
9	45.2	43.7	50.3	50.9
10	40.3	39.1	38.9	38.8
11	19.6	18.4	18.0	126.1
12	25.9	24.8	33.7	134.4
13	46.1	44.7	43.9	45.5
14	43.5	42.1	38.6	40.2
15	131.9	129.7	45.8	126.6
16	144.2	144.3	154.9	154.0
17	15.5	15.5	103.8	15.9
18	162	16.6	16.9	17.6
19	28.6	28.0	28.3	71.3
20	18.2	17.6	17.6	17.5
21	-	170.9	171.1	170.5
22	-	21.3	21.5	21.5

[a] CD$_3$OD, [b] CDCl$_3$.

Compound **4** was isolated as a light yellow oil. Its molecular formula was determined from the [M-AcOH+H]$^+$ observed at m/z 285.2251 (calculated for C$_{20}$H$_{29}$O, 285.2221, δ 10.5 ppm) in the HRESIMS spectrum acquired in positive ionization mode; the formula required seven degrees of unsaturation in the molecule. This additional unsaturation was quickly identified in the ^{1}H NMR spectrum as two olefinic signals at δ 5.36 (dd, J = 9.7, 3.5 Hz, 1H, H-11) and 6.25 (dd, J = 9.6, 6.5 Hz, H-12). The core of compounds **1** and **2** was conserved, but a methyl singlet was missing, and two oxygenated geminal protons were observed at δ 3.36 (d, J = 10.8 Hz, H-19a) and 3.04 (d, J = 10.8 Hz, 1H, H-19b). Oxidation at C-19 was confirmed by the HMBC correlations between H-19 and C-3/C-4/C-5/C-18. The acetyl group was positioned at C-7, as determined by the deshielding of H-7. This was further confirmed by the cross-peak at H-7/C-21 in the HMBC spectrum. Compound **4** was named 11,12-didehydrosiderol.

After an evaluation of the purity of the compounds, compounds **1** (97%), **3** (95%) and **4** (87%) were tested for cytotoxicity and activity against *Staphylococcus aureus* (ATCC 6538). Unfortunately, no antimicrobial activity was detected at the tested concentrations (data not shown). Compound **2** was indeed not tested for biological activity due to its low purity (<75%). Additionally, as shown in Figure 4, compound **3** was found to be cytotoxic to HaCaT cells at a concentration of 10 µg/mL (cell viability was reduced to ca. 60%), so it was excluded from subsequent testing for anti-inflammatory activity. It was previously reported that the exomethylene cyclopentanone moiety is beneficial for anticancer activity on cancer cell lines [16]. The *exo*-methylene group present in compound **3** and absent in compounds **1** and **4** may be therefore responsible for the cytotoxicity on the spontaneously immortalized HaCaT cell line.

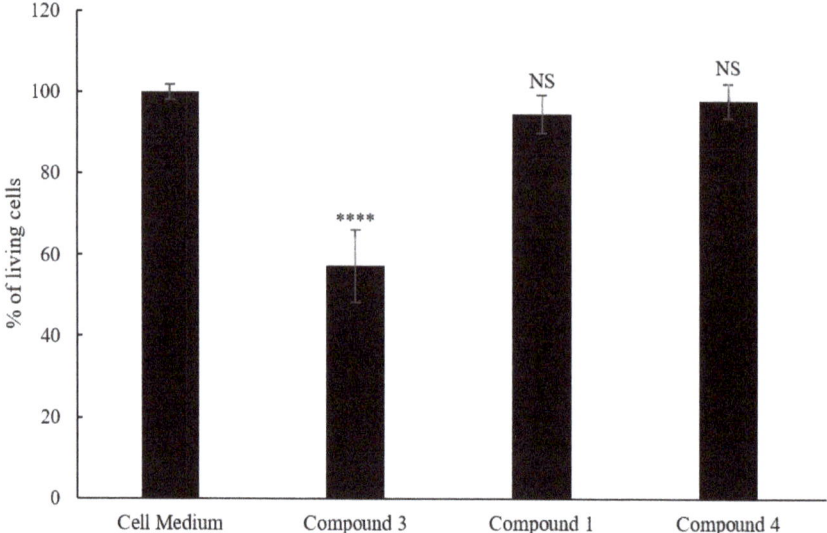

Figure 4. Viability of HaCaT cells after 6 h of incubation with compounds **1**, **3** and **4**. (NS: not significant; ****: $p < 0.0001$).

Compounds **1** and **4** were tested for potential anti-inflammatory activity by incubating human keratinocytes with the compounds for 24 hours, followed by stimulation of the cells with poly(I:C). As shown in Figure 5, poly(I:C) induced a marked elevation in the release of IL-1α (250-fold). Preincubation with compounds **1** and **4** significantly inhibited the release of IL-1α. These results demonstrate that two of the new diterpenoids extracted from *S. hyssopifolia* have anti-IL-1α effects on skin epithelial cells. Human keratinocytes constitutively synthesize proIL-1α and -β but they do not activate and secrete these proinflammatory cytokines under normal conditions [17]. Upon activation, IL-1 signalling is involved in many (auto)-inflammatory skin diseases like psoriasis [18], vitiligo [19] or melanoma [20]. The new diterpenoids extracted from *S. hyssopifolia* represent new therapeutic topical agents via the modulation of IL-1α secretion.

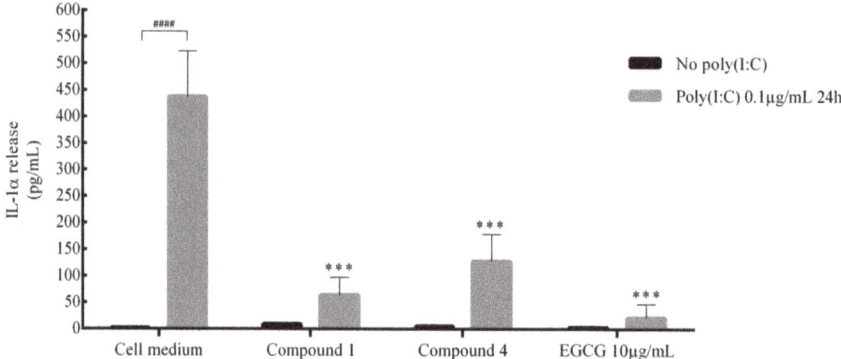

Figure 5. Anti-inflammatory activity of compounds **1** and **4** in HaCaT cells stimulated by poly(I:C). Compounds in ethanol were prepared at 1:100 dilution in cell medium to obtain a concentration of 10 μg/mL (***: $p < 0.001$ compared to cell medium with poly(I:C); ####: $p < 0.0001$).

3. Materials and Methods

3.1. General Experimental Procedures

Optical rotation was measured at the Na D-line (589.3 nm) with a 5 cm cell at 20 °C on a UniPol L1000 polarimeter (Schmidt + Haensch, Berlin, Germany) in methanol. UV and ECD data were obtained using a ChirascanTM V100 (Applied Photophysics, Leatherhead, UK) in acetonitrile. NMR experiments were performed using an Inova 500 MHz spectrometer (Varian, Palo Alto, CA, USA). Chemical shifts were referenced in ppm to the residual solvent signals (CD$_3$OD, at δ_H 3.31 and δ_C 49.00 ppm; CDCl$_3$, at δ_H 7.26 and δ_H 77.0 ppm). High-resolution mass spectra were obtained using a mass spectrometer (HRMS; Agilent 6540, Santa Clara, CA, USA). Preparative liquid chromatography was performed using a Jasco system (Tokyo, Japan) equipped with a PU-2087 pump and a UV-2075 detector, while semi-preparative purification was realized using a Waters 2690 system (Milford, MA, USA) equipped with the UV detector 2487.

3.2. Plant Material

Flowering tops of *S. hyssopifolia* were collected in the Alps, France, at an altitude of 1300 m. Botanical identification of the species was carried out by an ethnobotanist of Laboratoires Clarins. The samples were protected from direct light and air-dried at room temperature for three days. Two harvests were carried out (July 2016 and August 2017). After comparing the phytochemical composition, the harvests were gathered.

3.3. Extraction and Isolation

Dried powder of the aerial parts of *S. hyssopifolia* (300 g) was successively extracted three times with a methanol/dichloromethane mixture (1:1, *v/v*) for 15 min under sonication at room temperature. The crude extract (27 g) was further fractionated by reversed-phase (C$_{18}$) vacuum liquid chromatography (VLC) using a step gradient of H$_2$O/MeOH (100:0, 75:25, 50:50, 25:75, 0:100) followed by a step gradient of MeOH/DCM (50:50, 0:100) to yield seven fractions (F1: 4.56 g, F2: 3.67 g, F3: 2.76 g, F4: 5.93 g, F5: 5.47 g, F6: 3.33 g, and F7: 0.64 g). The methanolic fraction (F5, m = 860 mg) was purified by preparative reversed-phase high-performance liquid chromatography with a mixture of water and acetonitrile (flow: 12 mL/min; solvent A: H$_2$O; solvent B: acetonitrile; gradient: 0–3 min 72% B, 3–15 min 72 → 86% B, 15–20 min 86% B, 20–21 min 86% → 72% B, 21–25 min 72% B) to obtain 12 peaks (P1→P12). After ^{1}H NMR and MS analyses, only compound **1** was pure enough to be identified (6.43 mg, t_R = 11 min). The other compounds were identified after a second purification of peaks 4, 7, and 8 (see Supporting Information). Peak 4 (37 mg, 50 mg/mL) was subjected to preparative HPLC (column A, flow: 3.5 mL/min; solvent A: H$_2$O; solvent B: acetonitrile, isocratic 55% B, 31 min) to obtain three known molecules and compound **2** (2.5 mg, t_R = 11.6 min). Peak 7 (3.8 mg, 5 mg/mL) was subjected to semi-preparative HPLC (system: B, column B, flow: 1 mL/min; solvent A: H$_2$O; solvent B: acetonitrile, isocratic 47% B, 43 min) to obtain a known molecule and compound **3** (0.99 mg, t_R = 33.5 min). Peak 8 (7.5 mg, 5 mg/mL) was subjected to semi-preparative HPLC (system: B, column B, flow: 1 mL/min; solvent A: H$_2$O; solvent B: acetonitrile, isocratic 49% B, 40 min) to yield compound **4** (0.53 mg, t_R = 34 min).

3.4. Computational Details

All QM calculations were carried out using Gaussian 16. The GMMX package was used for the conformational analysis (force field: MMFF94). TD DFT calculations were performed using the B3LYP method at the 6-31G(d) level for 20 excited states. GaussView 6.0 was used to plot the ECD spectra.

3.5. Cell Experiments

HaCaT cells (spontaneously transformed human keratinocytes) were obtained from Cell Lines Service (CLS; Eppelheim, Germany). The cells were cultured in Dulbecco's Modified Eagle Medium

(DMEM; Gibco, France) supplemented with 10% fetal bovine serum, 2 mM glutamine, 50 IU/mL penicillin, and 50 IU/mL streptomycin (Gibco) at 5% CO_2 and 37 °C. When the HaCaT cells reached confluency, they were dispersed using trypsin and counted using a hematimeter. The cell suspension was diluted to a cell density of 100,000 cells/mL and seeded in 96-well microplates for 24 h. The compounds in ethanol were prepared at 1:100 dilution in culture medium and incubated for 24 h. Epigallocatechin gallate (EGCG) at 10 µg/mL was used as an anti-inflammatory control [21].

3.6. Cell Viability Evaluation

A cell viability assay was carried out using the resazurin salt assay. Briefly, after incubating the cells with compounds **1–4**, the medium was removed, and 200 µL of resazurin solution (9 mg/mL, m/v, Alfa Aesar by Thermo Fisher Scientific, Kandel, Germany) prepared in fresh medium was added to each well. Following 6 h of incubation, resorufin fluorescence was quantified at the respective excitation and emission wavelengths of 535 and 600 nm using a Tecan Spark microplate reader. The percentage of cell viability is expressed in relative fluorescence units (RFU) compared with the control cells (RFU × 100).

3.7. Interleukin Release Measurement

The potential anti-inflammatory effects of the compounds were evaluated by inducing cytokine release with poly(I:C), a synthetic analog of viral dsRNA (Sigma-Aldrich, Lyon, France) at 1 µg/mL for 24 hours in culture medium. The control group was incubated with culture medium. IL-1α release was quantified in supernatants by ELISA (DuoSet ELISA, R&D Systems, Minneapolis, MN) according to the manufacturer's instructions. The absorbance signal was read at 450 nm using a microplate reader (Spark).

3.8. Saponification of Compound 3

K_2CO_3 (50 mg, 0.36 mmol) was added to a methanol solution (1 mL) of compound **3** (0.53 mg, 0.0015 mmol) at room temperature. The reaction was monitored by TLC and quenched by pouring the reaction medium into brine. After extraction by ethylacetate, drying over anhydrous sodium sulfate, concentration under vacuum, and HPLC purification (heptane/ethylacetate, 1:1, v/v), the known compound *ent*-3β-7α-dihydroxykaur-16-ene (0.46 mg, 100%) was obtained. The spectral data of synthetic *ent*-3β-7α-dihydroxykaur-16-ene were identical to those of the natural compound [15].

3.9. Statistical Analyses

All statistical analyses were performed using R 3.5.0. Cell samples were analyzed by repeated measures (n = 3) one-way analysis of variance (ANOVA) followed by Dunnett's test. Significant differences for compounds **1–4** are relative to the control and indicated in the results (NS: not significant; ***: $p < 0.001$; ****: $p < 0.0001$).

3.10. Hyssopifoliol A (Compound 1)

Light yellow oil; $[\alpha]_D^{20}$ −35 (c 0.1, MeOH); CD (acetonitrile) λ_{max} ($\Delta\epsilon$) 210 (+0.11) nm; ^{1}H and ^{13}C NMR: see Tables 1 and 2; MS: (+)-HRESIMS m/z 305.2481 (calcd. for $C_{20}H_{33}O_2$, 305.2475, Δ +1.9 ppm).

3.11. Hyssopifoliol B (Compound 2)

Light yellow oil; $[\alpha]_D^{20}$ −26 (c 0.07, MeOH); CD (acetonitrile) λ_{max} ($\Delta\epsilon$) 210 (+0.06) nm; ^{1}H and ^{13}C NMR: see Tables 1 and 2; MS: (+)-HRESIMS m/z 287.2361 (calcd. for $C_{20}H_{31}O$, 287.2369, Δ −2.8 ppm).

3.12. 3-Acetoxy-ent-3β-7α-dihydroxykaur-16-ene (Compound 3)

Light yellow oil; $[\alpha]_D^{20}$ −18 (c 0.06, MeOH); CD (acetonitrile) λ_{max} ($\Delta\epsilon$) 210 (+0.05) nm; ^{1}H and ^{13}C NMR: see Tables 1 and 2; MS: (+)-HRESIMS m/z 347.2786 (calcd. for $C_{22}H_{34}O_3Na$, 347.2780, Δ +1.7 ppm).

3.13. 11,12-Didehydrosiderol (Compound 4)

Light yellow oil; $[\alpha]_D^{20}$ −23 (c 0.08, MeOH); CD (acetonitrile) λ_{max} ($\Delta\epsilon$) 215 (+0.07) nm; ^{1}H and ^{13}C NMR: see Tables 1 and 2; MS: (+)-HRESIMS m/z 285.2251 (calcd. for $C_{20}H_{29}O$, 285.2221, Δ +10.5 ppm).

4. Conclusions

The chemical study of *S. hyssopifolia* led to the isolation and identification of several diterpenoid compounds. Eight compounds are reported for the first time in this species, and four are new *ent*-kauranes, which are designated hyssopifoliol A, hyssopifoliol B, 3-acetoxy-*ent*-3β-7α-dihydroxykaur-16-ene, and 11,12-didehydrosiderol. Biological tests showed that two of these molecules have good anti-inflammatory properties. Further biological tests will be performed to find potential cosmetics applications.

Supplementary Materials: The Supplementary Materials are available online.

Author Contributions: compound purification A.A.; compound identification, K.C. and O.P.T.; DFT calculations, G.G.-J.; compound synthesis, E.R.; MS analyses, C.A. and O.L.; biological evaluation, P.B., E.O., M.D., P.R., and S.P.; writing—original draft preparation and editing, all the authors. All authors have read and agreed to the published version of the manuscript.

Funding: This research was funded by the ANRT under the CIFRE project N° 2016/1074 and NUIG start-up grant to O. Thomas.

Acknowledgments: We thank the Domaine Clarins for the plant sampling. The authors are also grateful to Roisin Doohan (NUIG) for recording NMR spectra.

Conflicts of Interest: The authors declare no conflict of interest.

References

1. González-Burgos, E.; Carretero, M.; Gómez-Serranillos, M. *Sideritis* spp.: Uses, chemical composition and pharmacological activities—A review. *J. Ethnopharmacol.* **2011**, *135*, 209–225. [CrossRef] [PubMed]
2. Piozzi, F.; Bruno, M.; Rosselli, S.; Maggio, A. The Diterpenoids from the Genus *Sideritis*. In *Studies in Natural Products Chemistry*; ur Rahman, A., Ed.; Elsevier: Amsterdam, The Netherlands, 2006; Volume 33, pp. 493–540.
3. Topçu, G.; Gören, A.C.; Yildiz, Y.K.; Tümen, G. *Ent*-Kaurene Diterpenes from *Sideritis athoa*. *Nat. Prod. Lett.* **1999**, *14*, 123–129. [CrossRef]
4. Ertaş, A.; Öztürk, M.; Boğa, M.; Topçu, G. Antioxidant and Anticholinesterase Activity Evaluation of *ent*-Kaurane Diterpenoids from *Sideritis arguta*. *J. Nat. Prod.* **2009**, *72*, 500–502. [CrossRef] [PubMed]
5. Ko, H.H.; Chang, W.L.; Lu, T.M. Antityrosinase and Antioxidant Effects of *ent*-Kaurane Diterpenes from Leaves of *Broussonetia papyrifera*. *J. Nat. Prod.* **2008**, *71*, 1930–1933. [CrossRef] [PubMed]
6. Zhang, M.; Zhao, C.; Dai, W.; He, J.; Jiao, S.; Li, B. Anti-inflammatory *ent*-kaurenoic acids and their glycosides from *Gochnatia decora*. *Phytochemistry* **2017**, *137*, 174–181. [CrossRef] [PubMed]
7. Rodríguez-Lyon, M.L.; Díaz-Lanza, A.M.; Bernabé, M.; Villaescusa-Castillo, L. Flavone glycosides containing acetylated sugars from *Sideritis hyssopifolia*. *Magn. Reson. Chem.* **2000**, *38*, 684–687. [CrossRef]
8. Adzet, T.; Cañigueral, S.; Monasterio, I.; Vila, R.; Ibáñez, C. The Essential Oil and Polyphenols of *Sideritis hyssopifolia* var *pyrenaica*. *J. Essent. Oil Res.* **1990**, *2*, 151–153. [CrossRef]
9. Piozzi, F.; Venturella, P.; Bellino, A.; Mondelli, R. Diterpenes from *Sideritis sicula* ucria. *Tetrahedron* **1968**, *24*, 4073–4081. [CrossRef]
10. Rodiguéz, B.; Peña, A.; Cuesta, R.; Peña, A. Diterpenes from three *Sideritis* species. *Phytochemistry* **1975**, *14*, 1670–1671. [CrossRef]
11. Venturella, P.; Bellino, A.; Marino, M.L. Siderone, a diterpene from *Sideritis syriaca*. *Phytochemistry* **1983**, *22*, 2537–2538. [CrossRef]
12. Rodriguez Gonzalez, B.; Valverde, S.R.J.M. Diterpenes from *Sideritis candicans* var *eriocephala*. *Anal. Quim.* **1970**, *66*, 503–511.
13. Piozzi, F.; Venturella, P. Structure of sideritriol. *Gazz. Chim. Ital.* **1969**, *99*, 582–587.

14. Piozzi, F.; Venturella, P.; Bellino, A.; Marino, M.L. Partial synthesis of *ent*-kaur-16-ene-15β,18-diol and ent-kaur-16-ene-7α,15β,18-triol. *J. Chem. Soc. Perkin Trans. 1 Organ. Bio-Organ. Chem.* **1973**, *1*, 1164–1166.
15. Halfon, B.; Ceyhan Gören, A.; Ertaş, A.; Topçu, G. Complete 13C NMR assignments for *ent*-kaurane diterpenoids from *Sideritis* species. *Magn. Reson. Chem.* **2011**, *49*, 291–294. [CrossRef] [PubMed]
16. Li, J.; Zhang, D.; Wu, X. Synthesis and biological evaluation of novel exo-methylene cyclopentanone tetracyclic diterpenoids as antitumor agents. *Bioorgan. Med. Chem. Lett.* **2011**, *21*, 130–132. [CrossRef] [PubMed]
17. Feldmeyer, L.; Keller, M.; Niklaus, G.; Hohl, D.; Werner, S.; Beer, H.D. The Inflammasome Mediates UVB-Induced Activation and Secretion of Interleukin-1β by Keratinocytes. *Curr. Biol.* **2007**, *17*, 1140–1145. [CrossRef] [PubMed]
18. Harden, J.L.; Krueger, J.G.; Bowcock, A.M. The immunogenetics of Psoriasis: A comprehensive review. *J. Autoimmun.* **2015**, *64*, 66–73. [CrossRef] [PubMed]
19. Jin, Y.; Mailloux, C.M.; Gowan, K.; Riccardi, S.L.; LaBerge, G.; Bennett, D.C.; Fain, P.R.; Spritz, R.A. NALP1 in Vitiligo-Associated Multiple Autoimmune Disease. *N. Engl. J. Med.* **2007**, *356*, 1216–1225. [CrossRef] [PubMed]
20. Okamoto, M.; Liu, W.; Luo, Y.; Tanaka, A.; Cai, X.; Norris, D.A.; Dinarello, C.A.; Fujita, M. Constitutively Active Inflammasome in Human Melanoma Cells Mediating Autoinflammation via Caspase-1 Processing and Secretion of Interleukin-1β. *J. Biol. Chem.* **2010**, *285*, 6477–6488. [CrossRef] [PubMed]
21. Audoin, C.; Zampalégré, A.; Blanchet, N.; Giuliani, A.; Roulland, E.; Laprévote, O.; Genta-Jouve, G. MS/MS-Guided Isolation of Clarinoside, a New Anti-Inflammatory Pentalogin Derivative. *Molecules* **2018**, *23*, 1237. [CrossRef] [PubMed]

Sample Availability: Samples of the compounds **1–4** are available from the authors.

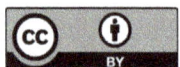

© 2020 by the authors. Licensee MDPI, Basel, Switzerland. This article is an open access article distributed under the terms and conditions of the Creative Commons Attribution (CC BY) license (http://creativecommons.org/licenses/by/4.0/).

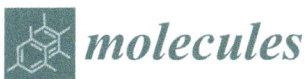

Article

Prenyleudesmanes and A Hexanorlanostane from the Roots of *Lonicera macranthoides*

Hui Lyu [1,2,†], Wenjuan Liu [3,†], Bai Bai [1], Yu Shan [1], Christian Paetz [2], Xu Feng [1,*] and Yu Chen [1,*]

1. Jiangsu Key Laboratory for the Research and Utilization of Plant Resources, The Jiangsu Provincial Platform for Conservation and Utilization of Agricultural Germplasm, Institute of Botany, Jiangsu Province and Chinese Academy of Sciences, Nanjing 210000, China; hlyu@ice.mpg.de (H.L.); baibai0924@126.com (B.B.); shanyu79@126.com (Y.S.)
2. Max Planck Institute for Chemical Ecology, D-07745 Jena, Germany; cpaetz@ice.mpg.de
3. Naval Compound Community Health Care Station, Beijing 100853, China; wenjuan9718@sina.com
* Correspondence: fengxucnbg@mail.cnbg.net (X.F.); yuchen1007@hotmail.com (Y.C.); Tel.: +86-25-84347158 (X.F.); +86-25-84347116 (Y.C.)
† These two authors contributed equally to this work.

Received: 22 October 2019; Accepted: 21 November 2019; Published: 23 November 2019

Abstract: Three previously undescribed compounds, two prenyleudesmanes (**1** and **2**), and one hexanorlanostane (**3**), were isolated from the roots of *Lonicera macranthoides*. Their structures were established based on 1D and 2D nuclear magnetic resonance (NMR) spectra and high-resolution electrospray ionization mass spectral (HR-ESI-MS) data. The absolute configurations of **1** and **3** were determined by X-ray diffraction. To the best of our knowledge, this is the first time that the absolute configuration of a prenyleudesmane with a *trans*-decalin system and a hexanorlanostane have been unambiguously confirmed by single-crystal X-ray diffraction with Cu Kα radiation. Thecompounds were tested for their antiproliferative activity on the cancer cell lines (HepG2 and HeLa). The compounds **1**–**3** exhibited moderate inhibitory effects against two human cancer cell lines.

Keywords: *Lonicera macranthoides*; Caprifoliaceae; Prenyleudesmanes; Hexanortriterpenes; Antiproliferative

1. Introduction

Lonicera macranthoides Hand.-Mazz., a plant of the genus *Lonicera* in the family Caprifoliaceae, is mainly distributed in the southwest of China [1]. The dried flower buds of *L. macranthoides* are commonly used as a raw material in traditional Chinese medicine for treating fever, inflammation, and infectious diseases [2]. Earlier phytochemical studies on the plant have shown the presence of various triterpenoid saponins (e.g., hederagenin saponins, oleanolic acid saponins, 18-oleanene saponins, and lupane saponins) [3–6], flavonoids [7], phenolic acids [8,9], and iridoids [8,9] in aerial parts and flowers of the plant. Because of our studies of *L. macranthoides*, we became interested in the diterpenes of this species. Recently, we reported the first known occurrence of diterpenes (e.g., labdane, aphidicolane, and *syn*-pimarane) in the roots of *L. macranthoides* [10–12]. To explore further unknown diterpenes, we reinvestigated the roots of *L. macranthoides*. Here, we report on the isolation and characterization of two new diterpenes, lonimacranthoidin C (**1**) and lonimacranthoidin D (**2**), and a novel hexanorlanostane, lonimacranthoidin E (**3**). Compounds **1**–**3** were screened for antiproliferative activity against two human cancer cell lines, HepG2 and HeLa.

2. Results and Discussion

An ethanolic extract of dried roots of *L. macranthoides* was suspended in water and partitioned sequentially between petroleum ether and ethyl acetate (EtOAc). The EtOAc fraction was subjected to repeated separation by column chromatography (CC) over silica gel and Sephadex LH-20. Selected fractions were further purified by preparative HPLC to yield three pure compounds, including the two prenyleudesmanes (**1**, **2**) and a hexanorlanostane (**3**), as seen in Figure 1. The structure elucidation was carried out by high-resolution mass spectrometry (HRMS), nuclear magnetic resonance (NMR) spectroscopy (^{1}H NMR, ^{13}C NMR, ^{1}H-^{1}H homonuclear chemical shift correlation spectroscopy (COSY), ^{1}H-^{13}C heteronuclear single quantum coherence (HSQC), ^{1}H-^{13}C heteronuclear multiple bond correlation (HMBC), and ^{1}H-^{1}H rotating frame Overhauser effect spectroscopy (ROESY)), and single-crystal X-ray diffraction analysis.

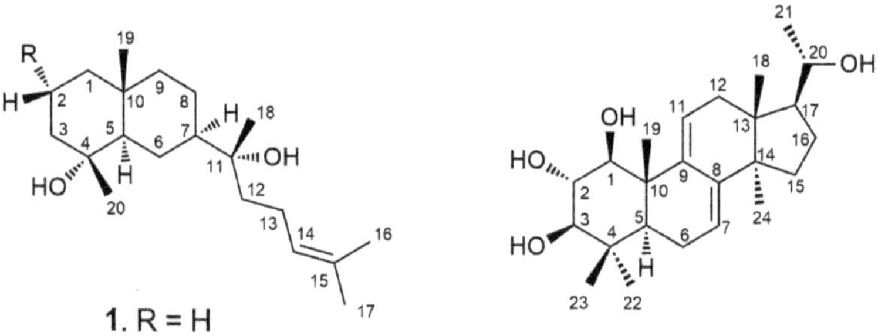

Figure 1. Chemical structures of the compounds 1–3.

Compound **1** was obtained as colorless crystals. The molecular formula of $C_{20}H_{36}O_2Na$ was determined by the pseudomolecular ion peak at m/z 331.2607 [M + Na]$^+$ (calculated: 331.2608) in positive HR-ESI-MS, corresponding to three unsaturations. The UV spectrum showed the absorption maximum at λ_{max} 201 nm. The compound showed a positive optical rotation of $[\alpha]_D^{25}$+26.4 (c 0.100 in methanol). The ^{1}H NMR spectrum of **1** displayed signals for one olefinic proton at δ_H 5.14 (1H, dd, J = 7.0/7.0, H-14), five methyl singlets at δ_H 0.86 (3H, s, H$_3$-19), δ_H 1.11 (3H, s, H$_3$-20), δ_H 1.16 (3H, s, H$_3$-18), δ_H 1.63 (3H, s, H$_3$-17), and δ_H 1.69 (3H, s, H$_3$-16), and overlapping aliphatic methylene and/or methine signals (δ_H 1.05–2.04). The assignment of the latter could be accomplished by a series of selective total correlation spectroscopy (SELTOCSY) experiments (see Supporting Information). The ^{13}C NMR and distortionless enhancement by polarization transfer (DEPT) NMR spectra of **1** showed the presence of 20 carbon resonances, including two signals of olefinic carbons at δ_C 124.6 (C-14) and δ_C 131.6 (C-15), five signals for methyl groups at δ_C 17.6 (C-16), δ_C 18.7 (C-19), δ_C 22.6 (C-20), δ_C 24.1 (C-18), and δ_C 25.7 (C-17), eight methylene signals at δ_C 41.0 (C-1), δ_C 20.1 (C-2), δ_C 43.5 (C-3), δ_C 21.4 (C-6), δ_C 21.8 (C-8), δ_C 44.6 (C-9), δ_C 39.7 (C-12), and δ_C 22.3 (C-13), two methine signals at δ_C 55.0 (C-5) and δ_C 48.3 (C-7), one signal for a quaternary carbon at δ_C 34.6 (C-10), and two signals of oxygenated tertiary carbons at δ_C 72.3 (C-4) and δ_C 74.5 (C-11). The interpretation of NMR spectra and the degree of unsaturation deduced from HRMS data suggested that compound **1** was a bicyclic diterpene possessing a trisubstituted double bond and two hydroxyl groups (OH-4 and OH-11). Analysis of the ^{1}H-^{1}H COSY and HSQC spectra of **1** provided three partial structures shown by bold lines in Figure 2. The interpretation of the HMBC spectrum of **1** showed correlations from H$_3$-17 to C-14, C-15, and C-16, and from H$_3$-16 to C-14, C-15, and C-17; these enabled the localization of the double bond at C-14. This spin system is further characterized by a coupling of H-12 to H-14. HMBC correlations from H-12 to C-11, and from H$_3$-18 to C-11 and C-12, eventually resulted in the definition of a side chain of eight carbons, including a trisubstituted double bond (Δ^{14}). A further HMBC correlation from H-12 to C-7 and from H$_3$-18 to C-7 indicated the linkage to C-7 of the decalin ring system. The two hydroxylated positions at C-4 and C-11, respectively, could be confirmed by the HMBC correlations from H$_3$-20 to C-3, C-4, and C-5, and from H$_3$-18 to C-11 and C-12, as seen in Figure 2. In summary, the NMR data analysis, as seen in Table 1, revealed a prenyleudesmane skeleton similar to dysokusone A [13], and the structure of **1** was determined as shown in Figure 1. The relative configuration of **1** was partially established by analyzing its ROESY correlations. Nuclear Overhauser effect (NOE) correlations between H$_3$-18, H$_3$-19, and H$_3$-20 suggested a cofacial arrangement. Finally, crystals of compound **1** were obtained and subjected to X-ray diffraction analysis, as seen in Figure 3. The absolute configuration of **1** was determined as (4*R*,5*R*,7*R*,10*R*)-4,10-dimethyl-7-(11*R*-hydroxy-11,15-dimethyl-14-ene-11-yl)-*trans*-decalin-4-ol by Cu X-ray crystallography (Flack parameter = −0.05 (11), Figure 3) [14,15] and named as lonimacranthoidin C (**1**). Ours was the first successful single-crystal X-ray analysis of a prenyleudesmane with a *trans*-decalin scaffold.

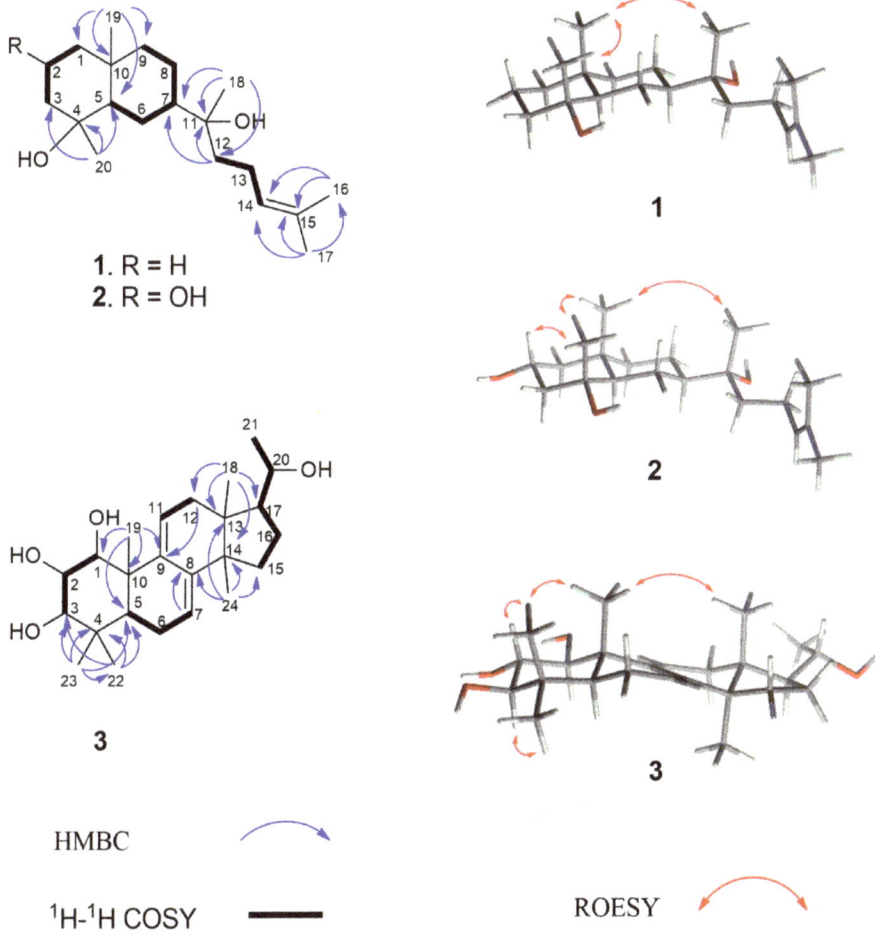

Figure 2. Key 2D NMR correlations of compounds **1**, **2**, and **3**.

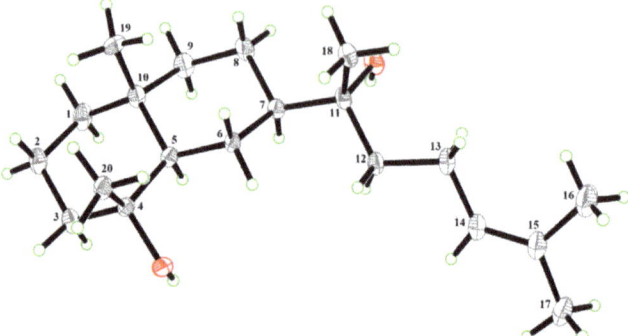

Figure 3. X-ray Oak Ridge thermal-ellipsoid plot program (ORTEP) drawing of compound **1**.

Table 1. ^{1}H and ^{13}C NMR spectral data of compounds **1**, **2**, and **3**.

Atom	1 [a,c]		2 [a,c]		3 [b,c]	
	δ_C	δ_H	δ_C	δ_H	δ_C	δ_H
1α	41.0	1.07 ddd 12.5/12.5/6.0	46.7	1.34 dd 14.0/3.2	78.4	3.57 d 10.0
1β		1.38 d 12.5		1.67 m		
2α	20.1	1.58 m	68.2	4.28 ddd 7.0/3.0/3.0	72.9	3.48 dd 10.0/10.0
2β		1.56 m				
3α	43.5	1.35 ddd 12.5/12.5/5.5	48.5	1.66 m	78.7	3.04 d 10.0
3β		1.79 d 12.5		2.01 d 14.0		
4	72.3		71.6		38.1	
5	55.0	1.19 d 12.5	54.4	1.29 dd 12.5/2.0	47.1	1.16 dd 5.0/12.0
6α	21.4	1.86 d 12.5	21.2	1.87 d 12.5	22.4	2.20 dd 12.0/17.0
6β		1.03 ddd 12.5/12.5/12.5		1.14 ddd 12.5/12.5/12.5		2.15 dd 5.0/5.0/17.0
7	48.3	1.41 dddd 12.5/12.5/3.0/3.0	48.5	1.42 dddd 12.5/12.5/3.0/3.0	119.5	5.49 d 5.0
8α	21.8	1.59 d 12.5	21.2	1.56 d 12.5	142.1	
8β		1.33 dddd 12.5/12.5/12.5/3.0		1.37 dddd 12.5/12.5/12.5/3.5		
9α	44.6	1.45 ddd 12.5/3.0/3.0	44.9	1.49 ddd 12.5/3.0/3.0	144.0	
9β		1.15 ddd 12.5/12.5/3.0		1.12 m		
10	34.6		34.0		43.2	
11	74.5		74.6		119.1	6.31 d 6.0
12α	39.7	1.53 dd 8.2/8.2	39.5	1.52 dd 8.1/8.1	36.4	2.18 d 17.0
12β						2.06 d 6.0/17.0
13	22.3	2.06 m	22.3	2.04 m	42.0	
14	124.6	5.14 dd 7.0/7.0	124.5	5.13 dd 6.7/6.7	49.9	
15α	131.6		131.6		31.1	1.68 ddd 7.5/11.5/11.5
15β						1.46 dd 9.0/11.5
16α	17.6	1.63 s	17.8	1.62 s	25.8	2.07 ddd 9.0/14.0/17.0
16β						1.60 dd 9.0/14.0
17	25.7	1.69 s	25.8	1.68 s	53.0	1.78 dd 9.0/17.0
18	24.1	1.16 s	24.2	1.16 s	15.4	0.57 s
19	18.7	0.86 s	20.3	1.14 s	15.9	1.06 s
20	22.6	1.11 s	25.0	1.33 s	70.4	3.62 dd 6.2/9.0
21					22.4	1.21 d 6.2
22					15.9	0.90 s
23					27.6	1.02 s
24					24.9	0.91 s

[a] Data were measured at 500 MHz for ^{1}H and 125 MHz for ^{13}C in CDCl$_3$, δ in ppm, J in Hz.; [b] Data were measured at 300 MHz for ^{1}H and 75 MHz for ^{13}C in CDCl$_3$:CD$_3$OD = 1:1, δ in ppm, J in Hz.; [c] Overlapping signals were assigned by HSQC, HMBC, COSY, and SELTOCSY experiments.

Compound **2** was obtained as milky oil with the molecular formula C$_{20}$H$_{36}$O$_3$ as determined by HR-ESI-MS (m/z 347.2551 [M + Na]$^+$, calculated: m/z 347.2557 for [C$_{20}$H$_{36}$O$_3$ + Na]$^+$). Similar to **1**, compound **2** showed three unsaturations. The UV spectrum of **2** showed an absorption at λ$_{max}$ 201 nm and a positive optical rotation of [α]$_D^{25}$ + 10.0 (c 0.100 in methanol) was determined. The assignment of all proton and carbon chemical shifts of **2** was achieved by analyzing the 1D and 2D NMR spectra, as seen in Table 1. Similar to **1**, the structure of **2** was also elucidated as a prenyleudesmane-type diterpene. Unlike the chemical shifts of position 2 in **1** (δ$_C$ 20.1 and δ$_H$ 1.56/1.58 (H-2β/H-2α, respectively)), the corresponding structural elements in **2** were an oxygenated methylene (δ$_C$ 68.2) and a hydroxymethine (δ$_H$ 4.28, H-2). Thus, **2** was determined as the C-2 hydroxylated derivative of **1**, as shown in Figure 1. The stereochemistry at C-2 was established by the occurrence of NOE correlations between H$_3$-19, H$_3$-20 H$_3$-18, and H-2 which indicated a cofacial orientation. Hence, the absolute configuration for C-2 was assigned, based on the X-ray determined configuration of **1**, as *R*-configured. Due to the occurrence of similar chemical shifts for C-4, C-5, C-7, C-10, and C-11, as seen in Table 1, similar NOESY correlations, as seen in Figure 2, similar values for the optical rotation, and the above defined configuration of C2, compound **2** was determined as (2*R*,4*R*,5*R*,7*R*,10*R*)-4,10-dimethyl-7-(11*R*-hydroxy-11,15-dimethyl-14-ene-11-yl)-*trans*-decalin-2,4-diol, and named lonimacranthoidin D (**2**).

The molecular formula of compound **3** was assigned as $C_{24}H_{38}O_4$ by its positive HR-ESI-MS data (*m/z* 413.2667, [M + Na]$^+$; calculated: 413.2662), which indicated six unsaturations in the molecule. Compound **3** was obtained as colorless crystals with an UV spectrum having an absorption maximum at λ_{max} 243 nm. The compound showed a positive optical rotation of $[\alpha]_D^{25}$ + 12.6 (c 0.100 in methanol). The ^{1}H NMR spectrum of **3** showed resonances of two olefinic protons at δ_H 6.31 (1H, d, *J* = 6.0 Hz, H-11) and δ_H 5.49 (1H, d, *J* = 5.0 Hz, H-7), six methyl resonances at δ_H 0.57 (3H, s, H$_3$-18), δ_H 1.06 (3H, s, H$_3$-19), δ_H 1.21 (3H, d, *J* = 6.2 Hz, H$_3$-21), δ_H 0.90 (3H, s, H$_3$-22), δ_H 1.02 (3H, s, H$_3$-23), and δ_H 0.91 (3H, s, H$_3$-24), four hydroxymethines at δ_H 3.57 (1H, d, *J* = 10.0 Hz, H-1), δ_H 3.48 (1H, dd, *J* = 10.0/10.0 Hz, H-2), δ_H 3.04 (1H, d, *J* = 10.0 Hz, H-3), and δ_H 3.62 (1H, dd, *J* = 6.2/9.0 Hz, H-20), and further overlapping aliphatic methylenes and/or methines in the range δ_H 1.10 to δ_H 2.30, which were assigned by means of SELTOCSY experiments (see Supporting Information). The ^{13}C NMR and DEPT spectra of **3** showed the presence of four olefinic carbons at δ_C 119.1 (C-7), δ_C 144.0 (C-8), δ_C 142.1 (C-9), and δ_C 119.1 (C-11). The remaining four MS-predicted unsaturations were assigned to a tetracyclic ring system. In addition, six methyl groups at δ_C 15.4 (C-18), δ_C 15.9 (C-19), δ_C 22.4 (C-21), δ_C 15.9 (C-22), δ_C 27.6 (C-23), and δ_C 24.9 (C-24), four methylenes at δ_C 22.4 (C-6), δ_C 36.4 (C-12), δ_C 31.1 (C-15), and δ_C 25.8 (C-16), two methines at δ_C 47.1 (C-5) and δ_C 53.0 (C-17), four oxygenated methines at δ_C 78.4 (C-1), δ_C 72.9 (C-2), δ_C 78.7 (C-3), and δ_C 70.4 (C-20), and four quaternary carbons at δ_C 38.1 (C-4), δ_C 43.2 (C-10), δ_C 42.0 (C-13), and δ_C 49.9 (C-14) were observed. Thus, **3** was assigned as a hexanortriterpene derivative with two trisubstituted double bonds (Δ^7 and Δ^9) and four hydroxyl groups (OH-1, OH-2, OH-3, and OH-20). Interpretation of the ^{1}H-^{1}H COSY data resulted in the identification of four spin systems: H-1/H-2/H-3, H-5/H-6/H-7, H-11/H-12, and H-15/H-16/H-17/H-20/H-21. The HMBC correlations from H$_3$-18 to C-12, C-13, C-14, and C-17; from H$_3$-19 to C-1, C-5, C-9, and C-10; from H$_3$-22 to C-3, C-4, C-5, and C-23; from H$_3$-23 to C-3, C-4, C-5, and C-22; and from H$_3$-24 to C-8, C-13, C-14, and C-15 allowed for the positioning of two methyl groups at C-4 and four methyl groups at C-10, C-13, C-14, and C-20, respectively. These data indicated that compound **3** was an unusual hexanorlanostane that had been described earlier as aglycon, from the saponins of the sea cucumber *Cucumaria koraiensis* [16,17]. The full assignment of all positions in the molecule was accomplished by the interpretation of the HSQC and HMBC data, as seen in Table 1, suggesting that **3** was 1,2,3,20-tetrahydroxy-hexanorlanostan-7, 9(11)-diene, as shown in Figure 1. In the ROESY spectrum of **3**, correlations between H$_3$-18/H$_3$-19/H$_3$-23/H-2 and H$_3$-22/H-3 indicated that H$_3$-18, H$_3$-19, H$_3$-23, and H-2 were on one side of the molecular plane, while H$_3$-22 and H-3 were located on the opposite side. Fortunately, crystals of compound **3** could be obtained and were subjected to single-crystal X-ray diffraction analysis, as seen in Figure 4. Based on our results, the absolute configuration of **3** was determined as (1*S*,2*S*,3*R*,5*S*,10*S*,13*R*,14*R*,17*S*,20*S*)-1,2,3,20-tetrahydroxy-hexanorlanostan-7, 9(11)-diene (**3**) by Cu X-ray crystallography (Flack parameter = 0.20 (6), Figure 4) and named lonimacranthoidin E.

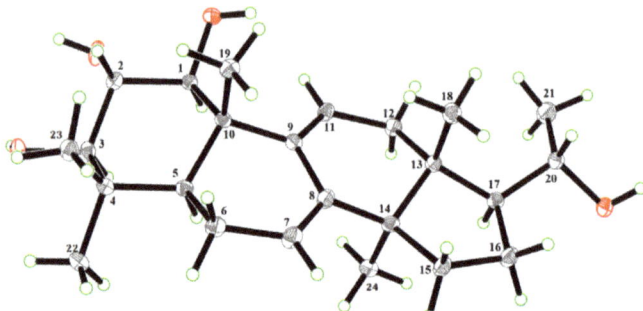

Figure 4. X-ray ORTEP drawing of compound **3**.

Compounds **1–3** were furthermore tested for their antiproliferative effect on the Human Hepatocellular Carcinoma Cell lines (HepG2), Human Cervical Carcinoma Cell line (HeLa), and the Human Aortic Smooth Muscle Cell line (HASMC). The results, as seen in Table 2, demonstrated that **1–3** showed moderate antiproliferative activities (IC$_{50}$ 12.5 ± 0.9 to 64.9 ± 3.5 μM) against the two tumor cell lines. No significant effect against HASMC was observed.

Table 2. Antiproliferative activities of compounds **1–3** against two cancer cells and one normal cell line. [a]

Cell Line	1	2	3	Etoposide
HepG2	36.3 ± 2.1	64.9 ± 3.5	46.0 ± 2.4	25.4 ± 1.7
HeLa	13.8 ± 1.1	27.1 ± 1.4	12.5 ± 0.9	21.2 ± 1.3
HASMC	>100	>100	>100	63.7

[a] Results are expressed as IC$_{50}$ values in μM.

Prenyleudesmanes are a rare class of diterpenes that were originally isolated from marine algae [18,19] and marine mollusks [20–24]. Prenyleudesmanes were also found in fungi [25] and plants of the genus *Dysoxylum* [13,26–28]. Our report on the isolation and full structure elucidation of lonimacranthoidin C (**1**) and lonimacranthoidin D (**2**) from *L. macranthoides* therefore suggests another source for prenyleudesmanes in nature. Interestingly, the hexanorlanostane **3** was initially found in sea creatures [16,17]. Lonimacranthoidin E (**3**) is the first example of a hexanorlanostane isolated from a terrestrial plant.

3. Materials and Methods

3.1. General Experimental Procedures

Thin-layer chromatography was carried out on silica gel 60 GF254 (Merck) plates. Preparative HPLC (LC-20AR, Shimadzu, Kyoto, Japan) was conducted on a Shim-pack GIS C$_{18}$ column (5 μm, 250 × 20 mm, Shimadzu). Column chromatography (CC) was performed on silica gel (200–300 mesh) and Sephadex LH-20. LC-HRMS spectra were obtained from an Agilent 1260 UPLC-DAD-6530 ESI Q-TOF MS (Agilent Technologies GmbH, Waldbronn, Germany). Optical rotation values were measured using a Jasco P-1020 polarimeter. NMR data were obtained using a Bruker Avance 500 MHz or Bruker Avance 300 MHz spectrometers (Bruker Biospin GmbH, Karlsruhe, Germany). Tetramethylsilane was used as an internal standard. The X-ray structures were solved by direct methods (SHELXL-97). The X-ray crystallographic data were collected on a Bruker SMART APEX-II CCD diffractometer using graphite monochromatic Cu K$_\alpha$ radiation.

3.2. Plant Material

The roots of *L. macranthoides* were collected from Longhui in the Hunan province of China in July 2015. The plants were taxonomically identified by Professor Changqi Yuan (Institute of Botany, Jiangsu province and Chinese Academy of Sciences). A voucher specimen (No. 20150701) has been deposited in the herbarium of the Institute of Botany, Jiangsu province, and Chinese Academy of Sciences.

3.3. Extraction and Isolation

The dried roots (4.0 kg) of *L. macranthoides* were milled and repeatedly extracted with 95% EtOH for 2 h under reflux (80 °C). After evaporation in vacuo, the crude extract (472.6 g) was resuspended in H_2O and partitioned with petroleum ether and ethyl acetate (EtOAc), in succession. The EtOAc fraction (94 g) was subjected to column chromatography (silica gel, CH_2Cl_2-MeOH 100:0–0:100) to produce six fractions (F1-F6) on the basis of TLC analysis. F2 (21 g) was purified by column chromatography on Sephadex LH-20 (CH_2Cl_2-MeOH, 1:1), followed by preparative HPLC using MeOH-H_2O (65:35, *v/v*, flow rate 1.0 mL/min) as an eluent to obtain the compounds **1** (11.0 mg) and **2** (6.0 mg). F5 (11 g) was purified by preparative HPLC with MeOH–H_2O (55:45, *v/v*, flow rate 3.0 mL/min) as an eluent to obtain compound **3** (13.0 mg).

3.4. Compound Characterization

Lonimacranthoidin C (**1**): colorless crystals (MeOH); $[\alpha]_D^{25}$ + 26.4 (c 0.100 in MeOH); UV (MeOH) λ_{max} 201 nm; mp 101–103 °C; HR-ESI-MS *m/z* 331.2607 [M + Na]$^+$ (calculated for $C_{20}H_{36}O_2$: 331.2608); ^{1}H NMR (500 MHz, CDCl$_3$) and ^{13}C NMR (125 MHz, CDCl$_3$) spectroscopic data, see Table 1. Lonimacranthoidin C (**1**) was recrystallized in methanol/ethyl acetate (3:1). A single-crystal X-ray diffraction analysis using Cu Kα radiation (1.54178 Å) was carried out to confirm the structure. M = 308.49, monoclinic, P2$_1$ 2$_1$ 2$_1$, *a* = 11.5498 (17) Å, *b* = 12.2435 (14) Å, *c* = 27.246 (3) Å, $\alpha = \gamma = \beta = 90.00°$, *V* = 3852.8 (9) Å^3, Z = 8, Dc = 1.064 mg mm^{-3}, T = 153 (2) K, F (000) = 1376.0. The crystallographic data centre has assigned the code Cambridge Crystallographic Data Centre (CCDC) 1,941,729 for the crystal structure of lonimacranthoidin C (**1**). The CCDC contains the supplementary crystallographic data for this paper. These data can be obtained free of charge via http://www.ccdc.cam.ac.uk/conts/retrieving.html.

Lonimacranthoidin D (**2**): milky oil (MeOH); $[\alpha]_D^{25}$ + 10.0 (c 0.100 in MeOH); UV (MeOH) λ_{max} 201 nm; HR-ESI-MS *m/z* 347.2551 [M + Na]$^+$ (calculated for $C_{20}H_{36}O_3$, 347.2557); ^{1}H NMR (500 MHz, CDCl$_3$) and ^{13}C NMR (125 MHz, CDCl$_3$) spectroscopic data are listed in Table 1.

Lonimacranthoidin E (**3**): colorless crystals (MeOH); $[\alpha]_D^{25}$ + 12.6 (c 0.100 in MeOH); UV (MeOH) λ_{max} 243 nm; mp 244–246 °C; HR-ESI-MS *m/z* 413.2667 [M + Na]$^+$ (calculated for $C_{24}H_{38}O_4$: 413.2662); ^{1}H NMR (300 MHz, in CDCl$_3$:CD$_3$OD = 1:1) and ^{13}C NMR (75 MHz, in CDCl$_3$:CD$_3$OD = 1:1), for NMR spectroscopic data, see Table 1. Lonimacranthoidin E (**3**) was re-crystallized in methanol/ethyl acetate (1:1). A single-crystal X-ray diffraction analysis using Cu Kα radiation (1.54178 Å) was carried out to confirm the structure. M = 390.54, monoclinic, P2$_1$ 2$_1$ 2$_1$, *a* = 6.0714 (4) Å, *b* = 13.2797 (8) Å, *c* = 28.6232 (17) Å, $\alpha = \gamma = \beta = 90.00°$, *V* = 2307.87 (2) Å^3, Z = 4, Dc = 1.124 mg mm^{-3}, T = 153 (2) K, F (000) = 856. The crystallographic data centre has assigned the code CCDC 1,941,730 for the crystal structure of lonimacranthoidin E (**3**) The CCDC contains the supplementary crystallographic data for this paper. These data can be obtained free of charge via http://www.ccdc.cam.ac.uk/conts/retrieving.html.

3.5. Biological Assay

HepG2, HeLa, and HASMC cell lines were cultured in Dulbecco's modified Eagle's medium (Gibco, Grand Island, NY, USA) supplemented with 10% fetal bovine serum (Gibco), 100 µg/mL penicillin, and 100 µg/mL streptomycin. The cells were cultivated in a humidified atmosphere of 5% CO_2 at 37 °C. Antiproliferative assays of the compounds **1**–**3** against the above-mentioned three cell lines were evaluated using the 3-(4,5-dimethylthiazol-2-yl)-2,5-diphenyltetrazoliumbromide (MTT) assay, carried out according to protocols [29] described previously.

Supplementary Materials: ^{1}H and ^{13}C NMR, ^{13}C-DEPT, ^{1}H-^{13}C HSQC, ^{1}H-^{13}C HMBC, ^{1}H-^{1}H COSY, ^{1}H-^{1}H ROESY, SELTOCSY, UV, and HR-ESI-MS data of compounds **1–3** are available in the Supporting Information.

Author Contributions: Funding acquisition, X.F. and Y.C.; Investigation, H.L., W.L., B.B., Y.S. and C.P.; Methodology, Y.C.; Project administration, Y.C.; Supervision, X.F. and Y.C.; Writing—original draft, H.L.; Writing—review & editing, C.P. and Y.C.

Acknowledgments: This research was supported financially by the National Natural Science Foundation of China (31770383, 31970375) and Research Project of 333 High-Level Talents Cultivation of Jiangsu Province (BRA2016463). We thank Emily Wheeler for editorial assistance.

Conflicts of Interest: The authors declare no conflict of interest.

References

1. FOC (Flora of China) Flora of China Website. 1988. Available online: http://frps.iplant.cn/frps/Lonicera%20macranthoides (accessed on 15 October 2019).
2. Chinese Pharmacopeia Commission. *Pharmacopeia of the People's Republic of China*; China Medical Science Press: Beijing, China, 2015; Volume 1, p. 30.
3. Chen, Y.; Zhao, Y.; Wang, M.; Wang, Q.; Shan, Y.; Guan, F.; Feng, X. A new lupane-type triterpenoid saponin from *Lonicera macranthoides*. *Chem. Nat. Compd.* **2014**, *49*, 1087–1090. [CrossRef]
4. Chen, Y.; Feng, X.; Jia, X.; Wang, M.; Liang, J.; Dong, Y. Triterpene glycosides from Lonicera. Isolation and structural determination of seven glycosides from flower buds of *Lonicera macranthoides*. *Chem. Nat. Compd.* **2008**, *44*, 39–43. [CrossRef]
5. Chen, Y.; Feng, X.; Wang, M.; Zhao, Y.Y.; Dong, Y.F. Triterpene glycosides from Lonicera. II. Isolation and structural determination of glycosides from flower buds of *Lonicera macranthoides*. *Chem. Nat. Compd.* **2009**, *45*, 514–518.
6. Chen, Y.; Shan, Y.; Zhao, Y.Y.; Wang, Q.Z.; Wang, M.; Feng, X.; Liang, J.Y. Two new triterpenoid saponins from *Lonicera macranthoides*. *Chin. Chem. Lett.* **2012**, *3*, 325–328. [CrossRef]
7. Sun, M.; Feng, X.; Yin, M.; Chen, Y.; Zhao, X.; Dong, Y. A biflavonoid from stems and leaves of *Lonicera macranthoides*. *Chem. Nat. Compd.* **2012**, *48*, 231–233. [CrossRef]
8. Sun, M.; Feng, X.; Lin, X.H.; Yin, M.; Zhao, X.Z.; Chen, Y.; Shan, Y. Studies on the chemical constituents from stems and leaves of *Lonicera macranthoides*. *J. Chin. Med. Mater.* **2011**, *34*, 218–220.
9. Liu, J.; Zhang, J.; Wang, F.; Chen, X.F. Chemical constituents from the buds of *Lonicera macranthoides* in Sichuan, China. *Biochem. Syst. Ecol.* **2014**, *54*, 68–70. [CrossRef]
10. Liu, W.J.; Chen, Y.; Ma, X.; Zhao, Y.Y.; Feng, X. Study on chemical constituents from roots of *Lonicera macranthoides*. *Chin. Med. Mat.* **2014**, *37*, 2207–2209.
11. Bai, B.; Chen, Y.; Liu, W.J.; Yin, M.; Wang, M.; Feng, X. Chemical constituents of petroleum ether fraction of *Lonicera macranthoides* roots. *J. Chin. Med. Mater.* **2015**, *38*, 518–520.
12. Lyu, H.; Liu, W.J.; Xu, S.; Shan, Y.; Feng, X.; Chen, Y. Two 9, 10-syn-pimarane diterpenes from the roots of *Lonicera macranthoides*. *Phytochem. Lett.* **2018**, *25*, 175–179. [CrossRef]
13. Fujioka, T.; Yamamoto, M.; Kashiwada, Y.; Fujii, H.; Mihashi, K.; Ikeshiro, Y.; Chen, I.S.; Lee, K.H. Novel cytotoxic diterpenes from the stem of *Dysoxylum kuskusense*. *Bioorg. Med. Chem. Lett.* **1998**, *8*, 3479–3482. [CrossRef]
14. Flack, H.D. On enantiomorph-polarity estimation. *Acta. Cryst. A Found. Crystallogr.* **1983**, *39*, 876–881. [CrossRef]
15. Flack, H.D.; Bernardinelli, G. Reporting and evaluating absolute-structure and absolute-configuration determinations. *J. Appl. Crystallogr.* **2000**, *33*, 1143–1148. [CrossRef]
16. Avilov, S.A.; Kalinovsky, A.I.; Kalinin, V.I.; Stonik, V.A.; Riguera, R.; Jiménez CKoreoside, A. A new nonholostane triterpene glycoside from the sea cucumber *Cucumaria koraiensis*. *J. Nat. Prod.* **1997**, *60*, 808–810. [CrossRef] [PubMed]
17. Kalinin, V.I.; Silchenko, A.S.; Avilov, S.A.; Stonik, V.A. Non-holostane aglycones of sea cucumber triterpene glycosides. Structure, biosynthesis, evolution. *Steroids* **2018**, *147*, 42–51. [CrossRef] [PubMed]

18. Sun, H.H.; Waraszkiewicz, S.M.; Erickson, K.L.; Finer, J.; Clardy, J. Dictyoxepin and dictyolene, two new diterpenes from the marine alga *Dictyota acutiloba* (Phaeophyta). *J. Am. Chem. Soc.* **1977**, *99*, 3516–3517. [CrossRef]
19. Takahashi, Y.; Suzuki, M.; Abe, T.; Masuda, M. Anhydroaplysiadiol from *Laurencia japonensis*. *Phytochemistry* **1998**, *48*, 987–990. [CrossRef]
20. Ojika, M.; Yoshida, Y.; Okumura, M.; Ieda, S.; Yamada, K. Aplysiadiol, A new brominated diterpene from the marine mollusc *Aplysia kurodai*. *J. Nat. Prod.* **1990**, *53*, 1619–1622. [CrossRef]
21. Matthée, G.F.; König, G.M.; Wright, A.D. Three new diterpenes from the marine soft coral *Lobophytum crassum*. *J. Nat. Prod.* **1998**, *61*, 237–240. [CrossRef]
22. Cheng, S.Y.; Chuang, C.T.; Wang, S.K.; Wen, Z.H.; Chiou, S.F.; Hsu, C.H.; Dai, C.F.; Duh, C.Y. Antiviral and anti-inflammatory diterpenoids from the soft coral *Sinularia gyrosa*. *J. Nat. Prod.* **2010**, *73*, 1184–1187. [CrossRef]
23. Li, L.; Sheng, L.; Wang, C.Y.; Zhou, Y.B.; Huang, H.; Li, X.B.; Li, J.; Molllo, E.; Gavagnin, M.; Guo, Y.W. Diterpenes from the Hainan soft coral *Lobophytum cristatum* Tixier-Durivault. *J. Nat. Prod.* **2011**, *74*, 2089–2094. [CrossRef] [PubMed]
24. Ye, F.; Zhu, Z.D.; Gu, Y.C.; Li, J.; Zhu, W.L.; Guo, Y.W. Further new diterpenoids as PTP1B inhibitors from the Xisha soft coral *Sinularia polydactyla*. *Mar. Drugs* **2018**, *16*, 103. [CrossRef] [PubMed]
25. Liu, D.Z.; Liang, B.W.; Li, X.F.; Liu, Q. Induced production of new diterpenoids in the fungus *Penicillium funiculosum*. *Nat. Prod. Commun.* **2014**, *9*, 607–608. [CrossRef] [PubMed]
26. Duh, C.Y.; Wang, S.K.; Chen, I.S. Cytotoxic prenyleudesmane diterpenes from the fruits of *Dysoxylum kuskusense*. *J. Nat. Prod.* **2000**, *63*, 1546–1547. [CrossRef]
27. Gu, J.; Qian, S.Y.; Zhao, Y.L.; Cheng, G.G.; Hu, D.B.; Zhang, B.H.; Liu, Y.P.; Luo, X.D. Prenyleudesmanes, rare natural diterpenoids from *Dysoxylum densiflorum*. *Tetrahedron* **2014**, *70*, 1375–1382. [CrossRef]
28. Zhang, P.; Lin, Y.; Wang, F.; Fang, D.; Zhang, G. Diterpenes from *Dysoxylum lukii* Merr. *Phytochem. Lett.* **2019**, *29*, 53–56. [CrossRef]
29. Alley, M.C.; Scudiero, D.A.; Monks, A.; Hursey, M.L.; Czerwinski, M.J.; Fine, D.L.; Abbott, B.J.; Mayo, J.G.; Shoemaker, R.H.; Boyd, M.R. Feasibility of drug screening with panels of human tumor cell lines using a microculture tetrazolium assay. *Cancer Res.* **1998**, *48*, 589–601.

Sample Availability: Samples of the compounds **1** and **3** are available from the authors.

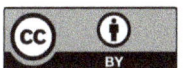

© 2019 by the authors. Licensee MDPI, Basel, Switzerland. This article is an open access article distributed under the terms and conditions of the Creative Commons Attribution (CC BY) license (http://creativecommons.org/licenses/by/4.0/).

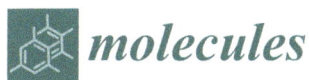

Article

Quantitative Analysis of Terpenic Compounds in Microsamples of Resins by Capillary Liquid Chromatography

H. D. Ponce-Rodríguez [1,2], R. Herráez-Hernández [1,*], J. Verdú-Andrés [1,*] and P. Campíns-Falcó [1]

1. MINTOTA Research Group, Department of Analytical Chemistry, Faculty of Chemistry, University of Valencia, Dr Moliner 50, 46100 Burjassot, Valencia, Spain; henrypon@alumni.uv.es (H.D.P.-R.); pilar.campins@uv.es (P.C.-F.)
2. Department of Chemical Control, Faculty of Chemistry and Pharmacy, National Autonomous University of Honduras, Ciudad Universitaria, 11101 Tegucigalpa, Honduras
* Correspondence: rosa.herraez@uv.es (R.H.-H); jorge.verdu@uv.es (J.V.-A)

Academic Editors: Pavel B. Drasar, Vladimir A. Khripach and Maria Carla Marcotullio
Received: 10 October 2019; Accepted: 8 November 2019; Published: 10 November 2019

Abstract: A method has been developed for the separation and quantification of terpenic compounds typically used as markers in the chemical characterization of resins based on capillary liquid chromatography coupled to UV detection. The sample treatment, separation and detection conditions have been optimized in order to analyze compounds of different polarities and volatilities in a single chromatographic run. The monoterpene limonene and the triterpenes lupeol, lupenone, β-amyrin, and α-amyrin have been selected as model compounds. The proposed method provides linear responses and precision (expressed as relative standard deviations) of 0.6% to 17%, within the 0.5–10.0 µg mL^{-1} concentration interval; the limits of detection (LODs) and quantification (LOQs) were 0.1–0.25 µg mL^{-1} and 0.4–0.8 µg mL^{-1}, respectively. The method has been applied to the quantification of the target compounds in microsamples. The reliability of the proposed conditions has been tested by analyzing three resins, white copal, copal in tears, and ocote tree resin. Percentages of the triterpenes in the range 0.010% to 0.16% were measured using sample amounts of 10–15 mg, whereas the most abundant compound limonene (≥0.93%) could be determined using 1 mg portions of the resins. The proposed method can be considered complementary to existing protocols aimed at establishing the chemical fingerprint of these kinds of samples.

Keywords: resins; limonene; triterpenes; microsamples; capillary liquid chromatography (Cap-LC)

1. Introduction

Natural resins are plant secretions formed by complex mixtures of organic molecules, being terpenoids the predominant components. The number and proportion of these substances highly depend on the botanical origin and age of the resins. For example, in resins derived from plants of the genera *Burseraceae*, commonly referred to as copal, monoterpenic compounds such as pinene and limonene are the most abundant compounds in the volatile fraction, whereas triterpenoids such as lupine compounds, α-amyrin, and β-amyrin are predominant in the non-volatile fraction [1]. Resins have important applications in the paint and cosmetic industries [1,2]. Very recently, some of their constituents have attracted the attention of researchers because of their pharmacological effects as anti-inflammatory, antipruritic, anti-fungal and others [2–6]. Besides their industrial applications, resins have been used from ancient times for a variety of purposes including religious ceremonies and decoration of artworks. For this reason, over the past years, the analysis of resins has attracted interest in the characterization of archaeological objects [7–9].

Different approaches have been described for the chemical analysis of resins in archeological items using gas chromatography (GC) coupled to mass spectrometry (MS) [7,9,10], liquid chromatography (LC) coupled to MS [10] or UV detection [9,11,12] and thin layer chromatography (TLC) [11]. Most of those studies were aimed at differentiating the samples according to their botanical origin through the comparison of the chromatographic profiles of the extracts obtained from the samples (chemical fingerprinting), often in combination with chemometric tools [8,10]. Interestingly, none of those methods reported the quantitative composition of the target compounds. This can be most probably explained by the lack of reliable quantitative methods that can be applied to microsamples, as the low amount of sample available is a major limitation in such studies. The quantitative composition of resins could be used not only to discriminate resins by their botanical origin but also to explore the age and storage conditions of the samples [1,6]. Thus, methods that can be used to provide a better knowledge of the amounts of (at least) the major components of resins are still needed [13].

Because of the bioactive properties of some triterpenes such as lupeol and amyrins, different methods have been recently proposed for their quantification in different plant materials [5,14–17]. The amount of sample in those studies was not limited, and therefore, the required sensitivity for quantification could be achieved after exhaustive sample treatments of large amounts of the samples, including multiple extractions, purification, solvent evaporation, and redissolution. Very recently, the quantification of the triterpenes lupeol, α-amyrin and β-amyrin in copal resins used in folk ceremonies was described using LC and UV detection, although the analytical performance of the method applied was not reported [12]; moreover, due to the large amount of resin needed (0.5 g), the method might be unsuitable for the analysis of microsamples.

On the other hand, several difficulties arise when analyzing resins by chromatographic methods. First, the samples contain a large number of compounds with very different chemical properties. Some of the most abundant high molecular triterpenes are highly apolar (octanol–water partition coefficients, $K_{ow} > 10^{9.0}$). Therefore, their separation under typical reversed-phase conditions is difficult because the choice of the mobile phase is rather limited [14]. When using absorbance detection, the lack of chromophores may be also a limitation, especially in the analysis of microsamples. As regards GC-based methods, most assays require a derivatization step before GC analysis, especially if low-volatile high-molecular triterpenes are going to be analyzed [7,9]. Because of the complexity of the samples, most assays have been focused only on one family of compounds, typically the triterpene fraction. Specific assays have also been developed to the characterization of volatile components of resins using GC [6]. Alternatively, different portions of the sample extract are analyzed under two or more different chromatographic conditions to obtain more exhaustive sample characterization [10,14].

In this work, we describe a method for the quantification of representative components of resins, both volatile and non-volatile using capillary chromatography. The method takes advantage of the high sensitivity attainable with miniaturized LC systems, which make them better suited for the analysis of microsamples [18,19]. The volatile monoterpene limonene and the high molecular triterpenes lupeol, lupenone, α-amyrin and β-amyrin have been selected as model compounds. Their structure and octanol-water partition coefficients are shown in Figure 1. The analytical performance of the proposed method has been tested. Examples of application to real samples are presented.

2. Results

2.1. Chromatographic Conditions

Initially, different acetonitrile–water mixtures were tested in order to optimize the separation and detection of the target compounds. In this study, the percentage of acetonitrile ranged from 60% to 95%; standard solutions of the analytes (10 μg mL^{-1}) prepared in methanol were used, and the injection volume was 5 μL.

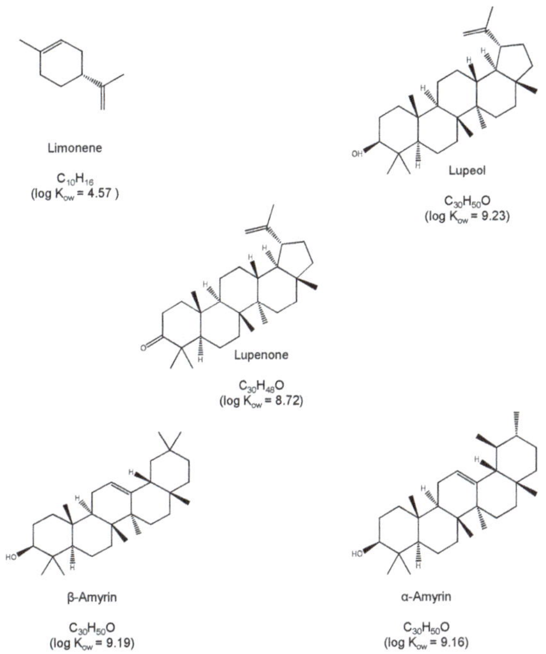

Figure 1. Chemical structures and log K_{ow} values of the tested compounds.

As expected, mobile phases with high contents of acetonitrile (>70%) were necessary for the analytes to be eluted at reasonable run times (<40 min). It must be noted that all the analytes presented decreasing absorbances within the 190–210 nm range and nearly null absorbance at higher wavelengths. Thus, 200 nm was selected as the working wavelength. Under most of the elution conditions assayed suitable separation of the analytes was obtained except for limonene. The isolation of this compound was particularly difficult due to the presence of an intense peak corresponding to the injection solvent (methanol). Because of its high intensity, such peak partially overlapped with that of limonene. The resolution between the two peaks could be improved by using a gradient elution program but at the expense of the total run time. For the rest of the compounds, a good resolution was obtained even with a mobile phase of 100% acetonitrile; with this eluent, the chromatographic run time was <20 min, as shown in Figure 2A. Besides the peaks of the solvent and analytes, two minor peaks were detected at 12.1 min and 15.3 min; those peaks were identified as impurities of β-amyrin. Tetrahydrofuran was also tested as it has an elution strength higher than that of acetonitrile. However, due to its significant absorbance at wavelengths <212 nm, the background noise at the wavelength necessary to detect the analytes was unacceptable. Therefore, this solvent was no longer used.

As an attempt to reduce the solvent peak and to improve the resolution of limonene, standard solutions of the analytes were prepared using different methanol-water mixtures as solvent, 0.1:9.9, 1:9 and 9:1 (v/v) [14]. Ideally, samples should be injected in an injection solvent with elution strength similar to or lower than that of the mobile phase. However, the presence of water in the processed solutions resulted in a decrement of the peaks areas of some of the analytes, especially α-amyrin. This suggested that at the working concentration the analytes were not completely dissolved in methanol–water, which is consistent with their high Kow values (see Figure 1). As an alternative, we tested if the introduction of an aliquot of water in the injection capillary before loading the sample could prevent peak broadening at the entrance of the chromatographic column. Variable volumes of water in the 5–25 μL range were loaded in the injection loop, before loading the samples (5 μL), and the chromatograms were compared with those observed for the same solution directly injected (Figure 2A).

The introduction of water into the injection capillary had a strong effect on the retention times of the analytes, as well as on peak shapes. As observed in Figure 2B, which shows the chromatogram obtained after the successive introduction of 5 µL of water and 5 µL of the working solution into the injection loop all the analytes eluted about 1.5 min later. This was particularly positive for the measurement of limonene, as it was completely separated from the solvent peak. The presence of water had also a positive effect on the peak shapes of the other analytes. Increasing the amount of water up to 25 µL did not modify substantially the chromatographic registers. Finally, the effect of the sample volume was evaluated with the range 5–25 µL. The absolute peak areas increased as the volume of the sample increased. However, the increment of the sample volume also resulted in wider peaks. As a result, the separation between lupeol and lupenone was unsuitable (data not shown).

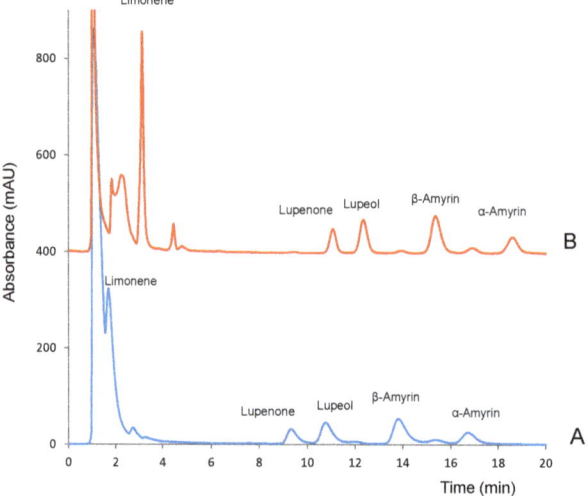

Figure 2. Obtained for standard solutions of the analytes (10 µg mL^{-1}) in methanol injected (**A**) directly and (**B**) after loading 5 µL of water in the injection loop. Sample volume, 5 µL; eluent, 100% acetonitrile; detection wavelength, 200 nm.

Based on the above results, the successive injection into the loop of 5 µL of water and 5 µL of the working solution was selected as the best option. As a compromise between resolution and chromatographic run time, a mobile phase of acetonitrile:water 85:15 (v/v) was selected for further work.

2.2. Method Validation

To study the analytical performance of the proposed method, working solutions of the target compounds at concentrations in the range 0.25–10 µg mL^{-1} were analyzed, and the linearity, limits of detection (LODs), limits of quantification (LOQs), accuracy and precision were studied [20]. The results obtained are summarized in Table 1.

Table 1. Analytical parameters of the proposed method.

Compound	Linearity *,** ($n = 15$) $y = (a \pm s_a) + (b \pm s_b) x$	R^2	Mean Found Concentration ** ($n = 3$)		Precision, rsd (%) ($n = 3$)						LOD ($\mu g \cdot mL^{-1}$)	LOQ ($\mu g \cdot mL^{-1}$)
					Intraday			Interday				
			$2.5\ \mu g\ mL^{-1}$	$7.5\ \mu g\ mL^{-1}$	$2.5\ \mu g\ mL^{-1}$	$7.5\ \mu g\ mL^{-1}$		$2.5\ \mu g\ mL^{-1}$		$7.5\ \mu g\ mL^{-1}$		
Limonene	$y = (-77 \pm 2) + (433 \pm 6)x$	0.997	2.3 ± 0.1	6.5 ± 0.4	2	0.6		3		4	0.1	0.4
Lupenone	$y = (-22 \pm 9) + (63.9 \pm 1.6)x$	0.994	2.4 ± 0.1	7.0 ± 0.1	4	0.8		7		7	0.25	0.8
Lupeol	$y = (-42 \pm 12) + (111 \pm 2)x$	0.996	2.6 ± 0.1	7.4 ± 0.2	1.4	2		7		8	0.25	0.8
β-Amyrin	$y = (-20 \pm 17) + (135 \pm 3)x$	0.995	2.3 ± 0.1	7.5 ± 0.6	3	8		8		8	0.25	0.8
α-Amyrin	$y = (72 \pm 42) + (313 \pm 8)x$	0.994	2.9 ± 0.2	8.4 ± 0.1	9	17		16		17	0.25	0.8

* within the range 0.25–10.0 $\mu g\ mL^{-1}$ for limonene and 0.5–10.0 $\mu g\ mL^{-1}$ for the rest of compounds (a: intercept; s_a: standard deviation of the intercept; b: slope; s_b: standard deviation of the slope; R^2: squared correlation coefficient; rsd: residual standard deviation); ** all values expressed with digits known plus the first uncertain digit.

As observed from Table 1, for all the compounds tested the peak areas showed a linear relationship with the concentration up to 10.0 μg mL^{-1}, with R^2 coefficients ranging from 0.994 to 0.997 (n = 15). In order to check the accuracy, the corresponding calibration equations were used to establish the concentration of the analytes in solutions containing mixtures of the tested analytes at low-intermediate (2.5 μg mL^{-1}) and high-intermediate (7.5 μg mL^{-1}) concentrations. The relative errors found ranged from −13% to +16%. It was therefore concluded that the accuracy was satisfactory according to the standards set for this kind of samples [21]. The precision was evaluated by calculating the relative standard deviations (RSDs) of the areas measured in three consecutive injections (intra-day RSD) and in three different working sessions (inter-day RSDs); both parameters were determined at two different concentrations levels. Although for α-amyrin the RSDs were slightly higher, values <8% were found. Finally, the LODs and LOQs were established. Although different options are available, in this study the LODs and LOQs were calculated as the concentrations that resulted in signal-to-noise ratios of 3 and 10, respectively [22]. These values were established by injecting solutions with decreasing concentrations of the analytes; before analyzing each solution, water was processed to confirm the absence of contaminants and/or memory effects. The LODs were 0.1 μg mL^{-1} for limonene and 0.25 μg mL^{-1} for the rest of compounds; the LOQs were 0.4 μg mL^{-1} for limonene and 0.8 μg mL^{-1} for the other analytes.

2.3. Analysis of Resins

2.3.1. Sample Preparation

The proposed conditions were applied to the analysis, to the target compounds in three resins, white copal, copal in tears and resin obtained from ocote trees. Different solubility studies were carried out by treating portions of 1–15 mg of the three resins with 1 mL of extracting solvent. Methanol, acetonitrile, ethyl acetate, isopropanol, and chloroform were tested as extraction solvents.

The chromatograms of the extracts obtained with ethyl acetate, isopropanol and chloroform were unsuitable due to the absorption of these solvents at 200 nm. It was concluded that the employment of such solvents would require the evaporation of the extracts followed by their redissolution in methanol or acetonitrile before the chromatographic analysis. In order to simplify the entire analytical process and to prevent possible losses of the volatile analyte limonene, these solvents were not used in further experiments. Examples of the extracts obtained with methanol are shown in Figure 3. As observed, the white copal (Figure 3a) and ocote (Figure 3b) samples were satisfactorily dissolved. However, significant amounts of solid matter were observed when 10–15 mg of the copal in tears resin was treated with 1 mL of methanol (Figure 3c), most probably due to the presence of highly polar gum compounds [8]. For the latter sample, a further study of the solid residue was carried out after centrifugation and separation of the liquid phase. The residue was treated with 1 mL of water, and complete dissolution was observed (Figure 3d), which confirmed the presence of a high percentage of gum in this sample. Therefore, it was concluded that the target compounds were satisfactorily extracted in methanol. As no significant differences between the chromatograms obtained with methanol and acetonitrile were observed, methanol was finally selected.

The effect of the sample matrix in the response was studied by spiking with known amounts of the analytes the extracts obtained from one of the resin samples (copal in tears) so that the concentration added of each of the analytes to extracts was 5 μg mL^{-1}. The increment on the peak areas between the spiked and unspiked extracts was used to calculate the added concentration, using the calibration equations of Table 1. The values obtained were then compared with the added concentrations (5 μg mL^{-1}) to calculate the recoveries. Values ranging from 52% to 103% were found, as listed in Table 2.

The minimum percentages of the analytes that could be measured were calculated for samples of 10 mg, taking into account the LOQs of Table 1 and the recoveries of Table 2. The values obtained ranged from 0.004% for limonene to 0.02% for β-amyrin. These values were considered low enough for most applications, making unnecessary extra pre-concentration operations.

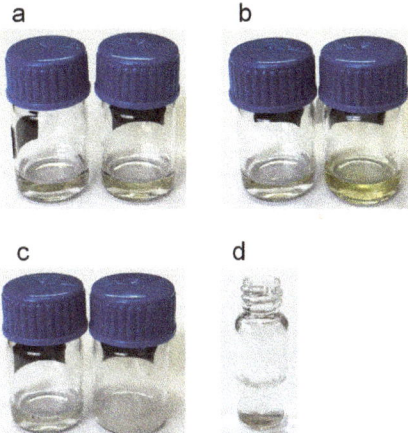

Figure 3. Images of the extracts obtained after adding 1 mL of methanol: (**a**) white copal, (**b**) ocote and (**c**) copal in tears; left vials in (**a–c**), 1 mg of samples; right vials in (**a–c**), 15 mg of the samples. (**d**) solution obtained after treating the residue insoluble in methanol of copal in tears (10 mg) with 1 mL of water. For other experimental details, see the text.

Table 2. Recoveries * obtained from the spiked extracts ($n = 3$).

Compound	Recovery (%)
Limonene	103 ± 4
Lupenone	101 ± 1
Lupeol	79 ± 9
β-Amyrin	52 ± 5
α-Amyrin	75 ± 3

(*) All values expressed with digits known plus the first uncertain digit.

2.3.2. Quantification Studies

Finally, the proposed method was applied to the quantitative analysis of the three resins tested. For this purpose, different portions of the samples ranging from 1 to 15 mg were analyzed under the conditions described above. The presence of the analytes in the samples was evaluated from the concordance between the retention times and UV spectra of the suspected peaks and those observed for the standard solutions. Additionally, the presence of a compound was confirmed by fortifying the extracts with standard solutions of such compound.

The only analyte found in the three resins analyzed was α-amyrin. Limonene was found in the white copal and ocote resins, whereas lupeol and β-amyrin were found in the copal in tears sample. As expected, besides the peaks of some of the analytes, peaks of unknown compounds were observed in the samples, particularly at retention times close to that of limonene. However, they could be easily differentiated from this compound through their respective UV spectra. The impurities found in the standard solutions of β-amyrin were not identified in the samples.

The percentages of each of the analytes found in the samples were established from the peak areas and the calibration equations of Table 1 and taking into account the recoveries of Table 2. The results are summarized in Table 3. As deduced from this table, the percentages of the triterpenic compounds were <1%.

Table 3. Percentages * of the analytes found in the analyzed resin samples ($n = 3$).

Sample		Percentage [a] (%), ($n = 3$)				
		Limonene	Lupenone	Lupeol	β-Amyrin	α-Amyrin
White copal	1 mg	0.9 ± 0.2	<LOD	<LOD	<LOD	<LOD
	15 mg	1.2 ± 0.2	<LOD	<LOD	<LOD	0.020 ± 0.002
Copal in tears	10 mg	<LOD	<LOD	0.034 ± 0.001	0.069 ± 0.002	0.011 ± 0.001
	10 mg [b]	<LOD	<LOD	0.033 ± 0.001	0.074 ± 0.001	0.010 ± 0.003
	10 mg [c]	<LOD	<LOD	0.035 ± 0.002	0.082 ± 0.005	0.010 ± 0.004
Ocote	1 mg	9.3 ± 0.2	<LOD	<LOD	<LOD	<LOQ
	10 mg	9.3 ± 0.1	<LOD	<LOD	<LOD	0.093 ± 0.003
	10 mg [b]	7.2 ± 0.1	<LOD	<LOD	<LOD	0.16 ± 0.01
	10 mg [c]	7.3 ± 0.3	<LOD	<LOD	<LOD	0.16 ± 0.02

([a]) All values expressed with digits known plus the first uncertain digit; ([b]) Exposed at ambient conditions for 5 days; ([c]) Dried at 40 °C until constant weight.

For the quantification of these compounds, a higher amount of sample was used (10–15 mg). For 1 mg of the sample, the concentration of α-amyrin in the white copal resin was below its LOD, and between its LOD and LOQ in the ocote resin sample. In the later resin, and even when processing 10 mg of the sample, the concentration of α-amyrin in the extract was close to its LOQ. Limonene was found in white copal and ocote resins at higher percentages. In fact, for the quantification of this analyte in the ocote resin, the extract of the sample had to be diluted with methanol (1:20, v/v) in order to adjust the analyte concentration to the linear working interval of Table 1. In Figure 4, representative chromatograms obtained for white copal are shown (Figure 4a), copal in tears (Figure 4b) and ocote (Figure 4c) resins; some of the pictures have been zoomed for better visualization of the peaks of interest.

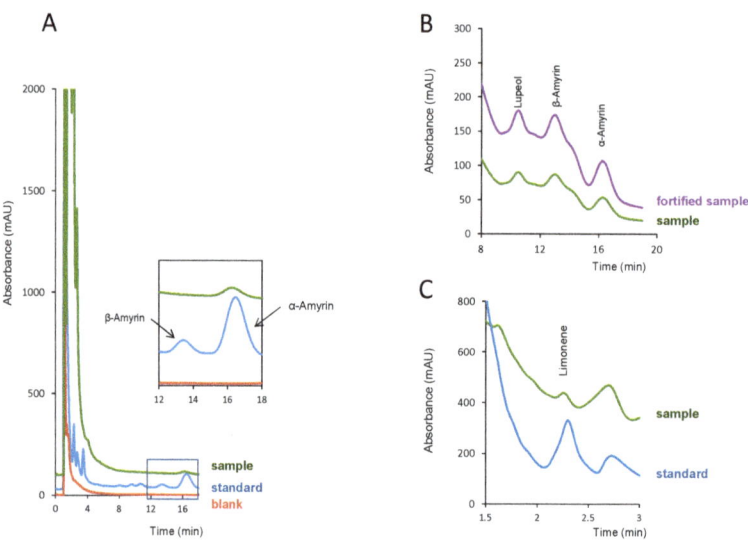

Figure 4. Chromatograms obtained in the analysis of the resin samples: (**a**) white copal, a standard solution of the analytes and a blank (methanol); (**b**) copal in tears (10 mg) and the same extract fortified with the analytes; (**c**) ocote resin diluted 1:20 with methanol and a standard solution of the analytes. Concentration of the analytes in the standard solution of (**a**) and (**c**), 5 µg mL^{-1}; amount of the analytes added in the fortified sample of (**b**), 5 µg mL^{-1}. For other experimental details, see the text.

It has to be noted that, because of its relative abundance in the samples, white copal and ocote (≥1%), the percentage of limonene could be established using both 1 mg and 10–15 mg of the samples. The values obtained by using different amounts of the samples were then compared. The $t_{calculated}$ were 2.01 and 0.17 for white copal and ocote resins, respectively ($t_{tabulated}$ at 95% confidence level = 2.776); in this calculation, equivalent variances were assumed, as $F_{calculated}$ were 1.15 and 4.86 for the white copal and ocote resins, respectively ($F_{tabulated}$ at 95% confidence level = 19.00). Therefore, it was concluded that the percentages obtained were not dependent on the sample size.

Finally, portions of two samples with different composition profiles, copal in tears and ocote, were subjected to different treatments in order to evaluate their effect on the sample composition. For this purpose, portions of the samples were spread on the surface of glass vials; then the vials were exposed at ambient conditions for five days before analysis. Additionally, portions of the samples were dried at 40 °C in an oven until constant weight and then processed. The results obtained are also listed in Table 3. As observed, the composition of the copal in tears sample was not significantly modified by any of the treatments applied. In contrast, both treatments led to lower contents of limonene in the ocote resin, whereas the percentage of α-amyrin increased. The results found for this sample indicate that limonene was partially volatilized both at ambient conditions and after drying at 40 °C; the loss of limonene, and possibly other volatile compounds, resulted in higher percentages of non-volatile compounds such α-amyrin. In the copal in tears resin, the absence of limonene suggests that volatile compounds had been previously lost, which is consistent with the fact that the percentages of the triterpenes remained approximately constant after exposing the sample at ambient conditions or after the thermal treatment applied.

3. Discussion

To date, several methods have been proposed for the classification of resins based on the comparison of the fingerprint profiles obtained by chromatographic [7–10] or spectroscopic techniques [23]. However, few data are available on the quantitative composition of this kind of samples [1,13]. Besides, most of the efforts have been focused on the triterpenoid fraction, while only a few studies have been focused on volatile compounds such as limonene even though this compound can play an important role in establishing the sample botanical origin and age [6].

In this work, we have developed a method for the chromatographic separation, identification, and quantification of compounds commonly found in resins, including the volatile monoterpene limonene and some long-chain non-volatile triterpenes in a single run. Despite the wide range of polarities of the target compounds, satisfactory separation in chromatographic times lower than 20 min was achieved and even under isocratic conditions, which is an additional advantage. As regards its analytical performance, the proposed method provides linear responses, RSDs of 0.6% to 17%, and adequate accuracy [22]. Moreover, because of the high sensitivity attainable with capillary LC, the method is compatible with the analysis of a low amount of the samples. As only a few mg of the samples is necessary, the sample treatment is very simple and avoids heating, multiple extractions or evaporation operations that could modify the content of volatile compound limonene [7,12].

Although significant fluctuations in the levels of the compounds tested can be expected in resins [1], according to the results obtained in our study (Table 3), the method can be applied to the accurate measurement of the analytes at percentages >1% using an amount of sample as low as 1 mg. If the amount of sample available is ≈10–15 mg, compounds present at percentages <0.1% can be also quantified. It is also remarkable that statistically equivalent percentages of the analytes are obtained regardless of the amount of sample (1–15 mg) provided that their concentrations in the corresponding extracts are above their respective LOQs. The percentages of triterpenic compounds found in this study are lower than those reported in other studies, although only few data are available [1]. Variations in the composition of resins can be mostly explained by the high number of species that are used in their production [9,10], although the age and the storage conditions of the samples can also be important sources of variability [6,13]. The proposed method could be used to obtain information relative to the evolution of the chemical composition of resins as a function of the external conditions. In this respect, systematic studies with resins of different botanical origin and age would be necessary. The method should be also tested for other terpenoids.

4. Materials and Methods

4.1. Chemicals and Solutions

All reagents were of analytical grade. Limonene, lupenone, β-amyrin and α-amyrin standards were obtained from Sigma-Aldrich (St. Louis, MO, USA), and lupeol from Cayman Chemical (Ann Arbor, MI, USA). Methanol and acetonitrile, both HPLC grade, were purchased from VWR Chemicals (Randnor, PA, USA). Ethyl acetate and chloroform super purity solvent were purchased from Romil (Cambridge, UK), and tetrahydrofuran (GPC grade) and isopropanol (HPLC grade) from Scharlau (Barcelona, Spain). Ultrapure water was obtained from an Adrona system (Riga, Latvia). Water was filtered through 0.22 μm nylon membranes purchased from GVS (Sandfor, ME, USA) before use.

Stock solutions of the analytes (1000 μg mL^{-1}) were prepared by dissolving the appropriate amounts of the commercial standards in methanol. Working solutions of the analytes and their mixtures were prepared by diluting the stock solutions with methanol (unless otherwise stated). All solutions were stored at 4 °C until use.

4.2. Instrumentation and Analytical Conditions

The chromatographic system consisted of a capillary pump (Agilent 1100 Series, Waldbronn, Germany) equipped with a Rheodyne model 7725 six-port injection valve and a photodiode array detector (Agilent 1200 Series). An Agilent HPLC ChemStation system was used for data acquisition and calculation.

A Zorbax SB C18 (150 mm × 0.5 mm id, 5 μm) column (Agilent) was used for the separation of the target compounds. Unless otherwise stated, the mobile phase was a mixture acetonitrile:water (85:15, v/v) at a flow rate of 10 μL min^{-1}. A 15-cm segment of 0.320 mm o.d. and 75 μm i.d. fused silica capillary (Análisis Vínicos, Tomelloso, Spain) was used as the injection loop; for connecting the capillary to the valve, 2.5-cm sleeves of 1/6 in polyether ether ketone (PEEK) tubing (1/6 in PEEK nuts and ferrules) from Teknokroma (Barcelona, Spain) were used. Working solutions were loaded into the loop employing a 25 μL precision syringe. The analytical signal was recorded between 190 and 400 nm and monitored at 200 nm.

4.3. Analysis of Resins

Samples of different commercial resins were analyzed, white copal and copal in tears, as well as a resin obtained from ocote trees. Samples were purchased in Sonora market (City of México, México) in the year 2010. Portions of the resins were homogenized mechanically in a mortar with a pestle. Next, accurately weighted portions of the pulverized samples (≈1–15 mg) were placed in 2 mL glass vials and treated with 1 mL of extraction solvent. Acetonitrile, methanol, chloroform, isopropanol, and ethyl acetate were tested as extraction solvents. The mixture was vortexed for 1 min and then filtered through 0.22 μm nylon membranes to remove any particulate that could be present. Finally, aliquots of 5 μL of the samples were chromatographed. All the experiments were carried out at room temperature by triplicate.

5. Conclusions

In this work, we have developed a method for the quantitative analysis of some relevant terpenoids typically used to characterize of resins, which is based on capillary LC with UV detection. Separation and chromatographic conditions have been optimized to make possible the analysis of volatile and non-volatile analytes within the same chromatographic run, with the adequate sensitivity to be applied when only small size samples are available (a few mg).

The results obtained throughout our study have proved that the quantitative performance of the proposed method is suitable. To the best of our knowledge, this is the first method validated for the quantification of limonene and representative triterpenes in microsamples of resins. Thus, it can be considered a useful tool to increase the knowledge about the chemical composition of resins, as most existing methods are limited to obtain their chemical fingerprints. Besides for classification purposes, the quantitative composition can be used to obtain information about the history (age and ambient conditions) of samples of similar origin.

Author Contributions: Data curation, H.D.P.-R., R.H.-H., J.V.-A., and P.C.-F.; formal analysis, H.D.P.-R., R.H.-H., J.V.-A., and P.C.-F.; funding acquisition, H.D.P.-R., R.H.-H., J.V.-A., and P.C.-F.; investigation, H.D.P.-R., R.H.-H., J.V.-A., and P.C.-F.; methodology, H.D.P.-R., R.H.-H., J.V.-A., and P.C.-F.; validation, H.D.P.-R., R.H.-H., J.V.-A., and P.C.-F.; writing—original draft, H.D.P.-R., R.H.-H., J.V.-A., and P.C.-F.

Funding: This research was funded by the EU FEDER and the Spanish Agencia Española de Investigación, AEI (project CTQ2017-90082-P), and the Generalitat Valenciana (PROMETEO 2016/109) for the financial support received. H.D.P.-R acknowledges a doctoral grant from the Universidad Nacional Autónoma de Honduras (Honduras).

Acknowledgments: The authors are grateful to M. L. Vázquez de Agredos Pascual for providing the resins used throughout the study.

Conflicts of Interest: The authors declare no conflict of interest.

References

1. Gigliarelli, G.; Becerra, J.X.; Curini, M.; Marcotullio, M.C. Chemical Composition and Biological Activities of Fragrant Mexican Copal (*Bursera spp.*). *Molecules* **2015**, *20*, 22383–22394. [CrossRef] [PubMed]
2. Rüdiger, A.L.; Siani, A.C.; Veiga Junior, V.V. The chemistry and pharmacology of the South America genus Protium Burm. f. (Burseraceae). *Phcog. Rev.* **2007**, *1*, 93–104.
3. Hernández Vázquez, L.; Palazon, J.; Navarro-Ocaña, A. The Pentacyclic Triterpenes α, β-amyrins: A Review of Sources and Biological Activities. In *Phytochemicals—A Global Perspective of Their Role in Nutrition and Health*; Venketeshwer-Estrada, R., Ed.; IntechOpen: Rijeka, Croatia, 2012; pp. 487–502. ISBN 978-953-51-0296-0.
4. Romero-Estrada, A.; Maldonado-Magaña, A.; González-Christen, J.; Bahena, S.M.; Garduño-Ramírez, M.L.; Rodríguez-López, V.; Alvarez, L. Anti-inflammatory and antioxidative effects of six pentacyclic triterpenes isolated from the mexican copal resin of bursera copallifera. *BMC Complement. Altern. Med.* **2016**. [CrossRef] [PubMed]
5. Schmidt, M.E.P.; Pires, F.B.; Bressan, L.P.; da Silva, F.B., Jr.; Lameira, O.; da Rosa, M.B. Some triterpenic compounds in extracts of Cecropia and Bauhinia species for different sampling years. *Rev. Bras. Farmacogn.* **2018**, *28*, 21–26. [CrossRef]
6. Villa-Ruano, N.; Pacheco-Hernández, Y.; Becerra-Martínez, Y.; Zárate-Reyes, J.A.; Cruz-Durán, R. Chemical profile and pharmacological effects of the resin and essential oil from Bursera slechtendalii: A medicinal "copal tree" of southern Mexico. *Fitoterapia* **2018**, *128*, 86–92. [CrossRef] [PubMed]
7. Stacey, R.J.; Cartwright, C.R.; McEwan, C.R. Chemical characterization of ancient Mesoamerican "copal" resins: Preliminary results. *Archaeometry* **2006**, *48*, 323–340. [CrossRef]
8. Lucero-Gómez, P.; Mathe, C.; Vieillescazes, C.; Bucio-Galindo, L.; Belio-Reyes, I.; Vega-Aviña, R. Archeobotanic: HPLC molecular profiles for the discrimination of copals in Mesoamerica Application to the study of resins materials from objects of Aztec offerings. *ArcheoSciences, revue d'archéométrie* **2014**, *38*, 119–133. [CrossRef]
9. Lucero-Gómez, P.; Mathe, C.; Vieillescazes, C.; Bucio-Galindo, L.; Belio-Reyes, I.; Vega-Aviña, R. Analysis of Mexican reference standards for Bursera spp. Resins by gas-chromatography-mass spectrometry and application to archaeological objects. *J. Archaeol. Sci.* **2014**, *41*, 679–690. [CrossRef]
10. Rhourrhi-Frih, B.; West, C.; Pasquier, L.; André, P.; Chaimbault, P.; Lafosse, M. Classification of natural resins by liquid chromatography-mass spectrometry and gas chromatography-mass spectrometry using chemometric analysis. *J. Chromatogr. A* **2012**, *1256*, 177–190. [CrossRef] [PubMed]

11. Hernández-Vázquez, L.; Mangas, S.; Palazón, J.; Navarro-Ocaña, A. Valuable medicinal plants and resins: Commercial phytochemicals with bioactive properties. *Ind. Crops. Prod.* **2010**, *31*, 476–480. [CrossRef]
12. Merali, Z.; Cayer, C.; Kent, P.; Liu, R.; Cal, V.R.; Harris, C.S.; Arnason, J.T. Sacred Maya incense, copal (Protium copal - Burseraceae), has antianxiety effects in animal models. *J. Ethnopharmacol.* **2018**, *216*, 63–70. [CrossRef] [PubMed]
13. Drzewicz, P.; Natkaniec-Nowak, L.; Czapla, D. Analytical approaches for studies of fossil resins. *Trends Anal. Chem.* **2016**, *85C*, 75–84. [CrossRef]
14. Martelanc, M.; Vovk, I.; Simonovska, B. Separation and identification of some common isomeric plant triterpenoids by thin-layer chromatography and high-performance liquid chromatography. *J. Chromatogr. A* **2009**, *1216*, 6662–6670. [CrossRef] [PubMed]
15. Ruiz-Montañez, G.; Ragazzo-Sánchez, J.A.; Calderón-Santoyo, M.; Velázquez-de la Cruz, G.; Ramírez de León, J.A.; Navarro-Ocaña, A. Evaluation of extraction methods for preparative scale obtention of mangiferin and lupeol from mango peels (Mangifera indica L.). *Food. Chem.* **2014**, *159*, 267–272. [CrossRef]
16. Bahadir-Acıkara, Ö.; Özbilgin, S.; Saltan-Iscan, G.; Dall'Acqua, S.; Rjašková, V.; Özgökçe, F.; Suchý, V.; Šmejkal, K. Phytochemical analysis of Podospermum and Scorzonera n-hexane extracts and the HPLC quantitation of triterpenes. *Molecules* **2018**, *23*, 1813. [CrossRef] [PubMed]
17. Herrera-López, M.G.; Rubio-Hernández, E.I.; Leyte-Lugo, M.A.; Schinkovitz, A.; Richomme, P.; Calvo-Irabién, L.M.; Peña-Rodríguez, L.M. Botanical Origin of Triterpenoids from Yucatecan Propolis. *Phytochem. Lett.* **2019**, *29*, 25–29. [CrossRef]
18. Nazario, C.E.D.; Silva, M.R.; Franco, M.S.; Lanças, F.M. Evolution in Miniaturized Column Liquid Chromatography Instrumentation and Applications: An Overview. *J. Chromatogr. A* **2015**, *1421*, 18–37. [CrossRef] [PubMed]
19. Jornet-Martínez, N.; Ortega-Sierra, A.; Verdú-Andrés, J.; Herráez-Hernández, R.; Campíns-Falcó, P. Analysis of Contact Traces of Cannabis by In-Tube Solid-Phase Microextraction Coupled to Nanoliquid Chromatography. *Molecules* **2018**, *23*, 2359. [CrossRef] [PubMed]
20. Magnusson, B.; Örnemark, U. (Eds.) *Eurachem Guide: The Fitness for Purpose of Analytical Methods: A Laboratory Guide to Method Validation and Related Topics*, 2nd ed. 2014, p. 57. Available online: https://www.eurachem.org/images/stories/Guides/pdf/MV_guide_2nd_ed_EN.pdf (accessed on 10 November 2019).
21. AOAC Official Methods of Analysis. *Appendix K: Guidelines for Dietary Supplements and Botanicals*; AOAC, International: Gaithersburg, MD, USA, 2013; p. 8.
22. Sanchez, J. Estimating detection limits in chromatography from calibration data: Ordinary least squares regression vs. weighted least squares. *Separations* **2018**, *5*, 49. [CrossRef]
23. Piña-Torres, C.; Lucero-Gómez, P.; Nieto, S.; Vázquez, A.; Bucio, L.; Belio, I.; Vega, R.; Mathe, C.; Vieillescazes, C. An analytical strategy based on Fourier transform infrared spectroscopy, principal component analysis and linear discriminant analysis to suggest the botanical origin of resins from Bursera. Application to archaeological Aztec Samples. *J. Cult. Herit.* **2018**, *33*, 48–59. [CrossRef]

Sample Availability: Samples of the compounds are not available from the authors.

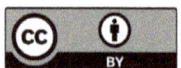

© 2019 by the authors. Licensee MDPI, Basel, Switzerland. This article is an open access article distributed under the terms and conditions of the Creative Commons Attribution (CC BY) license (http://creativecommons.org/licenses/by/4.0/).

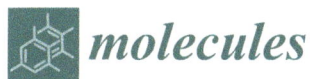

Article

High-Throughput ^{1}H-Nuclear Magnetic Resonance-Based Screening for the Identification and Quantification of Heartwood Diterpenic Acids in Four Black Pine (*Pinus nigra* Arn.) Marginal Provenances in Greece

Kostas Ioannidis [1,2,*], Eleni Melliou [2] and Prokopios Magiatis [2]

[1] Laboratory of Forest Genetics and Biotechnology, Institute of Mediterranean and Forest Ecosystems, Hellenic Agricultural Organization "Demeter", Ilissia, 11528 Athens, Greece
[2] Department of Pharmacognosy and Natural Products Chemistry, Faculty of Pharmacy, University of Athens, Panepistimiopolis Zografou, 15771 Athens, Greece; emelliou@pharm.uoa.gr (E.M.); magiatis@pharm.uoa.gr (P.M.)
* Correspondence: ioko@fria.gr; Tel.: +30-210-77-83-750; Fax: +30-210-77-84-602

Academic Editors: Pavel B. Drasar and Vladimir A. Khripach
Received: 30 August 2019; Accepted: 1 October 2019; Published: 7 October 2019

Abstract: A high-throughput quantitative Nuclear Magnetic Resonance ^{1}H-NMR method was developed and applied to screen the quantity of the diterpenic resin acids in the heartwood of black pine, due to the renewed scientific interest in their medicinal properties and use in various diseases treatment. The 260 samples were taken from *Pinus nigra* clones, selected from four provenances of the Peloponnese (Greece), participating in a 35-year-old clonal seed orchard. Total resin acids per dry heartwood weight (dhw) varied greatly, ranging from 30.05 to 424.70 mg/g_{dhw} (average 219.98 mg/g_{dhw}). Abietic was the predominant acid (76.77 mg/g_{dhw}), followed by palustric acid (47.94 mg/g_{dhw}), neoabietic acid (39.34 mg/g_{dhw}), and pimaric acid (22.54 mg/g_{dhw}). Dehydroabietic acid was at moderate levels (11.69 mg/g_{dhw}), while levopimaric, isopimaric, and sandaracopimaric acids were in lower concentrations. The resin acid fraction accounted for 72.33% of the total acetone extractives. Stilbenes were presented in significant quantities (19.70%). The resin acid content was composed mainly of the abietane type resin acids (83.56%). Peloponnesian *Pinus nigra* heartwood was found to be the richest source of resin acids identified to date and is considered the best natural source for the production of such bioactive extracts. The results indicate a high potential for effective selection and advanced breeding of pharmaceutical and high economic value bioactive substances from *Pinus nigra* clones.

Keywords: quantitative nuclear magnetic resonance; high-throughput screening; resin acids; diterpenes; *Pinus nigra*; provenances

---

1. Introduction

In Greece, as well as in other European countries, black pine constitutes extensive natural forests. Due to its advantages, it is considered one of the most important silvicultural coniferous species and it is extensively used in reforestation programs throughout the country [1]. Its significance lead to its planting outside its natural range, e.g., North and South America, Australia, and New Zealand. Furthermore, its importance is verified by its potential use for the production of high added value products, i.e., bioactive compounds produced from wood and wood waste materials [2,3]. Such bioactive substances are, inter alia, the resin acids occurring in pine's oleoresin.

Oleoresin consists of a non-volatile fraction, also referred as colophony or rosin, dissolved in a volatile monoterpenic part, the turpentine. Oleoresin, in coniferous species, is synthesized by the epithelial cells surrounding the resin canals, from which it is exuded as a response to mechanical wounds or biotic attacks, thus constituting a defense mechanism of living trees [4]. Resin acids, among other substances, are part of the non-volatile fraction, composed of a mixture of diterpenic resinous compounds. Diterpenic resin acids are the most common members of oleoresin [4] and the most abundant compounds in heartwood and knots [5–8]. Their fractions can vary among individual trees and species [9–11]. Many softwoods, and particularly *Pinus* species, contain relatively high oleoresin amounts, moving through the wood's extensive vertical and radial networks of resin canals.

Resin acids are mostly tricyclic compounds, arranged in two types depending on the presence or absence of double bonds in their aromatic rings. The first, called abietane-type, includes acids such as abietic acid (**1**), dehydroabietic acid (**2**), neoabietic acid (**3**), palustric acid (**4**) and levopimaric acid (**5**), and the second, named pimarane-type, includes acids such as pimaric acid (**6**), sandaracopimaric acid (**7**), and isopimaric acid (**8**) (Figure 1). The cyclic diterpene acids originate from a common acyclic biosynthetic precursor, geranylgeranyl diphosphate (GGPP) [12]. Diterpene synthase enzymes act on the 20-carbon GGPP substrate to form diterpenes, which are subsequently hydroxylated and then oxidized, in two independent transformations, by other enzymes to the diterpene acids [13].

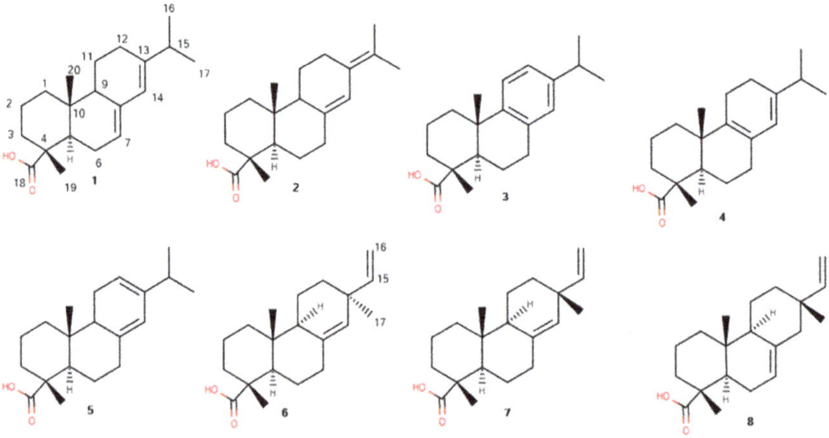

Figure 1. The structures and numbering of the diterpenic resin acids of the *Pinus nigra* heartwood extracts.

The diterpene synthase genes involved in resin acid formation prove their highly genetically-correlated heartwood properties [14,15]. Selection and breeding in *Pinus* species could result in doubling the oleoresin yields [16] and further genetic gains in extractive yield could be achieved [17]. Genetic control of extractive production has considerable economic potential in some species [18].

Pine resin has been highly applied in industry. Resin acids and their derivatives, apart from being used in intermediate chemical products, such as polymer additives, tackifiers, emulsifiers in synthetic rubber, paper sizing to control water absorptivity, and aroma industry, are also deployed in adhesives, surface coatings, printing inks, chewing gums, and in the Greek wine industry [19,20]. Furthermore, several medicinal uses concerning the treatment of abscesses, boils, cancers, toothache, and skin diseases, such as psoriasis and ringworm [19], have been reported even from antiquity. According to Dioscorides, during the first century A.D., a wine called retsina, i.e., wine that had been mixed with resin from *Pinus halepensis*, was used for lung and stomach disorders and as an antidote for cough [19].

In recent years, many studies have shown that several substances in rosin have antimicrobial properties [21], cardiovascular effects [22,23], antiallergic properties [24], anti-inflammatory properties [25,26], anticonvulsant effects [27], antiulcer-gastroprotective properties [28,29], and cytotoxic activity toward human fibroblasts [29]. Their medicinal properties, due to the bioactivity of natural abietane and pimarane diterpene acids, which have been reviewed by San Feliciano et al. [30] and Reveglia et al. [31] respectively, have caused a renewed scientific interest in pine extracts.

The aim of the present work was to analyze the resin acids composition and variability from the heartwood extractives of four *Pinus nigra* L. subsp. *pallasiana* marginal provenances from the Peloponnese, southern Greece, growing in a clonal seed orchard. The heartwood of these trees produced an exceptionally high extractive content, approximately 30% w/w [3], making it particularly interesting for the present analysis. The target compounds were the abietane-type resin acids: abietic, dehydroabietic, neoabietic, palustric, and levopimaric acids, and the pimarane-type: pimaric, isopimaric, and sandaracopimaric acids. The ^{1}H-NMR spectroscopy was used to analyze, qualitatively and quantitatively, the highly complex diterpenic acid mixtures of heartwood rosin.

Many studies have been carried out on pine oleoresin composition, some of which have demonstrated the potential of NMR spectroscopy, a modern analytical methodology with applications in complex mixtures [32,33]. The applied technique highlights its feasibility and wide practical applicability in characterizing various complex matrixes, from leaves [34] and walnuts [35] for profiling "green" extracts and different genotypes, respectively, to foodstuffs [36,37] for quality/safety or discrimination purposes, and biological [38] for lipid profiling. ^{13}C-NMR spectroscopy has already been used for the quantitation of resin acids in wood extracts from *Pinus radiata* [39] and *Pinus nigra* ssp. *laricio* [20,40]. Skakovskii et al. [41], through the use of high-field NMR spectrometers introduced the alternative ^{1}H-NMR analysis of resin acids, and this technique is here preferred as quicker and straightforward. Moreover, the possible simultaneous record of ^{1}H-NMR and ^{13}C-NMR experiments can pave the way to the robust analysis of resin acid by combined data as performed for other systems [42].

2. Results

^{1}H-NMR spectrum of black pine (P. nigra Arn.) heartwood extracts, showing the characteristic peaks of the studied resin acids and internal standard, are presented in Figure 2. The whole spectrum is available as supplementary Figure S1. Their chemical shifts are presented in Table 1. Recovery and intraday precision data are presented in Tables 2 and 3, respectively.

Table 1. ^{1}H-NMR proton's chemical shifts of the studied resin acids selected for quantitation (400 MHz, CDCl$_3$, δ-values in ppm).

Resin Acid	Abietane Type					Pimarane Type		
Proton	Abietic Acid (1)	Neoabietic Acid (2)	Dehydroabietic Acid (3)	Palustric Acid (4)	Levopimaric Acid (5)	Pimaric Acid (6)	Sandaracopimaric Acid (7)	Isopimaric Acid (8)
C(H)-15	-	-	-	-	-	5.67	-	5.84
C(H)-14	5.77	6.20	6.88	5.39	5.53	-	5.22	-

Table 2. Recovery data and their coefficient of variance for the studied resin acids.

	Abietic Acid (1)	Neoabietic Acid (2)	Dehydroabietic Acid (3)	Palustric Acid (4)	Levopimaric Acid (5)	Pimaric Acid (6)	Sandaracopimaric Acid (7)	Isopimaric Acid (8)
Recovery (%)	90.26	93.52	88.78	90.50	90.73	92.75	92.07	87.37
Coefficient of Variance (%)	1.06	1.82	0.85	2.39	8.40	1.93	3.82	1.48

Table 3. Intraday precision data for the studied resin acids, expressed as relative standard deviations (%).

ID	Abietic Acid (1)	Neoabietic Acid (2)	Dehydroabietic Acid (3)	Palustric Acid (4)	Levopimaric Acid (5)	Pimaric Acid (6)	Sandaracopimaric Acid (7)	Isopimaric Acid (8)
Sample 1	5.55	6.29	8.84	2.17	9.07	5.09	9.82	9.07
Sample 2	6.51	7.38	3.49	5.18	4.85	7.55	2.88	3.31
Sample 3	3.68	5.40	2.48	9.92	8.81	7.66	2.98	7.57
Average	5.25	6.36	4.93	5.76	7.58	6.77	5.22	6.65

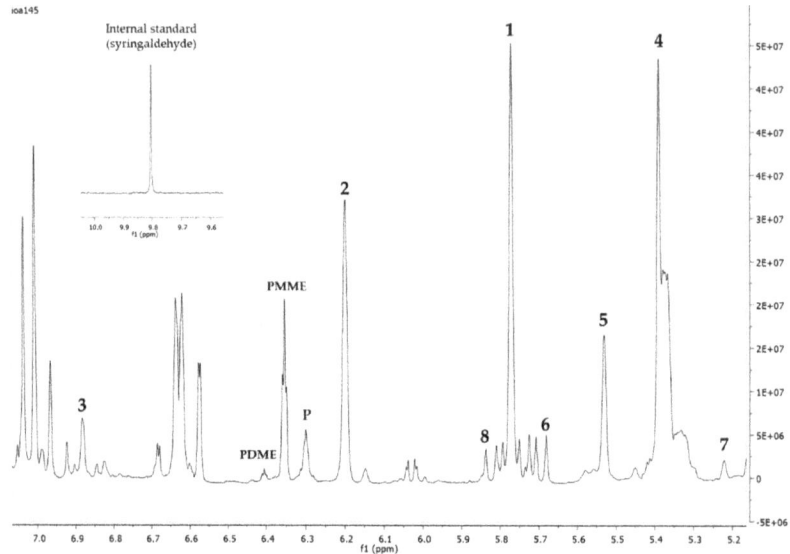

Figure 2. ^{1}H-NMR spectrum (400 MHz, CDCl$_3$, δ-values in ppm) of black pine (P. nigra Arn.) heartwood extracts, showing the characteristic peaks of studied resin acids and internal standard. The numbers indicate the corresponding resin acids' peaks used for quantitation: abietic acid (**1**), neoabietic acid (**2**), dehydroabietic acid (**3**), palustric acid (**4**), levopimaric acid (**5**), pimaric acid (**6**), sandaracopimaric acid (**7**), and isopimaric acid (**8**). Stilbenes' peaks are also indicated (P = pinosylvin, PMME and PDME = monomethylether and dimethylether of pinosylvin, respectively).

In the frame of this investigation 260 samples were analyzed. The heartwood of the studied trees was exceptionally rich in acetone extractive content (TAE), averaging 304.15 mg/g of dry heartwood (dhw), which contained high resin acid quantities. The mean resin acid fraction accounted for 72.33% of the total extractive content, while stilbenes were present in significant quantities, comprising 19.70%. The remaining 7.97% is referred to as other substances present in the TAE, i.e., minor unidentified resin acids, fatty acids, unsaponifiables, triglycerides, other phenols, waxes, sterols, etc.

The mean concentration of all studied diterpenic resin acids as their min and max values are presented in Table 4. The total resin acid (TRA) content showed an extent variation ranging from 30.05 to 424.70 mg/g$_{dhw}$, with an average of 219.98 mg/g$_{dhw}$ (±96.20). Abietic acid was the predominant acid (76.77 ± 37.39 mg/g$_{dhw}$), followed by palustric acid (47.94 ± 23.31 mg/g$_{dhw}$) and neoabietic acid (39.34 ± 21.21 mg/g$_{dhw}$), all belonging to the abietane-type resin acids. The next in abundance acid was the pimaric acid, with a mean concentration of 22.54 ± 11.28 mg/g$_{dhw}$. Dehydroabietic acid was found at moderate levels (11.69 ± 5.73 mg/g$_{dhw}$), while the rest, levopimaric acid, isopimaric acid, and sandaracopimaric acid, were observed in lower concentrations, i.e., 8.07 ± 211.38 mg/g$_{dhw}$, 10.91 ± 6.53 mg/g$_{dhw}$, and 2.72 ± 1.49 mg/g$_{dhw}$, respectively.

Table 4. The mean resin acid concentrations of *Pinus nigra* L. heartwood samples (*n* = 260) as determined by quantitative ^{1}H-NMR.

	Abietic Acid (1)	Neoabietic Acid (2)	Dehydroabietic Acid (3)	Palustric Acid (4)	Levopimaric Acid (5)	Pimaric Acid (6)	Sandaracopimaric Acid (7)	Isopimaric Acid (8)	Total Resin Acids
Average mg/g$_{dhw}$	76.77	39.34	11.69	47.94	8.07	22.54	2.72	10.91	219.98
Min. mg/g$_{dhw}$	7.00	2.91	2.56	9.76	0.08	2.20	0.16	0.50	30.05
Max. mg/g$_{dhw}$	181.75	101.82	38.59	105.22	64.91	59.42	6.67	34.09	424.70

In Table 5, the mean resin acid concentrations, the results from the analysis of variance (ANOVA), as well as Duncan's Multiple Range Test (MRT) results, of the four *Pinus nigra* L. provenances are presented. The ANOVA and MRT showed that there were statistically significant ($p < 0.001$) differences among clones for all examined acids (data not shown) and also among provenances in concentrations of both abietic acid ($p < 0.01$) and pimaric acid ($p < 0.01$).

Table 5. The mean resin acid concentrations (mg/g_{dhw}) of the four *Pinus nigra* L. provenances' heartwood after applying ANOVA and Duncan's MRT at $p = 0.05$, Zarouhla: 65 samples, Feneos: 85 samples, Parnonas: 45 samples, and Taigetos: 65 samples, total 260 samples.

Provenance	Abietic Acid (1)	Neoabietic Acid (2)	Dehydroabietic Acid (3)	Palustric Acid (4)	Levopimaric Acid (5)	Pimaric Acid (6)	Sandaracopimaric Acid (7)	Isopimaric Acid (8)	Total Resin Acids
Zarouhla	81.99 [a]	40.06 [a]	11.10 [a]	48.83 [a]	7.41 [a]	21.60 [ab]	2.61 [a]	11.45 [a]	224.46 [a]
Feneos	78.64 [a]	37.84 [a]	12.29 [a]	46.43 [a]	8.91 [a]	25.09 [a]	2.74 [a]	11.03 [a]	222.768 [a]
Parnonas	79.99 [ab]	41.87 [a]	11.74 [a]	49.86 [a]	6.88 [a]	23.57 [ab]	2.92 [a]	11.20 [a]	227.83 [a]
Taigetos	66.05 [b]	36.36 [a]	11.82 [a]	45.61 [a]	9.69 [a]	20.35 [b]	2.54 [a]	9.89 [a]	201.25 [a]

The means followed by the same letter (a, b as superscript) are not statistically different.

In Figure 3, the mean percentage of each individual resin acid to total resins, as well as their types, are presented. Abietic, palustric, and neoabietic acids, which were the most abundant resin acids, accounted for 34.90%, 21.79%, and 17.88%, respectively. Dehydroabietic and levopimaric acids comprised 5.32% and 3.67% of the TRA, respectively. Pimaric acid was in a fairly large quantity, corresponding to 10.25% of the total studied resin acids, while sandaracopimaric and isopimaric acids corresponded to 1.24% and 4.96%, respectively, of the total studied resin acids. The resin acid content was composed mainly of the abietane resin acid type ($\approx$84%), while the pimarane-type accounted only for the rest, $\approx$16%, so the abietane- to pimarane-type resin acids ratio was circa 5.2. In Figure 4, the mean percentage content of the constituents of black pine's heartwood acetone extraction from the Peloponnese is presented.

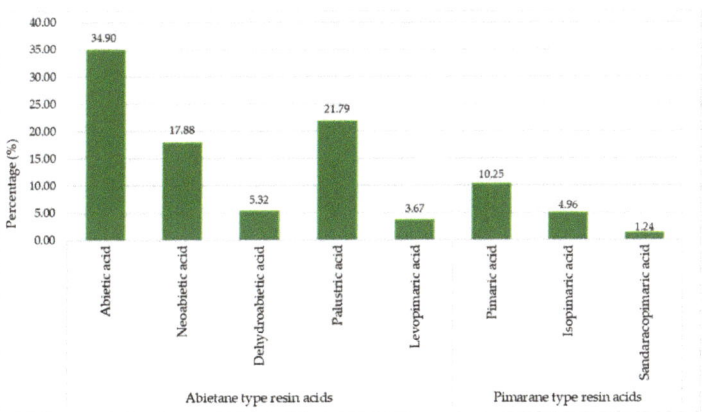

Figure 3. The mean percentage of abietane and pimarane types of resin acids.

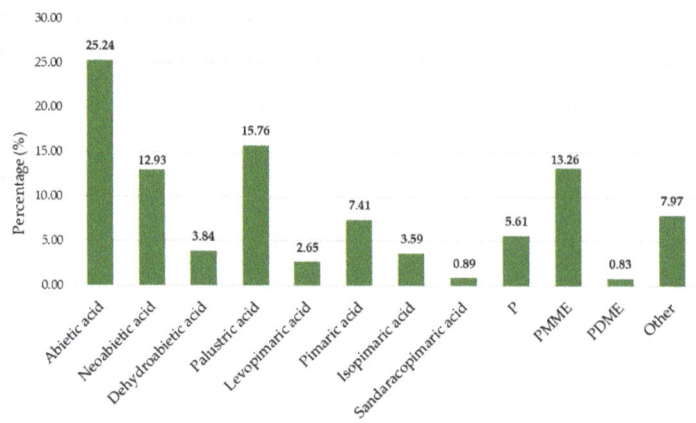

Figure 4. The mean percentage content of the constituents in the black pine's heartwood acetone extraction from the Peloponnese (P = pinosylvin, PMME and PDME = monomethylether and dimethylether of pinosylvin, respectively).

In Figure 5, the frequency distribution of the total resin acids (TRA) of black pine from the Peloponnese are presented.

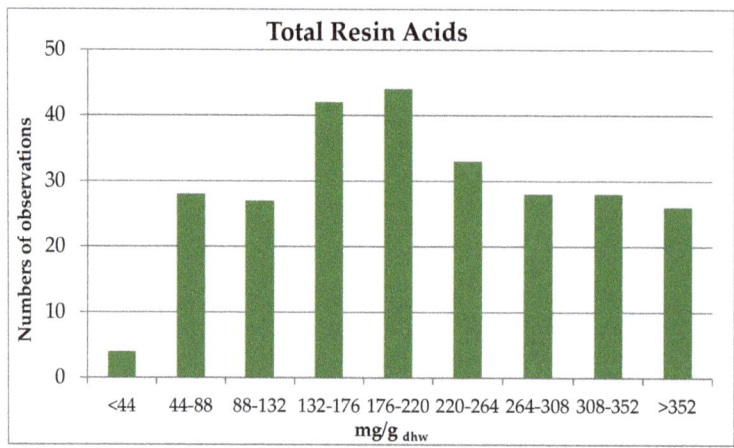

Figure 5. Total resin acids frequency distribution of black pine (*P. nigra* Arn.).

3. Discussion

The current study aimed to demonstrate that ^{1}H-NMR spectroscopy can be effectively used for the analysis of *Pinus nigra* heartwood resin acids although their spectra are complicated and partially overlapping. Despite the structural similarity of the terpenic acids included in the oleoresin, we were able to select non overlapping peaks, belonging to specific protons, that could lead to the identification and quantitation of the target resin acids. Using ^{1}H-NMR spectroscopy, we achieved to minimize time-consuming procedures of separation of every analyte before quantitation.

As it was previously shown in the cases of olive oil [43,44], beer [45], wine [33], and stilbenes from *Pinus nigra* heartwood [3], qNMR is the most appropriate method for quantitation. The developed methodology for the analysis of heartwood resin acids requires less than a minute to record the spectrum and perform the analytes quantitation, whereas using the previously reported ^{13}C-NMR methodology requires a considerably longer time, i.e., approximately two hours [40] or even more [46]. The advantage of the current methodology allowed the analysis of a very large amount of samples in a short period and led to reliable quantitative data.

The results indicated obvious individual tree and clone variation in heartwood resin acids content due to genetic and environmental factors affecting rosin production and secretion [4,47]. Venäläinen et al. [48] also reported high variation among trees in the resin acid concentrations of *Pinus sylvestris*. Heartwood resin acid contents present provenance variation as well (Table 5) because of the heterogeneity among populations [3]. In general, the southeastern provenance of Parnonas, grown at the most xerothermic environment [49] and subjected to the strongest winds [50], showed higher values of total resin acids, i.e., for neoabietic acid, palustric acid, and sandaracopimaric acid, while the southwestern of Taigetos had the lowest concentrations of all except for dehydroabietic and levopimaric acids. For the latter, Taigetos provenance showed the highest content of all provenances. Although Feneos provenance (northeastern origin) predominated in dehydroabietic acid and pimaric acid concentrations, only the latter acid statistically differed from Taigetos origin. The origin of Zarouhla presented the highest value for abietic and isopimaric acids, having a statistically significant difference only for the abietic acid found in Taigetos. Willför et al. [51] found similar results, mentioning that there were no significant differences between trees from the southern and northern regions, thus confirming Song's [52] view that the oleoresin of trees within several *Pinus* species show similar basic chemical characteristics, regardless of their geographic location.

The present study stated that acetone extractives of *Pinus nigra* heartwood mainly consisted of resin acids. These results were in accordance with those of Martínez-Inigo et al. [53], Willför et al. [51], and Belt et al. [54] for *Pinus sylvestris*. Hafizoğlu [55], in a review article, mentioned that several researchers have found that most of the oleoresin in *Pinus nigra* and *P. sylvestris* were comprised of resin acids. In the same direction were the results of Uprichard and Lloyd [56] in *P. radiata*, reporting that resin acids predominate in heartwood total extractives. Yildirim and Holmbom [57] have found a remotely lower percentage in stemwood extractives of *Pinus brutia*.

Lower resin acid concentrations compared to the present study were detected in *Pinus sylvestris* by Martínez-Inigo et al. [53], Hovelstad et al. [58], and Belt et al. [54]. Concerning *Pinus sylvestris* heartwood, Harju et al. [59], Venäläinen et al. [48], Willför et al. [51], and Arshadi et al. [60] estimated lower resin acid content, too. Moreover, in *Pinus nigra*, Yildirim and Holmbom [61] found similar results with the previous researchers. Correspondingly, medium resin acid concentrations were found in *P. radiata* by Lloyd [7]. On the contrary, Willför et al. [62] found in both *Pinus nigra* and *P. brutia* heartwood even lower amounts of resin acids than the present study, without referring to predominant acids or the fatty/resin and abietane/pimarane ratios. Low levels of resin acid were noted in *Pinus contorta* by Lewinsohn et al. [63] and Arshadi et al. [60]. Benouadah et al. [64] surprisingly found even lower concentrations in dry *Pinus halepensis* heartwood.

The fatty acid/resin acid ratio in the present study was estimated as very low due to the high presence of resin acids, as well as stilbenes, in total acetone extractives and could not exceed 0.18. Lower fatty/resin acid ratio in *Pinus sylvestris* was reported by Martínez-Inigo et al. [53] and Belt et al. [54], depending on the heartwood sample position, and in *P. radiata* by Uprichard and Lloyd [56]. Arshadi et al. [60] reported that in *Pinus sylvestris* and *Pinus contorta*, in general, the concentration of resin acids was higher than that of fatty acids. In *Pinus contorta* and *Pinus attenuata*, the results of Anderson et al. [65] confirmed the above findings as well as those of the present study. In contrast, Hafizoğlu's [55] review article reported that fatty/resin acid ratio was a multiple of the unit concerning *P. nigra* and *P. sylvestris*, and that only in *P. brutia* the resin acids were double the fatty ones. The results of Uçar and Fengel [66], as well as those of Uçar and Balaban [67], for *Pinus nigra* were in agreement with Hafizoğlu's. In both studies, the fatty/resin ratio depended on the *Pinus nigra* variety or provenance.

In the present study, the abietane-type dominated over the pimarane-type resin acids and the estimated (abietane/pimarane) ratio was calculated at 5.1. This is consistent with the results of

Harju et al. [68] and Willför et al. [51] in *Pinus sylvestris*, who estimated a little higher ratio values, as well as with Uçar and Fengel [66], who estimated a little lower ratio values, depending on variety. The common element in all studies was that the resin acids of abietane-type were multiples compared to the pimarane ones.

Abietic acid was the most abundant resin acid, which is in accordance with the findings of Martínez-Inigo et al. [53], Willför et al. [51,62], and Yildirim and Holmbom [61] in *Pinus sylvestris*, of Yildirim and Holmbom [57] in *Pinus brutia*, and of Anderson et al. [65] in *Pinus attenuata*. Hafizoğlu's review article [55] reported that, in most cases, abietic, mainly in *Pinus nigra*, and levopimaric, mainly in *Pinus sylvestris*, acids were the most abundant, followed by palustric acid though dependent on species and origins. Abietic acid was found to be the most abundant resin acid in Scots pine according to Harju et al. [68], but followed by the mixture of palustric/levopimaric acids and neoabietic or pimaric acids. Abietic acid was the most abundant resin acid in *P. radiata* too [56]. Different results were those of Rezzi et al. [20] who distinguished two clusters of *Pinus nigra* ssp. *laricio*. In the first one, levopimaric acid was the most abundant resin, whereas in the second, dehydroabietic acid and levopimaric acid were approximately in equal concentrations. Cannac et al. [46] identified *Pinus nigra* ssp. *laricio*, from Corsica too, as belonging to the first cluster.

In the examined *Pinus nigra* provenances, abietic acid was the most abundant one, followed by palustric acid, neoabietic acid, and pimaric acid. Similar results, but with a few differences in the classification of resin acid concentrations, were also those of Ekeberg et al. [69] in Scots pine and Benouadah et al. [64] in Aleppo pine. In both studies, abietic acid was the major acid though dehydroabietic acid was ranked second or third. Papajannopoulos et al. [70] reported that the basic composition of the oleoresin of three Greek pine species, *Pinus halepensis*, *P. brutia*, and *P. pinea*, were found to be similar concerning the abundance of several resin acids. The mixture of palustric/levopimaric acids were the most abundant followed by the abietic, in similar concentrations, and neoabietic or isopimaric acids. The above were in accordance with the results of Lange and Stefanovic Janezic [71] for *Pinus sylvestris* and Lloyd [7] for *Pinus radiata*.

Different were the results of Uçar and Fengel [66] who found palustric acid to be the richest resin acid in the stemwood of *Pinus nigra* varieties, followed by isopimaric acid or dehydroabietic acid (depending on the variety), while abietic acid was ranked third. Palustric acid was found to be the most abundant *Pinus nigra* resin acid by Uçar and Balaban [67] followed by abietic acid, neoabietic acid, or levopimaric acid, depending on the individual tree.

The results of Lewinsohn et al. [63] obtained in the case of *Pinus contorta* are in contrast with our results. They found that the total resin acids consisted mainly of levopimaric acid, followed by palustric, isopimaric, abietic, and neoabietic acids at moderate levels. The above composition resembled those of mature *Pinus contorta* rosin stated by Anderson et al. [65]. In *Pinus attenuata*, Anderson et al. [65] found that dehydroabietic acid was the major resin acid followed by the mixture of levopimaric/palustric acids, and finally by neoabietic acid.

The present study sets a framework for future research on a number of issues, which could lead to new scientific results. Exploiting the individual clone and provenance variation of the genetic material of *Pinus nigra* from the Peloponnese, its heartwood has been found to be the richest source in resin acids, as well as in stilbenes [3], identified to date. Effective selection and advanced breeding require further research towards the estimation of several genetic parameters (i.e., heritability, breeding values, and genetic gains for all the above mentioned traits) of the studied provenances and clones.

4. Materials and Methods

4.1. Plant Material

The plant material was sampled from a 10 hectares *Pinus nigra* Arnold clonal seed orchard (CSO), established in the western part of the Peloponnese in 1978. The CSO comprises 52 clones and a total number of 2700 grafts, derived from intensively selected plus trees, originating from four marginal provenances (Zarouhla, Feneos, Parnonas, and Taigetos) of the natural black pine forest of the Peloponnese (Figure 6). Clones (one ramet/clone) were randomly assigned at 6 m × 6 m spacing within replications (single tree plot design), without blocking, with the only restriction that no grafts of the same clone were planted closer than 30 m [72].

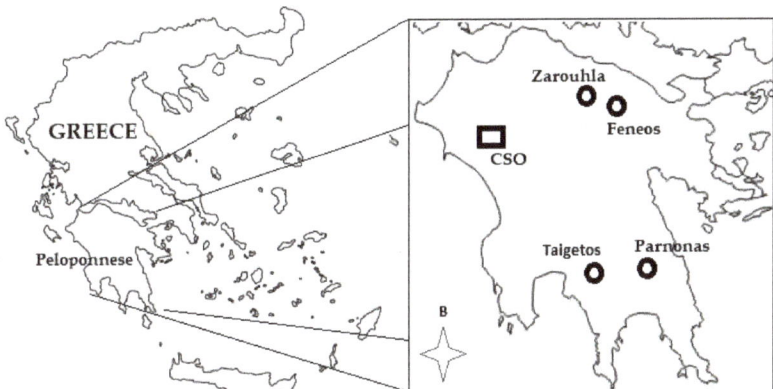

Figure 6. The positions of the provenances (circles) and the clonal seed orchard (CSO).

4.2. Sampling

Sampling, coring, heartwood discrimination and orientation, and extraction protocol are extensively described in Ioannidis et al. [3]. In brief, increment cores, approximately 30 cm above ground and in a north-south orientation, of 12 mm in diameter were extracted from a total of 260 healthy individuals that were sampled during October and November 2013 and covered all 52 clones participating in the seed orchard (five ramets per clone), and stored in darkness at −76 °C. Heartwood was separated from the rest of the core, using the benzidine discrimination method, and milled to produce ≤0.75 mm particles, which were freeze-dried for 48 h at −52 °C and 0.03 mbar pressure, to ensure almost complete removal of moisture and volatile compounds.

4.3. Extraction Protocol

In brief, resin acids were extracted with 12 ml acetone from 200 mg (±0.1 mg) of freeze-dried, ground heartwood. The mixture was first placed in an orbital shaker at 350 rpm (Edmund Bühler GmbH, Bodelshausen, Germany) in darkness at room temperature for 24 h, followed by its transfer to an ultrasonic bath (Semat, UK) for 1 h to complete the extraction. The liquid phase was separated by centrifuging (3075× g for 15 min) (Eppendorf 5810R, Germany) and the solvent was evaporated in a heated vacuum rotary evaporator (Buchi, Switzerland) at 40 °C to determine the weights. Recovery of the first extraction was calculated by employing successive extraction procedures and quantitation in each one.

4.3.1. H-NMR Spectral Analysis/Quantitation Methodology

The dried extractives were submitted to chemical analysis by ^{1}H-NMR using syringaldehyde as internal standard and deuterated chloroform ($CDCl_3$) as solvent. The extract of each sample obtained from the extraction procedure was dissolved in 600 μL deuterated chloroform ($CDCl_3$) (Euriso-Top) and the solution was transferred to a 5 mm NMR tube. ^{1}H-NMR spectra were recorded at 400 MHz (Bruker DRX400). Typically, 16 scans were collected into 32K data points over a spectral width of 0–16 ppm with a relaxation delay of 10 s. Prior to Fourier transformation (FT), an exponential weighting factor corresponding to a line broadening of 0.3 Hz was applied. The spectra were phase corrected automatically using TopSpin software (Bruker, Billerica, MA, USA). For the peaks of interest, accurate integration was performed manually. Quantitative determination of the resin acids (RA), i.e., the concentration C_{RA}, was obtained by comparing the area of the selected signals with that of the internal standard (IS), i.e., the relative integration (I_{RA}). The following formula was used, which include I_{RA} as well as the weight (m_{sample} = 200 mg), the molecular weight (MW_{RA}), and the average recovery of each resin acid (R_{RA}, Table 2) of the analyzed dry heartwood powder:

$$C_{RA} = [(0.002745 \times I_{RA} \times MW_{RA})/m_{sample}]/R_{RA}$$

The recovery was calculated as the ratio of successive extractions of heartwood samples for the studied resin acids. The samples contained different levels of extractives in order to obtain unbiased results. The intraday precision (i.e., the experimental error) was determined by analyzing three replicates of three random samples in the same day. Concentrations were based on freeze-dried heartwood (dhw) and expressed in mg/g_{dhw}. Syringaldehyde (Acros Organics) internal standard (IS) solution was prepared in acetonitrile at a concentration of 0.5 mg/mL. Prior to use, the IS solution reached room temperature and the solutions of all the extracted samples were mixed, before evaporation, with 1 mL of a syringaldehyde solution, i.e., 0.00274 moles of syringaldehyde.

The identity of all compounds was defined by the literature data [41,73–75]. Due to rather complicated resin acids' ^{1}H-NMR spectra, nonoverlapping, undoubtedly defined peaks of the olefinic or aromatic protons were selected for quantitation. Concerning the abietane-type resin acids, abietic acid (1), neoabietic acid (2), dehydroabietic acid (3), palustric acid (4), and levopimaric acid (5) were distinguished by their single C(H)-14 proton at 5.77 ppm, 6.20 ppm, 6.88 ppm, 5.39 ppm, and 5.53 ppm, respectively. For the pimarane-type resin acids, pimaric acid (6) and isopimaric acid (8) were distinguished by the C(H)-15 proton at 5.67 ppm and 5.84 ppm, respectively, and sandaracopimaric acid (7) was distinguished by the C(H)-14 proton at 5.22 ppm. It should be noted that for pimaric and isopimaric acids the selected signal for quantitation was only one of the four equivalent peaks of the corresponding doublet to avoid overlapping with other peaks. In these two cases, the integration value was multiplied by a factor of four before comparing the area with that of the internal standard in order to estimate the concentration.

To exclude the possibility of overlapping peaks we have performed 2D HMQC (2 Dimensional Heteronuclear Multiple Quantum Correlation) experiment presented in Supplementary Material Figures S2 and S3.

4.3.2. Statistical Analysis

Descriptive statistics, analysis of variance (ANOVA), as well as Duncan's Multiple Range Test (MRT), based on the 0.05 level of significance, were performed in order to check the hypothesis that there were statistically significant differences among the mean concentrations in the samples of all clones and among the four provenances, using SPSS v.20 software for Windows (IBM SPSS Statistics 2011, IBM Corp. New York, NY, USA).

5. Conclusions

The ^{1}H-NMR spectroscopy proved to be a fast, sensitive, accurate, and comfortable methodology for high-throughput identification and quantitation of resin acids. According to this study, the genetic material of black pine heartwood, originating from the Peloponnese, was proved to be the richest natural source of resin acids compared to any other European pine species/population referred to in the literature. The high resin acid concentrations, as well as differences among origins for some of them, can be attributed to their adaptation over time to individual environments that differ in bioclimatic and soil parameters. Such marginal populations growing in the edge of their natural range, under the pressure and impact of climate change, will be populations for further investigations and adaptability testing. Furthermore, the presence of great variation in resin acid concentrations among trees and origins from the Peloponnese, as well as the consensus of genetic control of resin acid production-segregation, highlight the great potential for effective selection and advanced breeding of the studied genetic material for pharmaceutical and high economic value bioactive substances derived from *Pinus nigra* L. heartwood.

Supplementary Materials: The supplementary materials are available online.

Author Contributions: Conceptualization, P.M., E.M., and K.I.; methodology, P.M., E.M., and K.I.; formal analysis, K.I.; investigation, K.I.; resources, P.M., E.M., and K.I.; data curation, K.I.; writing—original draft preparation, K.I.; writing—review and editing, K.I., P.M., and E.M..; supervision, P.M.; funding acquisition, P.M.

Funding: This research received no external funding.

Acknowledgments: We would like to express our appreciation to the Laboratory of Forest Genetics and Tree Improvement, Faculty of Forestry and Natural Environment, School of Agriculture, Forestry and Natural Environment, Aristotle University of Thessaloniki, Greece, for providing the increment borer in order to extract increment cores. The authors want to express their sincere thankfulness to the librarian of the Forest Research Institute of Athens, D. Panayiotopoulou (MSc Library and Information Science), for information seeking and retrieving processes as well as her additional proof reading service.

Conflicts of Interest: The authors declare no conflict of interest.

References

1. Matziris, D. Variation in growth and branching characters in black pine (*Pinus nigra* Arnold) of Peloponnesos. *Silvae Genet.* **1989**, *38*, 77–81.
2. Pietarinen, S.P.; Willför, S.M.; Ahotupa, M.O.; Hemming, J.E.; Holmbom, B.R. Knotwood and bark extracts: Strong antioxidants from waste materials. *J. Wood Sci.* **2006**, *52*, 436–444. [CrossRef]
3. Ioannidis, K.; Melliou, E.; Alizoti, P.; Magiatis, P. Identification of black pine (*Pinus nigra* Arn.) heartwood as a rich source of bioactive stilbenes by qNMR. *J. Sci. Food Agric.* **2017**, *97*, 1708–1716. [CrossRef] [PubMed]
4. Hillis, W.E. *Heartwood and Tree Exudates*; Springer Verlag: Berlin, Germany, 1987; p. 268.
5. Porter, L.J. The resin and fatty acid content of living *Pinus radiata* wood. *N. Z. J. For. Sci.* **1969**, *12*, 687–693.
6. Hemingway, R.W.; Hillis, W. Changes in fats and resins of *Pinus radiata* associated with heartwood formation. *Appita* **1971**, *24*, 439–443.
7. Lloyd, J.A. Distribution of extractives in *Pinus radiata* earlywood and latewood. *N. Z. J. For. Sci.* **1978**, *8*, 288–294.
8. Nisula, L. *Wood Extractives in Conifers: A Study of Stemwood and Knots of Industrially Important Species*; Åbo Akademi University Press: Åbo, Finland, 2018; p. 372.
9. Joye, N.M.; Lawrence, R.V. Resin acid composition of pine oleoresins. *J. Chem. Eng. Data* **1967**, *12*, 279–282. [CrossRef]
10. Conner, A.H.; Diehl, M.A.; Rowe, J.W. Tall oil precursors in three western pines: Ponderosa, Lodgepole, and Limber pine. *Wood Sci.* **1980**, *12*, 183–191.
11. Conner, A.; Diehl, M.; Rowe, J. Tall oil precursors and turpentine in jack and eastern white pine. *Wood Sci.* **1980**, *12*, 194–200.
12. Lichtenthaler, H.K. The 1-deoxy-d-xylulose-5-phosphate pathway of isoprenoid biosynthesis in plants. *Annu. Rev. Plant Physiol. Plant Mol. Biol.* **1999**, *50*, 47–65. [CrossRef]
13. Keeling, C.I.; Bohlmann, J. Diterpene resin acids in conifers. *Phytochemistry* **2006**, *67*, 2415–2423. [CrossRef] [PubMed]
14. Fries, A.; Ericsson, T.; Gref, R. High heritability of wood extractives in *Pinus sylvestris* progeny tests. *Can. J. For. Res.* **2000**, *30*, 1707–1713. [CrossRef]
15. Ericsson, T.; Fries, A.; Gref, R. Genetic correlations of heartwood extractives in *Pinus sylvestris* progeny tests. *For. Genet.* **2001**, *8*, 73–79.
16. Squillace, A.; Harrington, T. Olustee's high-yielder produces 487 bbls pine gum per crop for four straight years. *Nav. Stores Rev.* **1968**, *77*, 4–5.
17. Franklin, E.; Taras, M.; Volkman, D. Genetic gains in yields of oleoresin, wood extractives and tall oil. *Tappi* **1970**, *53*, 2302–2304.
18. Taylor, A.M.; Gartner, B.L.; Morre, J.I. Heartwood formation and natural durability—A review. *Wood Fiber Sci.* **2002**, *34*, 587–611.

19. Langenheim, J.H. *Plant Resins: Chemistry, Evolution, Ecology, and Ethnobotany*; Timber Press: Portland, OR, USA, 2003; p. 612. ISBN 0-88192-574-8.
20. Rezzi, S.; Bighelli, A.; Castola, V.; Casanova, J. Composition and chemical variability of the oleoresin of *Pinus nigra* ssp. *laricio* from Corsica. *Ind. Crops Prod.* **2005**, *21*, 71–79. [CrossRef]
21. Spessard, G.O.; Matthews, D.R.; Nelson, M.D.; Rajtora, T.C.; Fossum, M.J.; Giannini, J.L. Phytoalexin-like activity of abietic acid and its derivatives. *J. Agric. Food Chem.* **1995**, *43*, 1690–1694. [CrossRef]
22. De Oliveira, A.M.; Tirapelli, C.R.; Ambrosio, S.R.; da Costa, F.B. Diterpenes: A therapeutic promise for cardiovascular diseases. *Recent Patents Cardiovasc. Drug Discov.* **2008**, *3*, 1–8. [CrossRef]
23. Gonzalez, M.A.; Correa-Royero, J.; Agudelo, L.; Mesa, A.; Betancur-Galvis, L. Synthesis and biological evaluation of abietic acid derivatives. *Eur. J. Med. Chem.* **2009**, *44*, 2468–2472. [CrossRef]
24. Ulusu, N.N.; Ercil, D.; Sakar, M.K.; Tezcan, E.F. Abietic acid inhibits lipoxygenase activity. *Phytother. Res.* **2002**, *16*, 88–90. [CrossRef] [PubMed]
25. Fernandez, M.; Tornos, M.; Garcia, M.; De las Heras, B.; Villar, A.; Saenz, M. Anti-inflammatory activity of abietic acid, a diterpene isolated from *Pimenta racemosa* var. *grissea*. *J. Pharm. Pharmacol.* **2001**, *53*, 867–872. [CrossRef] [PubMed]
26. Takahashi, N.; Kawada, T.; Goto, T.; Kim, C.-S.; Taimatsu, A.; Egawa, K.; Yamamoto, T.; Jisaka, M.; Nishimura, K.; Yokota, K. Abietic acid activates peroxisome proliferator-activated receptor-γ (PPARγ) in RAW264.7 macrophages and 3T3-L1 adipocytes to regulate gene expression involved in inflammation and lipid metabolism. *FEBS Lett.* **2003**, *550*, 190–194. [CrossRef]
27. Talevi, A.; Cravero, M.S.; Castro, E.A.; Bruno-Blanch, L.E. Discovery of anticonvulsant activity of abietic acid through application of linear discriminant analysis. *Bioorg. Med. Chem. Lett.* **2007**, *17*, 1684–1690. [CrossRef] [PubMed]
28. Schmeda-Hirschmann, G.; Astudillo, L.; Rodríguez, J.; Theoduloz, C.; Yáñez, T. Gastroprotective effect of the Mapuche crude drug Araucaria araucana resin and its main constituents. *J. Ethnopharmacol.* **2005**, *101*, 271–276. [CrossRef]
29. Schmeda-Hirschmanna, G.; Astudillo, L.; Sepúlveda, B.; Rodríguez, J.A.; Theoduloz, C.; Yáñez, T.; Palenzuela, J.A. Gastroprotective effect and cytotoxicity of natural and semisynthetic labdane diterpenes from *Araucaria araucana* resin. *Z. Naturforschung C* **2005**, *60*, 511–522. [CrossRef]
30. San Feliciano, A.; Gordaliza, M.; Salinero, M.A.; del Corral, J.M.M. Abietane acids: Sources, biological activities, and therapeutic uses. *Planta Med.* **1993**, *59*, 485–490. [CrossRef] [PubMed]
31. Reveglia, P.; Cimmino, A.; Masi, M.; Nocera, P.; Berova, N.; Ellestad, G.; Evidente, A. Pimarane diterpenes: Natural source, stereochemical configuration, and biological activity. *Chirality* **2018**, *30*, 1115–1134. [CrossRef]
32. Simmler, C.; Napolitano, J.G.; McAlpine, J.B.; Chen, S.-N.; Pauli, G.F. Universal quantitative NMR analysis of complex natural samples. *Curr. Opin. Biotechnol.* **2014**, *25*, 51–59. [CrossRef]
33. Nikolantonaki, M.; Magiatis, P.; Waterhouse, A.L. Direct analysis of free and sulfite-bound carbonyl compounds in wine by two-dimensional quantitative proton and carbon nuclear magnetic resonance spectroscopy. *Anal. Chem.* **2015**, *87*, 10799–10806. [CrossRef]
34. Cerulli, A.; Masullo, M.; Montoro, P.; Hošek, J.; Pizza, C.; Piacente, S. Metabolite profiling of "green" extracts of *Corylus avellana* leaves by ^{1}H NMR spectroscopy and multivariate statistical analysis. *J. Pharm. Biomed. Anal.* **2018**, *160*, 168–178. [CrossRef] [PubMed]
35. Popescu, R.; Ionete, R.E.; Botoran, O.R.; Costinel, D.; Bucura, F.; Geana, E.I.; Alabedallat, Y.F.J.; Botu, M. ^{1}H-NMR profiling and carbon isotope discrimination as tools for the comparative assessment of walnut (*Juglans regia* L.) cultivars with various geographical and genetic origins—A preliminary study. *Molecules* **2019**, *24*, 1378. [CrossRef] [PubMed]
36. Merkx, D.W.H.; Hong, G.T.S.; Ermacora, A.; van Duynhoven, J.P.M. Rapid quantitative profiling of lipid oxidation products in a food emulsion by ^{1}H NMR. *Anal. Chem.* **2018**, *90*, 4863–4870. [CrossRef] [PubMed]
37. Fan, S.; Zhong, Q.; Fauhl-Hassek, C.; Pfister, M.K.-H.; Horn, B.; Huang, Z. Classification of Chinese wine varieties using ^{1}H NMR spectroscopy combined with multivariate statistical analysis. *Food Control* **2018**, *88*, 113–122. [CrossRef]
38. Barrilero, R.; Gil, M.; Amigó, N.; Dias, C.B.; Wood, L.G.; Garg, M.L.; Ribalta, J.; Heras, M.; Vinaixa, M.; Correig, X. LipSpin: A new bioinformatics tool for quantitative ^{1}H NMR lipid profiling. *Anal. Chem.* **2018**, *90*, 2031–2040. [CrossRef] [PubMed]

39. Suckling, I.D.; Ede, R. A quantitative ^{13}C nuclear magnetic resonance method for the analysis of wood extractives and pitch samples. *Appita J.* **1990**, *43*, 77–80.
40. Rezzi, S.; Bighelli, A.; Castola, V.; Casanova, J. Direct identification and quantitative determination of acidic and neutral diterpenes using ^{13}C-NMR spectroscopy. application to the analysis of oleoresin of *Pinus nigra*. *Appl. Spectrosc.* **2002**, *56*, 312–317. [CrossRef]
41. Skakovskii, E.D.; Tychinskaya, L.Y.; Gaidukevich, O.A.; Kozlov, N.G.; Klyuev, A.Y.; Lamotkin, S.A.; Shpak, S.I.; Rykov, S.V. NMR determination of the composition of balsams from Scotch pine resin. *J. Appl. Spectrosc.* **2008**, *75*, 439–443. [CrossRef]
42. Rotondo, A.; Mannina, L.; Salvo, A. Multiple assignment recovered analysis (MARA) NMR for a direct food labeling: The case study of olive oils. *Food Anal. Methods* **2019**, *12*, 1238–1245. [CrossRef]
43. Karkoula, E.; Skantzari, A.; Melliou, E.; Magiatis, P. Direct measurement of oleocanthal and oleacein levels in olive oil by quantitative ^{1}H NMR. Establishment of a new index for the characterization of extra virgin olive oils. *J. Agric. Food Chem.* **2012**, *60*, 11696–11703. [CrossRef]
44. Karkoula, E.; Skantzari, A.; Melliou, E.; Magiatis, P. Quantitative measurement of major secoiridoid derivatives in olive oil using qNMR. Proof of the artificial formation of aldehydic oleuropein and ligstroside aglycon isomers. *J. Agric. Food Chem.* **2014**, *62*, 600–607. [CrossRef] [PubMed]
45. Manoukian, P.; Melliou, E.; Liouni, M.; Magiatis, P. Identification and quantitation of benzoxazinoids in wheat malt beer by qNMR and GC–MS. *LWT Food Sci. Technol.* **2016**, *65*, 1133–1137. [CrossRef]
46. Cannac, M.; Barboni, T.; Ferrat, L.; Bighelli, A.; Castola, V.; Costa, J.; Trecul, D.; Morandini, F.; Pasqualini, V. Oleoresin flow and chemical composition of Corsican pine (*Pinus nigra* subsp. *laricio*) in response to prescribed burnings. *For. Ecol. Manag.* **2009**, *257*, 1247–1254. [CrossRef]
47. Zobel, B.; Jett, J. *Genetics of Wood Production*; Springer-Verlag: Berlin, Germany, 1995; 337p.
48. Venäläinen, M.; Harju, A.M.; Kainulainen, P.; Viitanen, H.; Nikulainen, H. Variation in the decay resistance and its relationship with other wood characteristics in old Scots pines. *Ann. For. Sci.* **2003**, *60*, 409–417. [CrossRef]
49. Matziris, D. Genetic variation in morphological and anatomical needle characteristics in the Black pine of Peloponnesos. *Silvae Genet.* **1984**, *33*, 164–169.
50. Ioannidis, K. Genetic Improvement of Multiple Traits in Black Pine (*Pinus nigra* Arn.). Ph.D. Thesis, Aristotle University of Thessaloniki, Thessaloniki, Greece, 2018.
51. Willför, S.; Hemming, J.; Reunanen, M.; Holmbom, B. Phenolic and lipophilic extractives in Scots pine knots and stemwood. *Holzforschung* **2003**, *57*, 359–372. [CrossRef]
52. Song, Z. *Characteristics of Oleoresin and Classification of Pinus in China*; China Forestry Publishing House: Beijing, China, 1998; 206p.
53. Martínez-Inigo, M.J.; Immerzeel, P.; Gutierrez, A.; del Río, J.C.; Sierra-Alvarez, R. Biodegradability of extractives in sapwood and heartwood from Scots pine by sapstain and white-rot fungi. *Holzforschung* **1999**, *53*, 247–252. [CrossRef]
54. Belt, T.; Keplinger, T.; Hänninen, T.; Rautkari, L. Cellular level distributions of Scots pine heartwood and knot heartwood extractives revealed by Raman spectroscopy imaging. *Ind. Crops Prod.* **2017**, *108*, 327–335. [CrossRef]
55. Hafizoglu, H. Wood extractives of *Pinus sylvestris* L., *Pinus nigra* Arn. and *Pinus brutia* Ten. with special reference to nonpolar components. *Holzforschung* **1983**, *37*, 321–326.
56. Uprichard, J.M.; Lloyd, J.A. Influence of tree age on the chemical composition of Radiata pine. *N. Z. J. For. Sci.* **1980**, *10*, 551–557.
57. Yildirim, H.; Holmbom, B. Investigations on the wood extractives of pine species from Turkey: III Non-volatile, nonpolar components in *Pinus brutia*. *Acta Acad. Abo.* **1977**, *B37*, 1–9.
58. Hovelstad, H.; Leirset, I.; Oyaas, K.; Fiksdahl, A. Screening analyses of pinosylvin stilbenes, resin acids and lignans in Norwegian conifers. *Molecules* **2006**, *11*, 103–114. [CrossRef] [PubMed]
59. Harju, A.M.; Venäläinen, M.; Anttonen, S.; Viitanen, H.; Kainulainen, P.; Saranpää, P.; Vapaavuori, E. Chemical factors affecting the brown-rot decay resistance of Scots pine heartwood. *Trees* **2003**, *17*, 263–268.
60. Arshadi, M.; Backlund, I.; Geladi, P.; Bergsten, U. Comparison of fatty and resin acid composition in boreal Lodgepole pine and Scots pine for biorefinery applications. *Ind. Crops Prod.* **2013**, *49*, 535–541. [CrossRef]
61. Yildirim, H.; Holmbom, B. Investigations on the wood extractives of pine species from Turkey: II Composition of fatty and resin acids in *Pinus sylvestris* and *Pinus nigra*. *Acta Acad. Abo.* **1977**, *B37*, 1–6.

62. Willför, S.; Hafizo-Glu, H.; Tümen, I.; Yazici, H.; Arfan, M.; Ali, M.; Holmbom, B. Extractives of Turkish and Pakistani tree species. *Holz Roh. Werkst.* **2007**, *65*, 215–221. [CrossRef]
63. Lewinsohn, E.; Savage, T.J.; Gijzen, M.; Croteau, R. Simultaneous analysis of monoterpenes and diterpenoids of conifer oleoresin. *Phytochem. Anal.* **1993**, *4*, 220–225. [CrossRef]
64. Benouadah, N.; Pranovich, A.; Aliouche, D.; Hemming, J.; Smeds, A.; Willför, S. Analysis of extractives from *Pinus halepensis* and *Eucalyptus camaldulensis* as predominant trees in Algeria. *Holzforschung* **2018**, *72*, 97–104. [CrossRef]
65. Anderson, A.B.; Riffer, R.; Wong, A. Monoterpenes, fatty and resin acids of *Pinus contorta* and *Pinus attenuata*. *Phytochemistry* **1969**, *8*, 2401–2403. [CrossRef]
66. Uçar, G.; Fengel, D. Variation in composition of extractives from wood of *Pinus nigra* varieties. *Phytochemistry* **1995**, *38*, 877–880. [CrossRef]
67. Uçar, G.; Balaban, M. Cyclohexane extracts of black pine wood naturally grown in eastern Thrace. *Holz Roh. Werkst.* **2002**, *60*, 34–40. [CrossRef]
68. Harju, A.M.; Kainulainen, P.; Venäläinen, M.; Tiitta, M.; Viitanen, H. Differences in resin acid concentration between brown-rot resistant and susceptible Scots pine heartwood. *Holzforschung* **2002**, *56*, 479–486. [CrossRef]
69. Ekeberg, D.; Flæte, P.-O.; Eikenes, M.; Fongen, M.; Naess-Andresen, C.F. Qualitative and quantitative determination of extractives in heartwood of Scots pine (*Pinus sylvestris* L.) by gas chromatography. *J. Chromatogr. A* **2006**, *1109*, 267–272. [CrossRef] [PubMed]
70. Papajannopoulos, A.D.; Song, Z.Q.; Liang, Z.Q.; Spanos, J.A. GC-MS analysis of oleoresin of three Greek pine species. *Holz Roh. Werkst.* **2001**, *59*, 443–446. [CrossRef]
71. Lange, W.; Stevanović Janežić, T. Chemical composition of some *Pinus sylvestris* L. oleoresins from southern Serbia, Bosnia and Makedonia: Two entities of Scotch Pine present on the Balkan peninsula. *Holzforschung* **1993**, *47*, 207–212. [CrossRef]
72. Matziris, D. Variation in cone production in a clonal seed orchard of black pine. *Silvae Genet.* **1993**, *42*, 136–141.
73. Landucci, L.L.; Zinkel, D.F. The ^{1}H and ^{13}C-NMR spectra of the abietadienoic resin acids. *Holzforschung* **1991**, *45*, 341–346. [CrossRef]
74. Muto, N.; Tomokuni, T.; Haramoto, M.; Tatemoto, H.; Nakanishi, T.; Inatomi, Y.; Murata, H.; Inada, A. Isolation of apoptosis- and differentiation-inducing substances toward human promyelocytic leukemia HL-60 cells from leaves of *Juniperus taxifolia*. *Biosci. Biotechnol. Biochem.* **2008**, *72*, 477–484. [CrossRef] [PubMed]
75. Olate, V.R.; Usandizaga, O.G.; Schmeda-Hirschmann, G. Resin diterpenes from *Austrocedrus chilensis*. *Molecules* **2011**, *16*, 10653–10667. [CrossRef] [PubMed]

Sample Availability: Samples of the extracts are available from the authors.

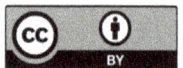

© 2019 by the authors. Licensee MDPI, Basel, Switzerland. This article is an open access article distributed under the terms and conditions of the Creative Commons Attribution (CC BY) license (http://creativecommons.org/licenses/by/4.0/).

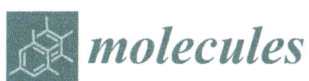

Article

Betulin Promotes Differentiation of Human Osteoblasts In Vitro and Exerts an Osteoinductive Effect on the hFOB 1.19 Cell Line Through Activation of JNK, ERK1/2, and mTOR Kinases

Magdalena Mizerska-Kowalska [1,*], Adrianna Sławińska-Brych [2], Katarzyna Kaławaj [1], Aleksandra Żurek [1], Beata Pawińska [1], Wojciech Rzeski [1,3] and Barbara Zdzisińska [1,*]

1 Department of Virology and Immunology; Maria Curie-Sklodowska University, Lublin 20-033, Poland
2 Department of Cell Biology, Maria Curie-Sklodowska University, Lublin 20-033, Poland
3 Department of Medical Biology, Institute of Rural Health, Lublin 20-090, Poland
* Correspondence: magdalena.mizerska-dudka@poczta.umcs.lublin.pl (M.M.-K.); basiaz@poczta.umcs.lublin.pl (B.Z.); Tel.: +48-81-537-59-42 (B.Z.)

Academic Editor: Vassilios Roussis
Received: 13 June 2019; Accepted: 17 July 2019; Published: 19 July 2019

Abstract: Although betulin (BET), a naturally occurring pentacyclic triterpene, has a variety of biological activities, its osteogenic potential has not been investigated so far. The aim of this study was to assess the effect of BET on differentiation of human osteoblasts (hFOB 1.19 and Saos-2 cells) in vitro in osteogenic (with ascorbic acid as an osteogenic supplement) and osteoinductive (without an additional osteogenic supplement) conditions. Osteoblast differentiation was evaluated based on the mRNA expression (RT-qPCR) of Runt-related transcription factor 2 (RUNX2), alkaline phosphatase (ALP), type I collagen-α1 (COL1A1), and osteopontin (OPN). Additionally, ALP activity and production of COL1A1 (western blot analysis) and OPN (ELISA) were evaluated. The level of mineralization (calcium accumulation) was determined with Alizarin red S staining. BET upregulated the mRNA level of RUNX2 and the expression of other osteoblast differentiation markers in both cell lines (except the influence of BET on ALP expression/activity in the Saos-2 cells). Moreover, it increased mineralization in both cell lines in the osteogenic conditions. BET also increased the mRNA level of osteoblast differentiation markers in both cell lines (except for ALP in the Saos-2 cells) in the osteoinductive conditions, which was accompanied with increased matrix mineralization. The osteoinductive activity of BET in the hFOB 1.19 cells was probably mediated via activation of MAPKs (JNK and ERK1/2) and mTOR, as the specific inhibitors of these kinases abolished the BET-induced osteoblast differentiation. Our results suggest that BET has the potential to enhance osteogenesis.

Keywords: betulin; osteoblasts; differentiation; mineralization

1. Introduction

Bone is an extremely heterogeneous tissue built up of cells and mineralized extracellular matrix [1]. It undergoes an unceasing process of remodeling that involves removal of old bone by osteoclasts and formation of new bone by osteoblasts. In physiological conditions, these events are balanced and provide tissue homeostasis [2]. However, in some cases, an imbalance in bone remodeling may lead to the development of bone diseases, e.g., osteopenia and osteoporosis. Osteoporosis is mainly associated with aging. Moreover, various diseases including rheumatoid arthritis, chronic inflammatory periodontal diseases, multiple myeloma, bone metastatic malignant cancers, or drugs adversely affect bone health and can contribute to the development of osteoporosis. Therefore, osteoporosis is considered as a global public health problem [3,4]. Currently, therapeutic options employed for managing of osteoporosis include antiresorptive agents whose actions is directed mainly to osteoclasts and bone anabolic drugs that regulate the function of osteoblasts. However, both types of therapies may have adverse side effects, especially upon long-term use in the elderly or patients having multimorbidity [5,6]. Therefore, new anti-osteoporotic agents are still being sought.

Differentiation of osteoblasts from mesenchymal stem cells to mature osteoblasts depositing mineralized matrix is regulated by extracellular signals that activate intracellular signaling pathways and regulate the action of several osteogenesis-related transcription factors, including Runt-related transcription factor 2 (RUNX2) [7]. RUNX2 is considered to be the master transcription factor, as it regulates the expression of genes linked with osteoblast maturation such as *ALPL* (alkaline phosphatase, ALP), *Col1A1* (collagen α1 type I, COL1), *SPP1* (osteopontin, OPN), *IBSP* (bone sialoprotein II, BSPII), and *BGLAP* (osteocalcin, OCN) [7]. Different signaling systems regulate bone formation, but mitogen-activated kinase (MAPK) and mammalian target of rapamycin (mTOR) pathways play a key role in this process, as they affect osteoblast differentiation [8,9]. MAP kinases, i.e., extracellular signal-regulated kinases (ERK1/2) and p38, have been identified as regulators of RUNX2 activation [10,11], while c-Jun N-terminal protein kinases (JNKs) regulate the expression of activating transcription factor 4 (ATF4) and are required for late-stage osteoblast differentiation [12]. Also, both mTOR complexes, i.e., mTORC1 and mTORC2, are involved in osteoblast differentiation [9]. More recently, it has been shown that mTORC1 promotes osteoblast differentiation through the regulation of RUNX2 expression [13].

At present, medicines or supplements derived from natural sources have aroused wide interest. Plant extracts are especially rich in diverse active compounds. One of them are pentacyclic triterpenes with a lupane skeleton, to which betulin (BET; lup-20(29)-ene-3β,28-diol) is included [14,15]. BET is found predominantly in the bark of trees of the genus Betula (Betulaceae), which are well known as a rich source of compounds with healing properties [15]. This triterpene exhibits a wide range of pharmacological effects [14], including anticancer [16–18], anti-viral [19,20], and anti-pathogenic [21] activities. Due to its anti-inflammatory and anti-oxidative activities, betulin may also exert hepato- or cardioprotective properties [22–25]. Moreover, BET exhibits analgesic [26] and anti-hyperlipidemic [27] activities. Betula bark and bark extracts have been known in traditional medicine and have been used for treatment of various diseases, including micro-fracture and dislocated bone [15]. Recently, it has been shown that pentacyclic triterpenoids such as ursolic, corosolic, and betulinic acid can influence bone formation as they enhance osteoblast differentiation [28–31]. However, to the best of our knowledge, the effect of betulin on osteogenesis has never been studied before. These all data prompted us to evaluate whether BET exerts anabolic activity by engagement in bone formation. To this end, we examined the effects of betulin on the differentiation and mineralization of osteoblasts of two human cell lines both in the presence of an osteogenic medium and without an osteogenic supplement such as ascorbic acid [32,33]. Moreover, some signaling mechanisms involved in the pro-osteogenic activity of BET were studied.

2. Results

2.1. Effect of BET on the Viability and Proliferation of Osteoblasts

Initially, to avoid the cytotoxicity of the compound towards osteoblasts, the effect of BET on the viability of hFOB 1.19 and Saos-2 cells was determined by the LDH assay. This test is one of the major methods for assessment of cell membrane integrity and, thus, the ability of the tested compound to disintegrate cells [34]. As shown in Figure 1A, BET decreased the viability of both osteoblast cell lines in a concentration-dependent manner. It was not toxic to the hFOB 1.19 cells up to 1 µM and to the Saos-2 cells up to 0.5 µM. Statistically significant LDH release appeared at 1 µM (Saos-2 cells) and 5 µM (hFOB 1.19 cells) of BET. The exposure of the osteoblasts to 25 µM of BET resulted in very high LDH leakage from the Saos-2 cells (more than six times higher than the control level), while only a minor cytotoxic effect was observed in the hFOB 1.19 cells. This revealed low toxicity of BET to the normal hFOB 1.19 osteoblasts, while the osteosarcoma Saos-2 cells were more sensitive to the compound.

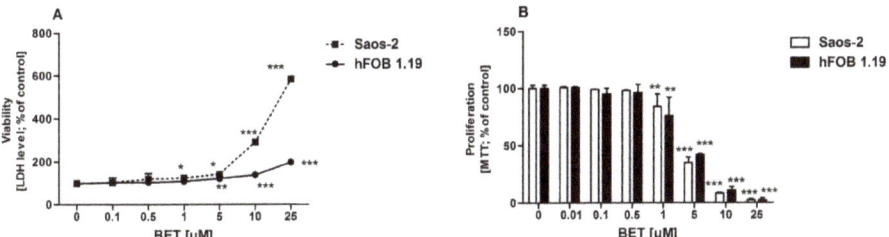

Figure 1. Effect of BET on hFOB 1.19 and Saos-2 cell viability (**A**) and proliferation (**B**). The osteoblasts were treated with the indicated concentrations of the compound and cell viability was estimated with the LDH assay after 24 h or cell proliferation was determined with the MTT method following the 96-h BET treatment. The results represent the mean ± SD of three independent experiments (n = 24 per concentration), * p < 0.05, ** p < 0.01, *** p < 0.001 in comparison to the control, one-way ANOVA with post hoc Dunnett's test.

As anabolic agents can increase bone formation either by increasing the proliferation and/or differentiation of osteoblast precursors [35], further investigation was undertaken to determine the effect of BET on osteoblast proliferation. As shown in Figure 1B, BET did not influence the proliferation of both cell lines up to 0.5 µM. However, at a concentration of 1 µM and higher doses, BET inhibited proliferation of osteoblasts in a concentration-dependent manner. BET used at the 25 µM concentration suppressed the proliferation of both osteoblast cell lines almost completely. Based on the viability/proliferation tests, only the non-toxic concentrations of BET, i.e., 0.01, 0.1, and 0.5 µM, were selected for further experiments.

2.2. BET Elevated the mRNA Level of RUNX2 and the Expression of other Osteoblast Differentiation Markers, and Enhanced the Level of Bone Matrix Mineralization in Osteogenic Conditions

The osteogenic potential of different compounds in osteoblast cultures in vitro is usually tested in the presence of osteogenic supplements. Therefore, we evaluated the influence of BET on differentiation of osteoblasts in osteogenic conditions, namely in a medium supplemented with ascorbic acid [32,33]. First, we determined whether BET was able to modulate the expression of *RUNX2* gene, as the product of this gene, i.e., RUNX2 a transcription factor that regulates the degree of expression of other osteoblast differentiation markers in human osteoblasts [7]. The RT-qPCR assay revealed that BET used at low concentrations such as 0.1 and 0.5 µM was able to increase *RUNX2* expression in both osteoblast cell lines. The statistically significant enhancement of the RUNX2 mRNA level in comparison with the control was detected at day 9 and 12 of culture (Figure 2A,B). BET also enhanced the expression of other differentiation markers such as ALP (marker of the early phase of osteoblast differentiation), COL1A1 (marker of the late stage of osteoblast differentiation), and OPN (marker of the terminal stage of osteoblast differentiation). As shown in Figure 2C, the triterpenoid (0.1 and 0.5 µM) significantly enhanced the *ALPL*, *COL1A1*, and *SPP1* (OPN) gene expression in the hFOB 1.19 cells, in comparison with the control cells. BET influenced especially the expression of *COL1A1* and *SPP1* and, to a lesser extent, the expression of *ALPL* in the hFOB 1.19 cells (Figure 2C). However, in the Saos-2 cells, BET did not influence the expression of the *ALPL* gene, but it enhanced significantly the expression of both other markers (*COL1A1* and *SPP1*) in a concentration-dependent manner (Figure 2D).

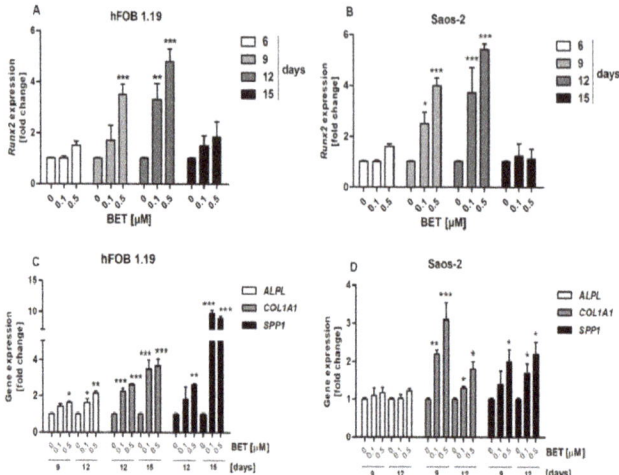

Figure 2. Effect of BET on the expression of *RUNX2* and other differentiation marker genes in osteoblasts in osteogenic conditions. The osteoblasts were cultured in an osteogenic medium supplemented with 0.1 or 0.5 μM of BET or without the compound (control). The expression of the *RUNX2* gene was determined in the hFOB 1.19 (**A**) and Saos-2 (**B**) cells by RT-qPCR after the indicated period of culture. The expression of osteogenic genes *ALPL*, *COL1A1* (type I collagen), and *SPP1* (OPN) was determined in the hFOB 1.19 (**C**) and Saos-2 (**D**) cells by RT-qPCR after the indicated period of culture. Mean ± SD from three independent experiments; * $p < 0.05$, ** $p < 0.01$, *** $p < 0.001$ in comparison to the control, one-way ANOVA with post hoc Dunnett's test.

Next, we evaluated the ALP activity and production of COL1A1 and OPN by osteoblasts to confirm additionally that BET promotes differentiation of osteoblasts. In this part of the study, BET was used in very low concentrations such as 0.01 and 0.1 μM. As shown in Figure 3A, the ALP activity in the hFOB 1.19 cell cultures started to increase at day 9 of incubation with 0.1 μM BET. Then, ALP reached maximal activity after treatment with 0.01 and 0.1 μM of BET at day 12 of culture. In contrast, a statistically significant decrease in the ALP activity was observed in the Saos-2 cell cultures at the same time points (Figure 3B). Moreover, western blot analysis revealed that BET enhanced the production of COL1A1 in the hFOB 1.19 and Saos-2 cells in a concentration-dependent manner, compared with the controls (Figure 3C,D). As shown in Figure 3E,F, the treatment of both cell lines with BET also enhanced the production of OPN after 12 days of incubation. In the case of the hFOB 1.19 cells, a similar effect of the triterpene treatment was also observed at day 15 of culture.

Finally, we conducted the ARS staining assay for qualitative and quantitative analysis of the mineralization process in the BET-treated hFOB 1.19 and Saos-2 cell cultures. The microscopic analysis of the ARS-stained osteoblast cultures revealed the appearance of evident nodules at day 12 of hFOB 1.19 and day 18 of Saos-2 differentiation (Figure 3G,H). Moreover, the ARS quantitative analysis indicated that calcium deposition was elevated by approx. 10% and 20% in the hFOB 1.19 cell cultures treated with 0.1 μM and 0.5 μM of BET, respectively, in comparison with the control. A similar increase in the level of mineralization was also observed in the Saos-2 cells at day 18 of the study.

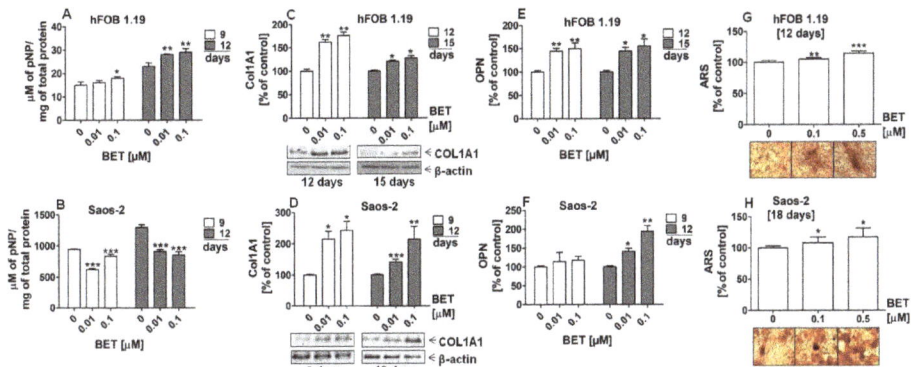

Figure 3. Effect of BET on the production of differentiation markers and the levels of mineralization in osteoblasts after the indicated period of culture in osteogenic conditions. The osteoblasts were cultured in an osteogenic medium supplemented with 0.01, 0.1, or 0.5 µM of BET or without the compound (control). ALP activity in the hFOB 1.19 (**A**) and Saos-2 cells (**B**) was measured with the colorimetric method. The levels of COL1A1 in the hFOB1.19 (**C**) and Saos-2 (**D**) cells were determined with the western blotting method. The levels of OPN in the culture media from the hFOB 1.19 (**E**) and Saos-2 (**F**) cells were evaluated with the ELISA method. The levels of calcium deposited in the extracellular matrix were determined in 24-well plates using Alizarin Red S staining. Representative micrographs (40×) of stained osteoblast cultures and mean levels of ARS extracted from the hFOB 1.19 (**G**) and Saos-2 cultures (**H**). Mean ± SD from three independent experiments; * $p < 0.05$, ** $p < 0.01$, *** $p < 0.001$ in comparison to the control, one-way ANOVA with post hoc Dunnett's test.

2.3. BET Elevated the mRNA Level of Osteoblast Differentiation Markers and Enhanced the Level of Bone Matrix Mineralization in Osteoinductive Conditions

Moreover, we carried out an assay of osteoblast differentiation in media without additional osteogenic supplements (ascorbic acid) to evaluate whether BET alone possesses the activity to regulate osteogenesis. As shown in Figure 4A and B, BET (0.1 and 0.5 µM) increased the expression of the *RUNX2* gene in both the hFOB1.19 and Saos-2 cells. Statistically significant increases in the RUNX2 mRNA levels in the BET-treated osteoblasts were detected at day 6, 9, and 12 of osteoblast cultures. Further investigations revealed that BET also induced the expression of other osteoblast differentiation marker genes and enhanced mineralization, i.e., the final step of this process. As shown in Figure 4C,D, at a concentration of 0.1 and/or 0.5 µM, BET elevated the expression of all tested differentiation makers, except *ALPL* in the Saos-2 cells, at the indicated culture time.

Especially, the expression of the *COL1A1* gene increased in comparison with the control and other markers in both BET-treated cell lines. In the hFOB 1.19 cells, the expression of *COL1A1* was 2.9 and 4.5 times higher after 0.1 and 0.5 µM BET treatment than in the control, respectively (Figure 4C). In turn, the COL1A1 mRNA levels increased about 1.9 and 3.8 times in the 0.1 µM and 0.5 µM BET-treated Saos-2 cells, respectively (Figure 4D). Moreover, the matrix mineralization in the BET-treated osteoblasts was also enhanced, as indicated by ARS staining (Figure 4E–G). The microscopic analysis showed that the hFOB 1.19 and Saos-2 cells cultured only in the basal medium (without ascorbic acid and β-glycerophosphate as a phosphate ion source) were able to form calcified matrix at the indicated culture time points, although at minimal levels. However, the addition of BET (0.01 and/or 0.1 µM) significantly enhanced mineralization in both BET-treated osteoblast cultures, compared with the control. This was evidenced by the ARS quantitative analysis and the microscopic and/or macroscopic (Figure 4G) observation of the bone nodule morphology in the hFOB 1.19 and Soas-2 cultures.

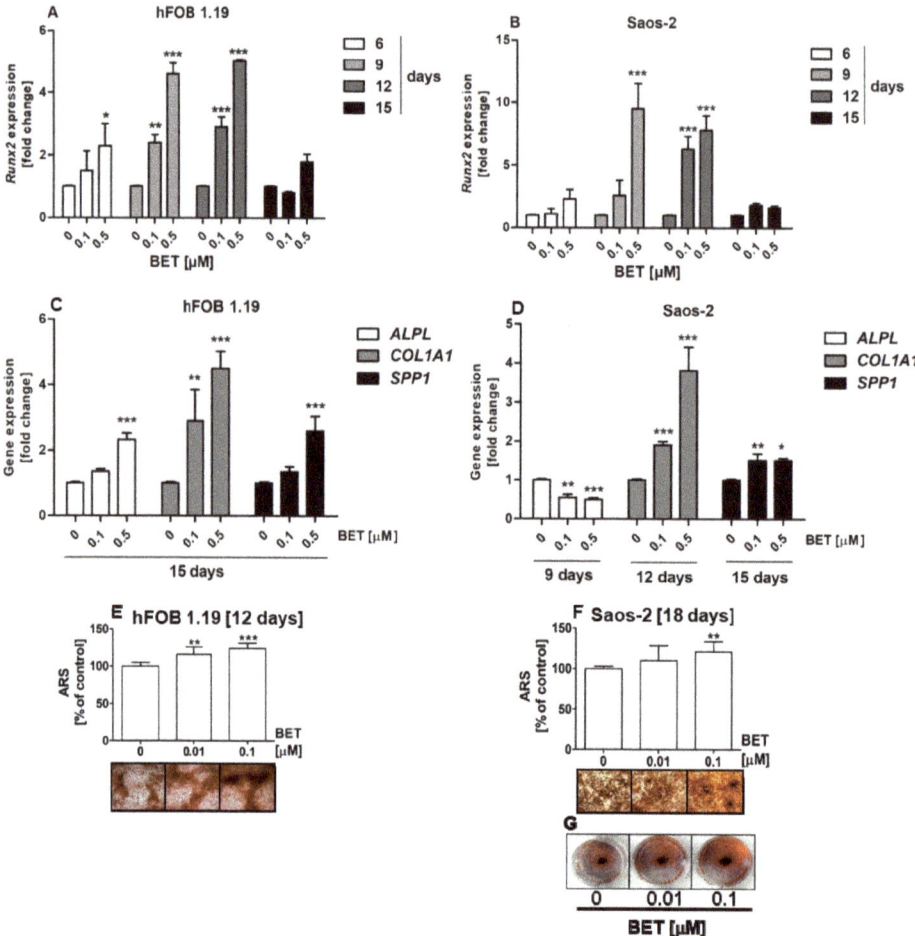

Figure 4. Effect of BET on the expression of *RUNX2* and other differentiation marker genes, and the levels of mineralization in osteoblasts in osteoinductive conditions. The osteoblasts were cultured in an osteoinductive medium supplemented with 0.01, 0.1, or 0.5 µM of BET or without the compound (control). The expression of the *RUNX2* gene was determined in the hFOB 1.19 (**A**) and Saos-2 (**B**) cells by RT-qPCR after the indicated period of culture. The expression of osteogenic genes *ALPL*, *COL1A1* (type I collagen), and *SPP1* (OPN) was determined in the hFOB 1.19 (**C**) and Saos-2 (**D**) cells by RT-qPCR after the indicated period of culture. The levels of calcium deposited in the extracellular matrix were determined in 24-well plates using Alizarin Red S staining. Representative micrographs (40×) of stained cultures and mean levels of ARS extracted from the hFOB 1.19 (**E**) and Saos-2 (**F**) cultures. Representative photographs of stained Saos-2 cultures (**G**). Mean ± SD from three independent experiments; * $p < 0.05$, ** $p < 0.01$, *** $p < 0.001$ in comparison to the control, one-way ANOVA with post hoc Dunnett's test.

2.4. BET Influences the Phosphorylation Status of JNK, ERK1/2, and mTOR Kinases

To explore the involvement of MAPKs and mTOR in BET-induced osteoblast differentiation, the phosphorylation status of all three members of MAP kinases, i.e., JNK, ERK1/2, and p38, as well as mTOR kinase was examined by the quantitative ELISA method. In this part of the study, we used the hFOB 1.19 cell line as a model of normal osteoblasts. As shown in Figure 5A–D, at a concentration of

0.5 µM, BET significantly increased the phosphorylation of JNK, ERK1/1, and mTOR (ser2481) kinases, but did not activate p38 kinase in the hFOB 1.19 cells. Especially, it influenced the activation of JNK and mTOR, and only slightly increased the phosphorylation of ERK1/2 kinase.

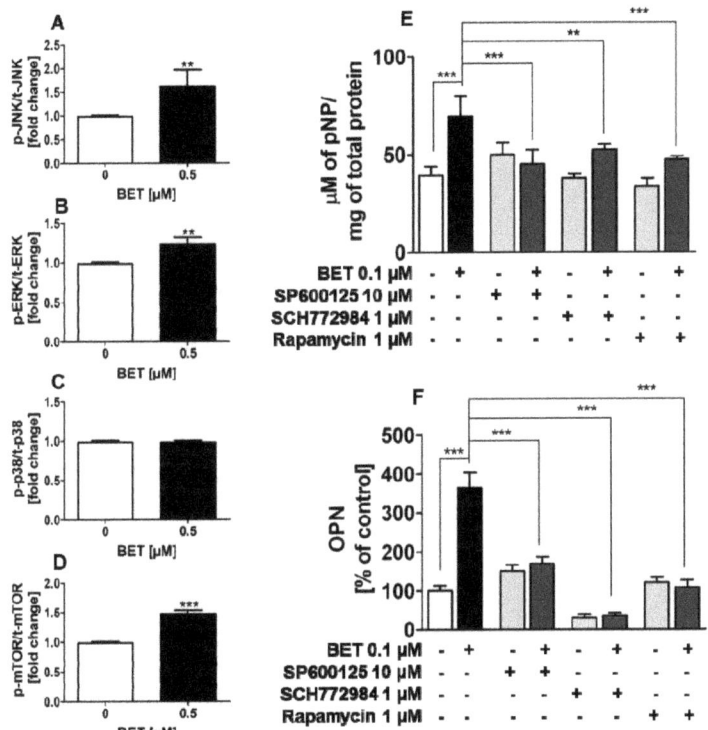

Figure 5. Effect of BET on the activation of JNK, ERK1/2, p38, and mTOR kinases in the hFOB 1.19 cells (**A–D**). Effects of JNK, ERK, and mTOR inhibitors on the levels of BET-induced ALP (**E**) and OPN (**F**). The cells were cultured in an osteoinductive medium with BET at a concentration of 0.5 µM or without the compound (control) for 6 h (JNK, ERK1/2, p38) or 24 h (mTOR). The levels of JNK (**A**), ERK1/2 (**B**), p38 (**C**), and mTOR (**D**) phosphorylation in the hFOB1.19 cells were evaluated with the ELISA method. The hFOB 1.19 cells were cultured in an osteoinductive medium with BET at a concentration of 0.1 µM or co-treated with SP600125 (5 µM), rapamycin (1 µM), or SCH772984 (1 µM). The osteoinductive medium supplemented with BET or BET plus the inhibitor was changed every three days. ALP activity was evaluated after 6 days with the colorimetric method with pNPP as a substrate for ALP. The OPN levels were measured after 9 days with the ELISA method. Mean ± SD from three independent experiments; ** $p < 0.01$, *** $p < 0.001$ in comparison to the control, one-way ANOVA with post hoc Dunnett's test (**A–D**) and Tukey's test (**E,F**).

2.5. BET-Induced Differentiation of hFOB 1.19 Cells Involves JNK, ERK1/2, and mTOR Activation

Since BET activated JNK, ERK1/2 and mTOR kinases in the normal human osteoblastic cell line hFOB 1.19 and all these kinases play an important role in osteoblast differentiation, further studies were undertaken to test whether the increased activity of these kinases is involved in BET-induced osteoblast differentiation. To this end, the hFOB 1.19 cells were treated with SP600125 (JNK inhibitor), SCH772984 (ERK1/2 inhibitor), or rapamycin (mTOR inhibitor) and co-treated with BET (0.1 µM). As shown in Figure 5E,F, all inhibitors significantly inhibited BET-induced ALP activity at day 6 of differentiation and OPN production at day 9 of hFOB 1.19 cell differentiation, i.e., an early and terminal marker of osteoblast differentiation, respectively. Thus, the results showed that the activation of JNK, ERK1/2, and mTOR is a critical factor in BET-induced differentiation of normal osteoblasts.

3. Discussion

Osteoporosis is now and will be a future health problem affecting Western countries due to the increasing longevity. Although new anti-osteoporotic agents with well-documented efficacy have been developed, there is a still need for a more effective anti-fracture strategy [36]. Therefore, new molecules that inhibit osteoclast formation and/or stimulate osteoblast differentiation and can be useful in the development of new anti-osteoporotic drugs are still being sought.

Betulin is a very interesting naturally occurring compound with a broad spectrum of biological activity [37]. Recently, it has been shown that BET possesses an ability to suppress osteoclast formation [38], which suggests that it has potential for prevention and/or therapeutic treatment of loss of bone mass. However, the osteogenic potential of BET has not been investigated so far. Moreover, only a few studies have been carried out on the osteogenic potential of some triterpenoids. For example, Lo et al. [30] showed the osteogenic potential of a betulin derivative, namely betulinic acid, in murine pre-osteoblast cell line MC3T3-E1. Moreover, Lee et al. [28] and Shim et al. [29] showed that ursolic acid and corosolic acid enhanced differentiation and mineralization of osteoblasts in the same murine osteoblast model (MC3T3-E1). Additionally, ursolic acid had bone-forming activity in vivo in a mouse calvarial bone formation model [28]. Thus, all these studies suggest that triterpenoids can stimulate osteoblast differentiation and enhance new bone formation. However, in all of these studies, only murine osteoblast models were used and the osteogenic potential of these compounds was tested in vitro in media with additional supplementation of ascorbic acid, i.e., a compound with well-established osteogenic activity [32,33].

In this study, we used two human osteoblast cell lines, i.e., a normal osteoblast cell line hFOB 1.19 and a neoplastic osteoblast-like cell line Saos-2. These commonly used models of osteoblast differentiation for in vitro research [39] were used to evaluate the effect of BET on osteoblast differentiation and mineralization in the osteogenic conditions. Moreover, the osteoinductive potential of BET in both models of osteoblasts and the underlying mechanism of its action in hFOB 1.19 cells were investigated. First, we evaluated the cytotoxic effect of BET in both cell lines. Although the results showed that BET exerted low cytotoxic activity against the hFOB 1.19 cells and higher cytotoxic activity against the Saos-2 cells, it significantly inhibited proliferation of both cell lines at such a low concentration as 1 µM. There are some reports indicating that BET exerted low cytotoxicity against human normal cells. For example, at concentrations below 10 µM, BET exerted no toxicity against human skin fibroblasts (HSF) [16]. Also, low cytotoxicity towards immortalized human epithelial cells (hTERT-RPE1 cell line) and human umbilical vein endothelial cells (HUVEC) with the IC_{50} value > 45 µM has been shown [40]. On the other hand, BET has been shown to exert a significant anti-proliferative effect against both human normal cells and neoplastic cells. For example, BET inhibited proliferation of human normal skin fibroblasts (WS1 cell line) with the IC_{50} value of 3.6 µM [41,42] and human neuroblastoma cells (SK-N-AS cell line) with the IC_{50} value of 2.5 µM [16]. Thus, the results of our study on the effect of BET on osteoblast proliferation are consistent with the results of other studies.

Given the significant anti-proliferative activity of BET towards human osteoblasts, in the studies on the osteogenic/osteoinductive potential of this compound, BET was tested only at low concentrations. Our present study showed a stimulatory effect of BET on the differentiation of osteoblasts in both the osteogenic and osteoinductive conditions.

During osteoblast differentiation in vitro, three phases of osteoblast phenotype development leading to bone formation can be distinguished: (1) cell proliferation; (2) extracellular matrix synthesis and maturation; (3) terminal differentiation with matrix mineralization. During these steps, the expression of appropriate genes/markers occurs temporally and sequentially, and the levels of expression of these genes are often used to monitor the progression of differentiation [43]. The induction of osteoblast differentiation is closely related to the positive regulation of RUNX2. Both, overexpression and/or elevated transcriptional activity of RUNX2 influence osteoblastic differentiation at the early stage [7,44]. It is detected in pre-osteoblasts and its expression is upregulated in immature osteoblasts, but downregulated in mature osteoblasts [7]. In our experiments, BET up-regulated *RUNX2* gene expression especially at day 9 and 12 of culture in both cell lines in the osteogenic and osteoinductive conditions. Consistently, BET significantly increased the production and/or mRNA expression of markers of osteoblast maturation and differentiation such as ALP, type I collagen and OPN, in both the osteogenic and osteoinductive conditions, except the ALP expression/activity in the Saos-2 cells. These results indicated indirectly that BET positively regulated RUNX2 because *ALPL*, *COL1A1* and *OPN* are target genes of this transcription factor [7,45]. However, as we did not examine the protein level of RUNX2 in the BET-treated osteoblasts, we can only suppose that BET could stimulate/induce osteoblast differentiation by increasing the level of this transcription factor or by increasing its transcriptional activity. It is well known that post-translational modifications such as phosphorylation and acetylation affect the transcriptional activity of RUNX2 [46]. For example, phosphorylation and activation of RUNX2 has been shown to be mediated by different kinases including ERK, protein kinases A and Cδ (PKA, PKCδ), Akt, homeodomain-interacting protein kinase 3 (HIPK3) or cyclin-dependent kinase-1 (CDK1). Also, ERK signaling-dependent acetylation results in stimulatory effect on RUNX2 activation and stability [46]. Given the multiple possible ways of RUNX2 regulation [46], this issue needs separate studies to determine the detailed mechanism of regulation of this transcription factor by BET in human osteoblasts.

The appearance of ALP activity is an early phenotypic marker of osteoblast maturation and synthesis of this enzyme is enhanced along the process of cell differentiation [47]. In our study, BET increased the expression of the *ALP* gene in the hFOB 1.19 cells in both the osteogenic and osteoinductive conditions, which suggests that the triterpene influenced an early stage of differentiation of these cells. In contrast, BET decreased the expression of the *ALP* gene in the Saos-2 cells at day 9 of culture in the osteoinductive conditions and ALP activity in these cells at the same time point in the osteogenic conditions. However, in contrast to hFOB 1.19 pre-osteoblasts, Saos-2 cells have a mature osteoblast phenotype with a high endogenous level of ALP activity [39]. Thus, the phenomenon observed may suggest that BET accelerated the differentiation of the Saos-2 cells.

Type I collagen is the main protein of bone matrix and acts as a scaffold for the nucleation of hydroxyapatite crystals. It is a phenotypic marker for a late stage of osteoblast differentiation. In turn, OPN is a non-collagenous bone matrix protein synthesized and secreted by osteoblastic cells in the terminal stage of differentiation [43]. In our experiments, the treatment of the hFOB1.19 and Saos-2 cells with BET increased the expression of *COL1A1* and *SPP1* (OPN) genes in both the osteogenic and osteoinductive conditions, which additionally correlated directly to the protein level of these markers in the osteogenic conditions. Thus, our results proved that BET stimulated the late stages of osteoblast differentiation as well. Moreover, the osteogenic/osteoinductive activity of BET was further proved, as the treatment of both the hFOB 1.19 and Saos-2 cells with BET enhanced the formation of mineralized nodules significantly, which is a morphological manifestation of osteogenesis.

There are reports indicating that BET has ability to interact with melanocortin receptors [48], which are also detected on osteoblasts [49]. However, BET itself did not stimulate cyclic adenosine 3′,5′-monophosphate (cAMP), i.e., second messenger, generation after melanocortin receptor ligation [48]. On the other hand, BET is a compound with high cell permeability [50], which suggests that it can directly activate different signaling pathways after entering into cells. For example, it has been shown that BET activates the signal transducer and activator of transcription 3 (STAT3) pathway [51]. For this reason, we can suppose that BET had osteogenic activity through direct activation of some kinases.

Since osteogenesis is mediated among others by JNK, ERK1/2, and p38 signaling pathways [8], we evaluated the activation of these kinases in order to elucidate the mechanism by which BET acts on osteoblasts. Considering the osteoblast differentiation, ERK has been reported to regulate the process by regulating the activity of RUNX2 [52]. It was described that numerous bone-active factors, including fibroblast growth factor (FGF), insulin-like growth factors (IGFs), or estrogen, induce ERK signaling in osteoblasts [8,53]. The p38 signaling in turn is activated by TGF-β and bone morphogenetic proteins (BMPs), and controls RUNX2 activity as well. However, recent evidence suggests that ERK and p38 may be responsible for different osteoblast responses [8]. The JNK signaling is activated by cytokines, including BMPs, and different kinds of stress [53]. This pathway is involved in osteoblast differentiation through activation of the osteogenesis-related transcription factors such as AP-1 or ATF4 [12,54]. In the present study, BET enhanced ERK1/2 and JNK phosphorylation in the hFOB 1.19 cells although it did not affect p38 activation. Moreover, pretreatment of these cells with the JNK inhibitor (SP600125) or ERK inhibitor (SCH772984) abolished the BET-induced increase in the ALP activity and OPN production. These data suggest an essential role of the JNK and ERK signaling pathways in BET-induced osteoblast differentiation.

mTOR kinase is a component of two distinct multi-protein complexes, mTORC1 and mTORC2, which can be distinguished by their essential factors such as Raptor for mTORC1 and Rictor for mTORC2 [55]. mTOR is a central coordinator of fundamental biological processes such as cell growth, cell-cycle progression, and cell differentiation. It is activated by a multitude of intracellular end extracellular signals [55]. Both mTOR complexes are activated by various growth factors including bone anabolic signals such as IGF-1, Wnt, or BMP-2 [56–60]. Recent studies have established that mTORC1 and mTORC2 are implicated in regulating osteoblast differentiation and function [9]. Moreover, it has been shown that rapamycin, a specific inhibitor of mTOR, significantly reduced the levels of the Runx2 protein and the expression of other osteoblast differentiation markers in differentiating osteoblasts [61]. Our present study demonstrated for the first time that BET at low concentrations induced phosphorylation of mTOR in human osteoblasts. Moreover, pretreatment of these cells with rapamycin abolished the BET-induced increase in the ALP activity and OPN production, indicating the importance of the mTOR pathway in BET-induced osteoblast differentiation.

3.1. Reagent

Betulin (BET) was purchased from Sigma-Aldrich Chemicals (St. Louis, MO, USA). A stock solution of BET was prepared in DMSO (Sigma) and stored at 4 °C until use. The final concentration of DMSO in all experiments was lower than 0.01%, and all treatment conditions were compared with vehicle controls. The triterpenoid stock solution was diluted in a culture medium immediately before use.

3.2. Cell Cultures

The human fetal osteoblastic cell line hFOB 1.19 (CRL-11372^{TM}) was obtained from the American Type Culture Collection (ATCC, Manassas, VA, USA). The cells were maintained in a growth medium containing a 1:1 mixture of Dulbecco's Modified Eagle's Medium without phenol red and Ham's F12 medium, supplemented with 2.5 mM of L-glutamine, 0.3 mg/mL of G418, antibiotic/antimycotic solution (all from Sigma), and 10% of fetal bovine serum, FBS (Thermo Fisher Scientific, Gibco, Waltham, MA, USA) in a humidified 5% CO_2 atmosphere at a permissive temperature of 34 °C. The human osteoblast-like cell line of osteosarcoma Saos-2 (HTB-85^{TM}) was purchased in ATCC. Saos-2 cells were maintained in McCoy's 5A Modified Medium (Sigma) supplemented with an antibiotic/antimycotic solution and 10% FBS in a humidified 5% CO_2 atmosphere at a temperature of 37 °C.

The modulatory influence of BET on differentiation of osteoblasts was examined in cells cultivated in osteogenic media, which consisted of the basal medium for each cell line supplemented with 1% (hFOB 1.19) or 2% (Saos-2) FBS and additionally 10 mM of β-glycerophosphate (Sigma) (hFOB 1.19) and 50 µg/mL of ascorbic phosphate-magnesium salt (Sigma) (both cell lines). The osteoinductive activity of BET was examined in cells cultivated in basal medium with 1% (hFOB1.19) or 2% (Saos-2) FBS and without any osteogenic supplements (osteoinductive medium). During the osteoblast differentiation experiments, the media were changed every three days and the cells were cultured for up to 18 days.

3.3. Cytotoxicity Assay

The cytotoxicity of BET towards osteoblasts was estimated by measurement of lactate dehydrogenase (LDH) activity (Tox-7, Sigma). The cells were seeded in 96-well microplates at a density of 3×10^4 cells/well (hFOB 1.19) or 5×10^4 cells/well (Saos-2) in 100 µL of a complete growth medium. The next day, the medium was changed to a new one containing 1% FBS and the cells were exposed to various concentrations of BET (0.1–25 µM). After 24 h of incubation, LDH activity was examined in culture supernatants according to the manufacturer's instruction. The absorbance measurement was performed at a wavelength of 450 nm using an E-max Microplate Reader (Molecular Devices Corporation, Menlo Park, CA, USA).

3.4. Cell Proliferation Assay

The cells were seeded into 96-well plates at a density of 3×10^3 cells/well (hFOB 1.19) or 5×10^3 cells/well (Saos-2) in 100 µL of a complete growth medium. After 24 h, the culture medium was removed and the cells were exposed to BET (0.01–25 µM). Cell proliferation was measured after 96 h of incubation by the MTT assay. The cells were incubated for 3 h with 20 microliters of 5 mg/mL 3-(4,5-dimethylthiazol-2-yl)-2,5-diphenyltetrazolium bromide solution (MTT, Sigma). Next, formazan crystals were solubilized overnight in SDS buffer (10 % SDS in 0.01 N HCl) and absorbance of the product was measured at a wavelength of 570 nm using the E-max Microplate Reader (Molecular Devices Corporation, Menlo Park, CA, USA).

The expression of *ALPL*, *COL1A1*, *SPP1*, *Runx2*, and β-actin (*ACTB*) genes were analyzed by quantitative real-time PCR (RT-qPCR). After cell harvesting, total cellular RNA from each sample was isolated using the QIAamp® RNA Blood Mini Kit (QIAGEN® GmbH, Hilden, Germany) according to the manufacturer's protocol. cDNA was synthesized by reverse transcription of 1 µg of total RNA for 30 min at 42 °C using a QuantiTect®Reverse Transcription Kit (QIAGEN®) according to the manufacturer's protocol. RT-qPCR was performed using a TaqMan Gene Expression Assay probe/primer specific for each analyzed marker (*ALPL* – Hs01029144, *COL1A1* – Hs00164004, *SPP1* – Hs00959010, *Runx2* - Hs00231692) and internal control β-actin (human ACTB Endogenous Control VIC/MGB Probe, Applied Biosystems, Carlsbad, CA, USA). The real-time PCR was performed using 1 µL of cDNA template of each sample and 2.5 µL of the specific primer in 50 µL of the reaction mixture. The amplification was performed on a CFX96™ Real-Time PCR Detection System C1000 Touch™ (Bio-Rad Laboratories, Hercules, CA, USA) using the following cycle parameters: 95 °C for 10 min followed by 40 cycles (or 60 cycles in the case of Runx2) at 95 °C for 15 s and 60 °C for 1 min. All reactions were run in triplicate, and data were analyzed using the threshold cycle (CT) and the $2^{-\Delta CT}$ method. The mRNA level in the control (untreated cells; 0 µM) was considered as 1. The results of gene expression were presented as a fold change in comparison with the control.

3.5. Alkaline Phosphatase Activity Assay

The ALP activity was assessed using the colorimetric method. To this end, the cells were plated on 96-well microplates (5×10^3 cells/well) in the growth medium and cultivated for 2-3 days to obtain a confluent monolayer. Then, the cells were grown in the osteogenic medium without or with BET (0.01 and 0.1 µM). In some experiments, the hFOB 1.19 cells were exposed to BET (0.1 µM) without or in combination with SCH772984 (an ERK1/2 inhibitor, 1 µM, Selleck Chemicals LLC, Houston, TX, USA), SP600125 (a JNK inhibitor, 5 µM, Sigma), or rapamycin (an mTOR inhibitor, 1 µM, Sigma) in osteoinductive conditions. ALP activity was assayed as previously described [58]. The absorbance was determined at a wavelength of 405 nm using an E-max Microplate Reader (Molecular Devices Corporation, Menlo Park, CA, USA). The total protein concentration in the cell lysates was determined by incubation with a bicinchoninic acid protein assay reagent (Pierce® BCA Protein Assay Kit; Thermo Fisher Scientific, Rockford, IL, USA). ALP activity was calibrated with a p-nitrophenol (pNP) standard curve and calculated as µM of pNP/mg of total protein concentration.

3.6. Western Blot Analysis of Type I Collagen Level

The collagen type 1A1 (Col1A1) level was determined by western blot analysis as previously described [62]. Briefly, the cells were seeded into 25 cm^2 plastic flasks (Nunc, Roskilde, Denmark). After 2–3 days of incubation, the growth medium was removed and the osteogenic medium without or with BET (0.01 and 0.1 µM) was added. After an appropriate incubation time, cells were harvested, lysed in RIPA buffer (Sigma) supplemented with protease and phosphatase inhibitor cocktail (Sigma), and centrifuged (14,000 rpm for 10 min at 4 °C). The total protein concentrations were determined using a Pierce BCA Protein Assay Kit (Thermo Fisher Scientific) according to the manufacturer's instructions. Primary rabbit polyclonal antibodies against collagen α1 type I (COL1A1) of human origin (1:500; sc8784-R) were purchased from Santa Cruz Biotechnology Inc. (Dallas, TX, USA). The primary antibodies were detected by horseradish peroxidase (HRP)-conjugated goat anti-rabbit secondary antibodies (Amersham™ GE Healthcare, Buckinghamshire, UK). The enhanced chemiluminescence method (ECL™ Western Blotting Analysis System, Amersham Bioscience) was used to detect protein bands according to the manufacturer's protocol. After incubation with the substrate, membranes were visualized and analyzed by means of Molecular Imager®ChemiDoc™ XRS+ (Bio-Rad Laboratories, Hercules, CA, USA) equipped with Image Lab™ Version 3.0 Software for measurement of protein band intensity. The COL1A1 bands were determined on the basis of molecular mass using Precision Plus Protein™ Standards (Bio-Rad Laboratories, Hercules, CA, USA). The blots used for collagen detection were stripped and reprobed with anti β-actin antibodies (1:500, AC-74, Sigma) used as a load control. The COL1A1 band densities were normalized to that of β-actin. The changes in the COL1A1 level were expressed as a % of the control level (100%).

3.7. Assay of Osteopontin Production

The concentrations of OPN in the cell culture media were estimated by the ELISA method. Cells were seeded into 24-well plates in the growth medium. After 24 h, the culture medium was removed and the osteogenic medium without or with BET (0.01 and 0.1 µM) was added. In some experiments, hFOB 1.19 cells were exposed to BET (0.1 µM) without or in combination with SCH772984 (an ERK inhibitor, 1µM), SP600125 (a JNK1/2 inhibitor, 5 µM), or rapamycin (1 µM) in osteoinductive conditions. After the indicated time of incubation, the cell culture media were collected, centrifuged, and stored at −80 °C. The OPN level was measured using a RayBio® Human Osteopontin ELISA kit (RayBiotech, Inc., Atlanta, GA, USA) according the manufacturer's protocol. The OPN concentration in control samples (without BET) was considered as 100%. The OPN level in samples collected from the BET and/or inhibitors-treated cell cultures were expressed as a % of control.

3.8. Alizarin Red S Staining

The degree of the extracellular matrix mineralization was determined using Alizarin Red S (ARS, Sigma) staining of cultured osteoblasts to detect bone nodules (calcium precipitates) as previously described [63]. The ARS-stained cell cultures were examined under a light microscope. Finally, the incorporated ARS dye was extracted from the cell cultures with 10% cetylpiridinium chloride in 10 mM sodium phosphate (pH = 7) for 1 h at 37 °C. The extracted stain was transferred to a 96-well plate and the absorbance at 562 nm was measured using an E-max Microplate Reader. The level of ARS stain extracted from the control cell cultures was considered as 100%. The calcium deposition level in the BET-treated cell cultures was expressed as % of control.

3.9. ELISA Assay of MAP Kinases and mTOR Activation

The quantification of the intracellular levels of total and phosphorylated JNK, ERK1/2, p38, and mTOR kinases in the BET-treated hFOB 1.19 cells was carried out using the following PathScan® ELISA kits: phospho-SAPK/JNK (Thr183/Tyr185), total SAPK/JNK, phospho-p44/42 MAPK (Thr202/Tyr204), total p44/42 (ERK 1/2), phospho-p38 MAPK (Thr180/Tyr182), phospho-mTOR (Ser2448) and total mTOR

Sandwich ELISA Kit (Cell Signaling Technology, Danvers, MA, USA), and p38 MAPK alpha ELISA Kit (Abcam, Cambridge, UK), according to the manufacturer's instructions. Briefly, hFOB 1.19 cells were seeded into 10-cm diameter plastic plates and cultured in the growth medium until confluency. Then, the medium was removed and the osteoinductive medium supplemented (or not) with BET (0.5 µM) was added. After 6 or 24 h of exposure, the media were removed and the cells were lysed in lysis buffer supplemented with PMSF (Sigma) and protease and phosphatase inhibitor cocktail (Sigma) according to the manufacturer's protocol. The cell lysates were centrifuged at 14,000 rpm for 5 min at 4 °C and stored at −80 °C until analysis. Before the assay, the total protein concentrations in the cell lysates were determined with a Pierce BCA Protein Assay Kit (Thermo Fisher Scientific), and samples containing equal amounts of total proteins per 100 µL of sample diluent were subjected to ELISA.

3.10. Statistical Analyses

Each experiment was repeated at least three times. Statistical analyses were performed using GraphPAD Prism v5 (GraphPAD Software Inc., San Diego, CA, USA). The data were analyzed by one-way ANOVA followed by Dunnett's or Tukey's tests for multiple comparisons between pairs. The p values < 0.05 were considered statistically significant.

4. Conclusions

In summary, the present study demonstrated that betulin promoted osteogenesis in vitro in human osteoblasts models in osteogenic conditions. Moreover, our studies suggest that BET can induce osteoblast differentiation via JNK, ERK1/2 and mTOR kinase-dependent signaling pathways. Noteworthy, BET exerted a pro-osteogenic effect at the low, non-toxic concentrations. Given the satisfactory bioavailability of BET at the diverse routes of administration [64,65], we can conclude that this compound has the potential to be used as a medicine or supplement in treatment of bone osteoporotic lesions, especially since the recent studies [38] indicated the anti-osteoclastic activity of BET. However, further in vivo studies in animal models are necessary to confirm the potential of BET to enhance osteogenesis.

Author Contributions: Conceptualization, M.M.-K. and B.Z.; methodology and investigations, M.M.-K., A.S.-B., K.K., A.Ż., B.P., B.Z.; formal analysis, M.M.-K. and B.Z.; writing—original draft preparation, B.Z. and M.M.-K.; writing—review & editing, W.R. and B.Z.

Funding: This study was supported by Maria Curie-Sklodowska University funds.

Conflicts of Interest: The authors declare that there is no conflict of interests.

References

1. Florencio-Silva, R.; Sasso, G.R.D.S.; Sasso-Cerri, E.; Simões, M.J.; Cerri, P.S. Biology of Bone Tissue: Structure, Function, and Factors That Influence Bone Cells. *Biomed Res. Int.* **2015**, *2015*, 1–17. [CrossRef] [PubMed]
2. Eriksen, E.F. Cellular mechanisms of bone remodeling. *Rev. Endocr. Metab. Disord.* **2010**, *11*, 219–227. [CrossRef] [PubMed]
3. Rodan, G.A.; Martin, T.J. Therapeutic approaches to bone diseases. *Science* **2000**, *289*, 1508–1514. [CrossRef] [PubMed]
4. Curtis, E.M.; Moon, R.J.; Harvey, N.C.; Cooper, C. The impact of fragility fracture and approaches to osteoporosis risk assessment worldwide. *Bone* **2017**, *104*, 29–38. [CrossRef] [PubMed]
5. Skjødt, M.K.; Frost, M.; Abrahamsen, B. Side effects of drugs for osteoporosis and metastatic bone disease. *Br. J. Clin. Pharmacol.* **2018**, *85*, 1063–1071. [CrossRef] [PubMed]
6. Rossini, M.; Adami, G.; Adami, S.; Viapiana, O.; Gatti, D. Safety issues and adverse reactions with osteoporosis management. *Expert Opin. Drug Saf.* **2016**, *15*, 321–332. [CrossRef] [PubMed]
7. Komori, T. Regulation of bone development and extracellular matrix protein genes by RUNX2. *Cell Tissue Res.* **2010**, *339*, 189–195. [CrossRef]
8. Franceschi, R.T.; Ge, C. Control of the Osteoblast Lineage by Mitogen-Activated Protein Kinase Signaling. *Curr. Mol. Biol. Rep.* **2017**, *3*, 122–132. [CrossRef]

9. Chen, J.; Long, F. mTOR signaling in skeletal development and disease. *Bone Res.* **2018**, *6*, 1. [CrossRef]
10. Ge, C.; Xiao, G.; Jiang, D.; Yang, Q.; Hatch, N.E.; Roca, H.; Franceschi, R.T. Identification and Functional Characterization of ERK/MAPK Phosphorylation Sites in the Runx2 Transcription Factor. *J. Biol. Chem.* **2009**, *284*, 32533–32543. [CrossRef]
11. Greenblatt, M.B.; Shim, J.-H.; Zou, W.; Sitara, D.; Schweitzer, M.; Hu, D.; Lotinun, S.; Sano, Y.; Baron, R.; Park, J.M.; et al. The p38 MAPK pathway is essential for skeletogenesis and bone homeostasis in mice. *J. Clin. Investig.* **2010**, *120*, 2457–2473. [CrossRef]
12. Matsuguchi, T.; Chiba, N.; Bandow, K.; Kakimoto, K.; Masuda, A.; Ohnishi, T. JNK Activity Is Essential for Atf4 Expression and Late-Stage Osteoblast Differentiation. *J. Bone Miner. Res.* **2009**, *24*, 398–410. [CrossRef]
13. Dai, Q.; Xu, Z.; Ma, X.; Niu, N.; Zhou, S.; Xie, F.; Jiang, L.; Wang, J.; Zou, W. mTOR/Raptor signaling is critical for skeletogenesis in mice through the regulation of Runx2 expression. *Cell Death Differ.* **2017**, *24*, 1886–1899. [CrossRef]
14. Alakurtti, S.; Mäkelä, T.; Koskimies, S.; Yli-Kauhaluoma, J. Pharmacological properties of the ubiquitous natural product betulin. *Eur. J. Pharm. Sci.* **2006**, *29*, 1–13. [CrossRef]
15. Rastogi, S.; Pandey, M.M.; Kumar Singh Rawat, A. Medicinal plants of the genus Betula–traditional uses and a phytochemical-pharmacological review. *J. Ethnopharmacol.* **2015**, *159*, 62–83. [CrossRef]
16. Rzeski, W.; Stepulak, A.; Szymański, M.; Juszczak, M.; Grabarska, A.; Sifringer, M.; Kaczor, J.; Kandefer-Szerszeń, M. Betulin Elicits Anti-Cancer Effects in Tumour Primary Cultures and Cell Lines In Vitro. *Basic Clin. Pharmacol. Toxicol.* **2009**, *105*, 425–432.
17. Mullauer, F.B.; Kessler, J.H.; Medema, J.P. Betulin Is a Potent Anti-Tumor Agent that Is Enhanced by Cholesterol. *PLoS ONE* **2009**, *4*, e1. [CrossRef]
18. Król, S.K.; Kiełbus, M.; Rivero-Müller, A.; Stepulak, A. Comprehensive Review on Betulin as a Potent Anticancer Agent. *Biomed Res. Int.* **2015**, *2015*, 1–11. [CrossRef]
19. Pavlova, N.I.; Savinova, O.V.; Nikolaeva, S.N.; Boreko, E.I.; Flekhter, O.B. Antiviral activity of betulin, betulinic and betulonic acids against some enveloped and non-enveloped viruses. *Fitoterapia* **2003**, *74*, 489–492. [CrossRef]
20. Gong, Y.; Raj, K.; Luscombe, C.; Gadawski, I.; Tam, T.; Chu, J.; Gibson, D.; Carlson, R.; Sacks, S. The synergistic effects of betulin with acyclovir against herpes simplex viruses. *Antiviral Res.* **2004**, *64*, 127–130. [CrossRef]
21. Copp, B.R.; Pearce, A.N. Natural product growth inhibitors of Mycobacterium tuberculosis. *Nat. Prod. Rep.* **2007**, *24*, 278–297. [CrossRef]
22. Zdzisińska, B.; Rzeski, W.; Paduch, R.; Szuster-Ciesielska, A.; Kaczor, J.; Wejksza, K.; Kandefer-Szerszeń, M. Differential effect of betulin and betulinic acid on cytokine production in human whole blood cell cultures. *Pol. J. Pharmacol.* **2003**, *55*, 235–238.
23. Szuster-Ciesielska, A.; Kandefer-Szerszeń, M. Protective effects of betulin and betulinic acid against ethanol-induced cytotoxicity in HepG2 cells. *Pharmacol. Rep.* **2005**, *57*, 588–595.
24. Szuster-Ciesielska, A.; Plewka, K.; Daniluk, J.; Kandefer-Szerszeń, M. Betulin and betulinic acid attenuate ethanol-induced liver stellate cell activation by inhibiting reactive oxygen species (ROS), cytokine (TNF-α, TGF-β) production and by influencing intracellular signaling. *Toxicology* **2011**, *280*, 152–163. [CrossRef]
25. Xia, A.; Xue, Z.; Li, Y.; Wang, W.; Xia, J.; Wei, T.; Cao, J.; Zhou, W. Cardioprotective effect of betulinic Acid on myocardial ischemia reperfusion injury in rats. *Evid. Based Complement. Altern. Med.* **2014**, *2014*. [CrossRef]
26. de Souza, M.T.; Buzzi, F.D.C.; Cechinel Filho, V.; Hess, S.; Della Monache, F.; Niero, R. Phytochemical and antinociceptive properties of Matayba elaeagnoides Radlk. barks. *Z. Naturforsch. C* **2007**, *62*, 550–554. [CrossRef]
27. Tang, J.-J.; Li, J.-G.; Qi, W.; Qiu, W.-W.; Li, P.-S.; Li, B.-L.; Song, B.-L. Inhibition of SREBP by a Small Molecule, Betulin, Improves Hyperlipidemia and Insulin Resistance and Reduces Atherosclerotic Plaques. *Cell Metab.* **2011**, *13*, 44–56. [CrossRef]
28. Lee, S.; Park, S.; Kwak, H.; Oh, J.; Min, Y.; Kim, S. Anabolic activity of ursolic acid in bone: Stimulating osteoblast differentiation in vitro and inducing new bone formation in vivo. *Pharmacol. Res.* **2008**, *58*, 290–296. [CrossRef]
29. Shim, K.S.; Lee, S.-U.; Ryu, S.Y.; Min, Y.K.; Kim, S.H. Corosolic acid stimulates osteoblast differentiation by activating transcription factors and MAP kinases. *Phyther. Res.* **2009**, *23*, 1754–1758. [CrossRef]

30. Lo, Y.-C.; Chang, Y.-H.; Wei, B.-L.; Huang, Y.-L.; Chiou, W.-F. Betulinic Acid Stimulates the Differentiation and Mineralization of Osteoblastic MC3T3-E1 Cells: Involvement of BMP/Runx2 and β-Catenin Signals. *J. Agric. Food Chem.* **2010**, *58*, 6643–6649. [CrossRef]
31. Choi, H.; Jeong, B.-C.; Kook, M.-S.; Koh, J.-T. Betulinic acid synergically enhances BMP2-induced bone formation via stimulating Smad 1/5/8 and p38 pathways. *J. Biomed. Sci.* **2016**, *23*, 45. [CrossRef]
32. Franceschi, R.T.; Iyer, B.S.; Cui, Y. Effects of ascorbic acid on collagen matrix formation and osteoblast differentiation in murine MC3T3-E1 cells. *J. Bone Miner. Res.* **2009**, *9*, 843–854. [CrossRef]
33. Takamizawa, S.; Maehata, Y.; Imai, K.; Senoo, H.; Sato, S.; Hata, R.-I. Effects of ascorbic acid and ascorbic acid 2-phosphate, a long-acting vitamin C derivative, on the proliferation and differentiation of human osteoblast-like cells. *Cell Biol. Int.* **2004**, *28*, 255–265. [CrossRef]
34. Legrand, C.; Bour, J.M.; Jacob, C.; Capiaumont, J.; Martial, A.; Marc, A.; Wudtke, M.; Kretzmer, G.; Demangel, C.; Duval, D. Lactate dehydrogenase (LDH) activity of the cultured eukaryotic cells as marker of the number of dead cells in the medium [corrected]. *J. Biotechnol.* **1992**, *25*, 231–243. [CrossRef]
35. Hsu, Y.-L.; Kuo, P.-L. Diosmetin Induces Human Osteoblastic Differentiation Through the Protein Kinase C/p38 and Extracellular Signal-Regulated Kinase 1/2 Pathway. *J. Bone Miner. Res.* **2008**, *23*, 949–960. [CrossRef]
36. Anagnostis, P.; Gkekas, N.K.; Potoupnis, M.; Kenanidis, E.; Tsiridis, E.; Goulis, D.G. New therapeutic targets for osteoporosis. *Maturitas* **2019**, *120*, 1–6. [CrossRef]
37. Dzubak, P.; Hajduch, M.; Vydra, D.; Hustova, A.; Kvasnica, M.; Biedermann, D.; Markova, L.; Urban, M.; Sarek, J. Pharmacological activities of natural triterpenoids and their therapeutic implications. *Nat. Prod. Rep.* **2006**, *23*, 394–411. [CrossRef]
38. Kim, K.-J.; Lee, Y.; Hwang, H.-G.; Sung, S.; Lee, M.; Son, Y.-J. Betulin Suppresses Osteoclast Formation via Down-Regulating NFATc1. *J. Clin. Med.* **2018**, *7*, 154. [CrossRef]
39. Czekanska, E.M.; Stoddart, M.J.; Richards, R.G.; Hayes, J.S. In search of an osteoblast cell model for in vitro research. *Eur. Cell. Mater.* **2012**, *24*, 1–17. [CrossRef]
40. Hwang, B.Y.; Chai, H.-B.; Kardono, L.B.S.; Riswan, S.; Farnsworth, N.R.; Cordell, G.A.; Pezzuto, J.M.; Kinghorn, A.D. Cytotoxic triterpenes from the twigs of Celtis philippinensis. *Phytochemistry* **2003**, *62*, 197–201. [CrossRef]
41. Gauthier, C.; Legault, J.; Lebrun, M.; Dufour, P.; Pichette, A. Glycosidation of lupane-type triterpenoids as potent in vitro cytotoxic agents. *Bioorg. Med. Chem.* **2006**, *14*, 6713–6725. [CrossRef]
42. Gauthier, C.; Legault, J.; Lavoie, S.; Rondeau, S.; Tremblay, S.; Pichette, A. Synthesis and Cytotoxicity of Bidesmosidic Betulin and Betulinic Acid Saponins. *J. Nat. Prod.* **2009**, *72*, 72–81. [CrossRef]
43. Neve, A.; Corrado, A.; Cantatore, F.P. Osteoblast physiology in normal and pathological conditions. *Cell Tissue Res.* **2011**, *343*, 289–302. [CrossRef]
44. Shui, C.; Spelsberg, T.C.; Riggs, B.L.; Khosla, S. Changes in Runx2/Cbfa1 Expression and Activity During Osteoblastic Differentiation of Human Bone Marrow Stromal Cells. *J. Bone Miner. Res.* **2003**, *18*, 213–221. [CrossRef]
45. Weng, J.; Su, Y. Nuclear matrix-targeting of the osteogenic factor Runx2 is essential for its recognition and activation of the alkaline phosphatase gene. *Biochim. Biophys. Acta Gen. Subj.* **2013**, *1830*, 2839–2852. [CrossRef]
46. Bruderer, M.; Richards, R.G.; Alini, M.; Stoddart, M.J. Role and regulation of RUNX2 in osteogenesis. *Eur. Cell Mater.* **2014**, *28*, 269–286. [CrossRef]
47. Marom, R.; Shur, I.; Solomon, R.; Benayahu, D. Characterization of adhesion and differentiation markers of osteogenic marrow stromal cells. *J. Cell. Physiol.* **2005**, *202*, 41–48. [CrossRef]
48. Muceniece, R.; Saleniece, K.; Riekstina, U.; Krigere, L.; Tirzitis, G.; Ancans, J. Betulin binds to melanocortin receptors and antagonizesα-melanocyte stimulating hormone induced cAMP generation in mouse melanoma cells. *Cell Biochem. Funct.* **2007**, *25*, 591–596. [CrossRef]
49. Zhong, Q.; Sridhar, S.; Ruan, L.; Ding, K.; Xie, D.; Insogna, K.; Kang, B.; Xu, J.; Bollag, R.; Isales, C. Multiple melanocortin receptors are expressed in bone cells. *Bone* **2005**, *36*, 820–831. [CrossRef]
50. Zhao, X.; Wang, W.; Zu, Y.; Zhang, Y.; Li, Y.; Sun, W.; Shan, C.; Ge, Y. Preparation and characterization of betulin nanoparticles for oral hypoglycemic drug by antisolvent precipitation. *Drug Deliv.* **2014**, *21*, 467–479. [CrossRef]

51. Zhang, S.-Y.; Zhao, Q.-F.; Fang, N.-N.; Yu, J.-G. Betulin inhibits pro-inflammatory cytokines expression through activation STAT3 signaling pathway in human cardiac cells. *Eur. Rev. Med. Pharmacol. Sci.* **2015**, *19*, 455–460.
52. Xiao, G.; Jiang, D.; Thomas, P.; Benson, M.D.; Guan, K.; Karsenty, G.; Franceschi, R.T. MAPK Pathways Activate and Phosphorylate the Osteoblast-specific Transcription Factor, Cbfa1. *J. Biol. Chem.* **2000**, *275*, 4453–4459. [CrossRef]
53. Chau, J.F.L.; Leong, W.F.; Li, B. Signaling pathways governing osteoblast proliferation, differentiation and function. *Histol. Histopathol.* **2009**, *24*, 1593–1606.
54. Jensen, E.D.; Gopalakrishnan, R.; Westendorf, J.J. Regulation of gene expression in osteoblasts. *Biofactors* **2010**, *36*, 25–32. [CrossRef]
55. Saxton, R.A.; Sabatini, D.M. mTOR Signaling in Growth, Metabolism, and Disease. *Cell* **2017**, *168*, 960–976. [CrossRef]
56. Chen, J.; Tu, X.; Esen, E.; Joeng, K.S.; Lin, C.; Arbeit, J.M.; Rüegg, M.A.; Hall, M.N.; Ma, L.; Long, F. WNT7B Promotes Bone Formation in part through mTORC1. *PLoS Genet.* **2014**, *10*, e1004145. [CrossRef]
57. Karner, C.M.; Long, F. Wnt signaling and cellular metabolism in osteoblasts. *Cell. Mol. Life Sci.* **2017**, *74*, 1649–1657. [CrossRef]
58. Xian, L.; Wu, X.; Pang, L.; Lou, M.; Rosen, C.J.; Qiu, T.; Crane, J.; Frassica, F.; Zhang, L.; Rodriguez, J.P.; et al. Matrix IGF-1 maintains bone mass by activation of mTOR in mesenchymal stem cells. *Nat. Med.* **2012**, *18*, 1095–1101. [CrossRef]
59. Esen, E.; Chen, J.; Karner, C.M.; Okunade, A.L.; Patterson, B.W.; Long, F. WNT-LRP5 Signaling Induces Warburg Effect through mTORC2 Activation during Osteoblast Differentiation. *Cell Metab.* **2013**, *17*, 745–755. [CrossRef]
60. Shi, Y.; Chen, J.; Karner, C.M.; Long, F. Hedgehog signaling activates a positive feedback mechanism involving insulin-like growth factors to induce osteoblast differentiation. *Proc. Natl. Acad. Sci. USA* **2015**, *112*, 4678–4683. [CrossRef]
61. Singha, U.K.; Jiang, Y.; Yu, S.; Luo, M.; Lu, Y.; Zhang, J.; Xiao, G. Rapamycin inhibits osteoblast proliferation and differentiation in MC3T3-E1 cells and primary mouse bone marrow stromal cells. *J. Cell. Biochem.* **2008**, *103*, 434–446. [CrossRef]
62. Sławińska-Brych, A.; Zdzisińska, B.; Dmoszyńska-Graniczka, M.; Jeleniewicz, W.; Kurzepa, J.; Gagoś, M.; Stepulak, A. Xanthohumol inhibits the extracellular signal regulated kinase (ERK) signalling pathway and suppresses cell growth of lung adenocarcinoma cells. *Toxicology* **2016**, *357–358*, 65–73. [CrossRef]
63. Żurek, A.; Mizerska-Kowalska, M.; Sławińska-Brych, A.; Kaławaż, K.; Bojarska-Junak, A.; Kandefer-Szerszeń, M.; Zdzisińska, B. Alpha ketoglutarate exerts a pro-osteogenic effect in osteoblast cell lines through activation of JNK and mTOR/S6K1/S6 signaling pathways. *Toxicol. Appl. Pharmacol.* **2019**, *374*, 53–64. [CrossRef]
64. Jäger, S.; Laszczyk, M.; Scheffler, A. A Preliminary Pharmacokinetic Study of Betulin, the Main Pentacyclic Triterpene from Extract of Outer Bark of Birch (Betulae alba cortex). *Molecules* **2008**, *13*, 3224–3235. [CrossRef]
65. Pozharitskaya, O.N.; Karlina, M.V.; Shikov, A.N.; Kosman, V.M.; Makarov, V.G.; Casals, E.; Rosenholm, J.M. Pharmacokinetics and Tissue Disposition of Nanosystem-Entrapped Betulin After Endotracheal Administration to Rats. *Eur. J. Drug Metab. Pharmacokinet.* **2017**, *42*, 327–332. [CrossRef]

Sample Availability: Not available.

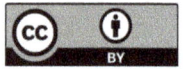

© 2019 by the authors. Licensee MDPI, Basel, Switzerland. This article is an open access article distributed under the terms and conditions of the Creative Commons Attribution (CC BY) license (http://creativecommons.org/licenses/by/4.0/).

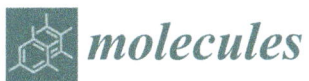

Communication

New 11,20-Epoxybriaranes from the Gorgonian Coral *Junceella fragilis* (Ellisellidae)

Chia-Cheng Lin [1], Jui-Hsin Su [2,3], Wu-Fu Chen [1,4], Zhi-Hong Wen [4], Bo-Rong Peng [2], Lin-Cyuan Huang [2,3,*], Tsong-Long Hwang [5,6,7,8,9,10,*] and Ping-Jyun Sung [2,3,4,11,12,*]

[1] Department of Neurosurgery, Kaohsiung Chang Gung Memorial Hospital and Chang Gung University College of Medicine, Kaohsiung 833, Taiwan
[2] National Museum of Marine Biology and Aquarium, Pingtung 944, Taiwan
[3] Graduate Institute of Marine Biology, National Dong Hwa University, Pingtung 944, Taiwan
[4] Department of Marine Biotechnology and Resources, National Sun Yat-sen University, Kaohsiung 804, Taiwan
[5] Research Center for Chinese Herbal Medicine, College of Human Ecology, Chang Gung University of Science and Technology, Taoyuan 333, Taiwan
[6] Research Center for Food and Cosmetic Safety, College of Human Ecology, Chang Gung University of Science and Technology, Taoyuan 333, Taiwan
[7] Graduate Institute of Healthy Industry Technology, College of Human Ecology, Chang Gung University of Science and Technology, Taoyuan 333, Taiwan
[8] Graduate Institute of Natural Products, College of Medicine, Chang Gung University, Taoyuan 333, Taiwan
[9] Chinese Herbal Medicine Research Team, Healthy Aging Research Center, Chang Gung University, Taoyuan 333, Taiwan
[10] Department of Anaesthesiology, Chang Gung Memorial Hospital, Taoyuan 333, Taiwan
[11] Graduate Institute of Natural Products, Kaohsiung Medical University, Kaohsiung 807, Taiwan
[12] Chinese Medicine Research and Development Center, China Medical University Hospital, Taichung 404, Taiwan
* Correspondence: bigpa830123@gmail.com (L.-C.H.); htl@mail.cgu.edu.tw (T.-L.H.); pjsung@nmmba.gov.tw (P.-J.S.); Tel.: +886-8-882-5001 (ext. 1384) (L.-C.H.); +886-3-211-8800 (ext. 5523) (T.-L.H.); +886-8-882-5037 (P.-J.S.); Fax: +886-8-882-5087 (L.-C.H. & P.-J.S.); +886-3-211-8506 (T.-L.H.)

Academic Editors: Pavel B. Drasar and Vladimir A. Khripach
Received: 14 June 2019; Accepted: 5 July 2019; Published: 7 July 2019

Abstract: Two new 11,20-epoxybriaranes, fragilides P (**1**) and Q (**2**), as well as two known analogues, robustolide F (**3**) and juncin Z (**4**), were obtained from the gorgonian coral *Junceella fragilis*. The structures, including the absolute configurations of briaranes **1** and **2**, were elucidated by using spectroscopic methods and comparing the spectroscopic and rotation data with those of known related analogues. Briarane **4** decreased the generation of superoxide anions by human neutrophils. The propionate group in **1** is rarely found.

Keywords: *Junceella fragilis*; fragilide; briarane; superoxide anion

1. Introduction

Since the first structure elucidation of a briarane-type natural product, briarein A, in 1977 by single-crystal X-ray diffraction analysis [1], over 700 marine origin briaranes have been isolated and reported from various octocorals, especially from genera *Briareum* (family Briareidae) [2] and *Junceella* (family Ellisellidae) [3–5]. Among these compounds, 11,20-epoxybriaranes were proven to be a chemical marker for the gorgonian corals belonging to family Ellisellidae [6]. During the course of our research on new natural substances from the marine invertebrates distributed in the waters of

Taiwan, a series of briarane-type diterpenoids were isolated from various octocorals belonging to the genera *Junceella* [7] and *Briareum* [8], and the compounds of this type were proven to possess various interesting bioactivities. Recently, we focused our ongoing studies on a gorgonian coral identified as *Junceella fragilis*. From the results of our studies on this species, we report herein the isolation, structural determination, and bioactivity of two new briaranes, fragilides P (**1**) and Q (**2**), along with two known metabolites, robustolide F (**3**) [9,10] and juncin Z (**4**) [11] (Figure 1).

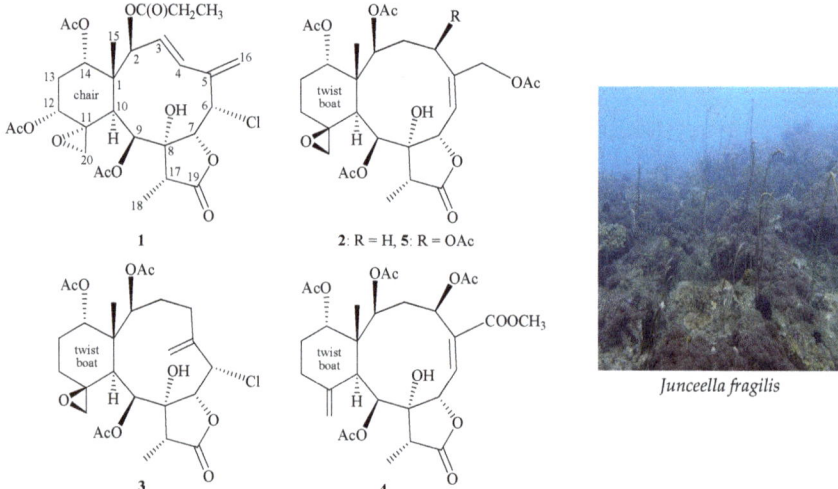

Figure 1. Structures of fragilides P (**1**), Q (**2**), juncins Z (**4**), X (**5**), and robustolide F (**3**) and a picture of *Junceella fragilis*.

2. Results and Discussion

Fragilide P (**1**) has the molecular formula $C_{29}H_{37}ClO_{12}$ as deduced by (+)-ESIMS—which showed a pair of peaks at *m/z* 635/637 (3:1) [M + H$^+$], suggesting a chlorine atom in **1**—and further confirmed by (+)-HRESIMS at *m/z* 635.18683 (calcd. for $C_{29}H_{37}{}^{35}ClO_{12}$ + Na, 635.18658). The IR spectrum of **1** indicated the presence of hydroxy (3466 cm^{-1}), γ-lactone (1783 cm^{-1}), and ester carbonyl (1735 cm^{-1}) groups. The ^{13}C-NMR spectral data (Table 1) showed the presence of a disubstituted olefin (δ_C 132.7, CH-4; 130.4, CH-3) and an exomethylene (δ_C 142.0, C-5; 115.1, CH$_2$-16). Moreover, five carbonyl resonances at δ_C 174.6, 173.3, 170.3, 169.9, and 169.6 in the ^{13}C spectrum confirmed the presence of a γ-lactone and four other ester groups. In the ^{1}H NMR spectrum, three acetate methyls (δ_H 2.11, 2.09, 2.06, each 3H × s) and a propionate (δ_H 2.31, 2H, q, *J* = 7.6 Hz; 1.11, 3H, t, *J* = 7.6 Hz) were observed. An exocyclic epoxy group was elucidated from the signals of two oxygenated carbons at δ_C 57.3 (C-11) and 49.2 (CH$_2$-20). The proton chemical shifts at δ_H 2.77 (1H, dd, *J* = 3.2, 1.2 Hz, H-20a) and 2.64 (1H, d, *J* = 3.2 Hz, H-20b) confirmed the presence of this group. Moreover, a methyl singlet, a methyl doublet, two aliphatic protons, a pair of aliphatic methylene protons, five oxymethine protons, a chlorinated methine proton, and a hydroxy proton were observed in the ^{1}H-NMR spectrum of **1** (Table 1).

Table 1. ^{1}H and ^{13}C-NMR data for **1** and **2**.

C/H	1		2	
	δ_H ^{a} (J in Hz)	δ_C, ^{b} Mult.	δ_H ^{c} (J in Hz)	δ_C, ^{d} Mult.
1		49.2, C		46.9, C
2	5.73 d (9.6)	75.6, CH	4.80 d (5.0)	74.8, CH
3	6.00 dd (15.6, 9.6)	130.4, CH	2.44 m; 1.68 m	32.3, CH$_2$
4	6.89 d (15.6)	132.7, CH	2.47 m; 2.01 m	24.9, CH$_2$
5		142.0, C		139.8, C
6	5.07 d (4.0)	65.0, CH	5.53 d (10.5)	119.2, CH
7	4.16 d (4.0)	80.6, CH	5.20 d (10.5)	77.0, CH
8		82.8, C		80.4, C
9	5.19 d (2.0)	72.2, CH	5.61 d (6.0)	67.6, CH
10	3.84 br s	33.8, CH	2.29 d (6.0)	39.6, CH
11		57.3, C		62.4, C
12	4.52 dd (2.4, 2.4)	73.7, CH	2.28 m; 1.16 m	23.6, CH$_2$
13α/β	2.32 m; 2.06 m	29.0, CH$_2$	1.77 ddd (15.5, 10.0, 10.0); 2.16 m	24.5, CH$_2$
14	4.96 dd (2.4, 2.4)	73.1, CH	4.90 d (5.0)	72.9, CH
15	1.18 s	14.4, CH$_3$	1.01 s	14.9, CH$_3$
16a/b	5.34 s; 5.26 s	115.1, CH$_2$	5.26 dd (16.0, 2.0); 4.23 d (16.0)	67.1, CH$_2$
17	2.84 q (7.2)	50.1, CH	2.34 q (7.0)	42.3, CH
18	1.25 d (7.2)	6.9, CH$_3$	1.16 d (7.0)	6.7, CH$_3$
19		174.6, C		176.4, C
20a/b	2.77 dd (3.2, 1.2); 2.64 d (3.2)	49.2, CH$_2$	2.82 d (4.5); 3.23 br d (4.5)	59.0, CH$_2$
2-OCOEt	2.31 q (7.6) 1.11 t (7.6)	173.3, C 27.7, CH$_2$ 8.8, CH$_3$		
Acetate methyls	2.11 s 2.09 s 2.06 s	21.4, CH$_3$ 21.1, CH$_3$ 21.0, CH$_3$	2.22 s 2.14 s 2.04 s 2.01 s	21.0, CH$_3$ 20.9, CH$_3$ 20.9, CH$_3$ 20.9, CH$_3$
Acetate carbonyls		170.3, C 169.9, C 169.6, C		170.8, C 170.8, C 170.2, C 169.5, C
8-OH	3.07 s		5.19 s	

^{a} Spectra recorded at 400 MHz in CDCl$_3$ at 25 °C. ^{b} Spectra recorded at 100 MHz in CDCl$_3$ at 25 °C. ^{c} Spectra recorded at 500 MHz in CDCl$_3$ at 25 °C. ^{d} Spectra recorded at 125 MHz in CDCl$_3$ at 25 °C.

Analyses of 2D-NMR (COSY and Heteronuclear Multiple Bond Correlation (HMBC)) data established a tetracyclic nucleus. This assignment was evident from the spin systems from H-2 to H-3, H-3 to H-4, H-6 to H-7, H-9 to H-10, H-12 to H$_2$-13, H$_2$-13 to H-14, and H-17 to H$_3$-18 (Figure 2), while the HMBC between protons and quaternary carbons, such as H-2, H-10, H$_3$-15/C-1; H-3, H-6, H-16b/C-5; H-6, H-9, H-10, H-17, H$_3$-18, OH-8/C-8; H-9, H-10, H-20b/C-11; and H-17, H$_3$-18/C-19 revealed the carbon skeleton (Figure 2). The epoxy group positioned at C-11/20 was further confirmed by the HMBC between H-20b to C-11 and C-12. The C-15 methyl group was positioned at C-1 from the HMBC between H$_3$-15 to C-1 and C-14. The HMBC spectrum also revealed that the carbon signal at δ_C 173.3 (C) was correlated with the signals of the methylene and methyl protons of propionate at δ_H 2.31 and 1.11, and it was assigned to the carbon atom of the propionate carbonyl group. The propionate at C-2 was confirmed from the connectivity between H-2 and the carbonyl carbon of the propionate group. The HMBC revealed that an acetoxy group is attached to C-9. The hydroxy group at C-8 was deduced from the HMBC of a hydroxy proton (δ_C 3.07) to C-7, C-8, and C-9. Thus, the remaining acetoxy groups were positioned at C-12 and C-14 by analysis of the characteristic NMR signals (δ_H 4.52, 1H, dd, J = 2.4, 2.4 Hz; δ_C 73.7, CH-12; δ_H 4.96, 1H, dd, J = 2.4, 2.4 Hz; δ_C 73.1, CH-14), although no HMBC was observed between H-12 and H-14 and the acetate carbonyl carbons.

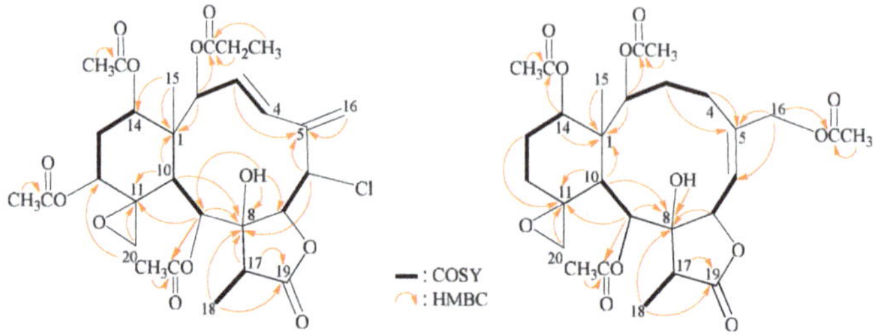

Figure 2. The COSY correlations and selective HMBC of **1** and **2**.

According to a summary of the chemical shifts of 11,20-epoxy groups in briarane derivatives, with ^{13}C-NMR data for C-11 and C-20 at δ_C 55–61 and 47–52 ppm, respectively, the epoxy group was α-oriented and the cyclohexane ring existed in a chair conformation [12]; hence, the configuration of the 11,20-epoxy group in **1** (δ_C 57.3, C-11; 49.2, CH$_2$-20) should be α-oriented, and the cyclohexane ring should be in a chair conformation. The *E* configuration of the C-3/4 double bond was determined from the large proton coupling constant (J = 15.6 Hz) between H-3 and H-4. The stereochemistry of the 11 stereogenic centers of **1** was established by analysis of NOE correlations observed in a NOESY experiment and further supported by molecular mechanics 2 (MM2) force field analysis [13], as shown in Figure 3. In the NOESY spectrum, NOE correlations were observed between H-10 and H-2/H-9/OH-8, while no NOE correlation was seen with Me-15, suggesting that H-2, H-9, H-10, and OH-8 were all α-oriented; meanwhile, a NOE correlation of Me-15 with H-14 indicated that H-14 was β-oriented. In addition, H-12 was found to correlate with H-13α/β and one proton of C-20 methylene (δ_H 2.77, H-20a), indicating that the C-12 acetoxy group was α-oriented. H$_3$-18 showed a NOE correlation with OH-8, indicating that Me-18 was α-oriented at C-17. H-7 exhibited NOE correlations with H-6 and H-17, suggesting that H-6 and H-7 were positioned on the β face. Furthermore, H-3 showed a NOE correlation with H$_3$-15; and H-4 showed NOE correlations with H-2 and OH-8, demonstrating the *E*-configuration of Δ^3 and establishing the *s-cis* diene moiety. As briaranes **1** and **2** were isolated along with a known metabolite **3** (robustolide F) from the same organism, and the absolute configuration of **3** was determined by single-crystal X-ray diffraction analysis [10], it is reasonable on biogenetic grounds and supported by the equal sign of optical rotation of **1**, **2**, and **3** to assume that **1** and **2** have the same absolute configurations as **3**. Therefore, based on the above findings, the configurations of the stereogenic carbons of **1** were determined as 1*R*, 2*S*, 6*S*, 7*R*, 8*R*, 9*S*, 10*S*, 11*R*, 12*R*, 14*S*, and 17*R* (see Figures S1–S10). It is interesting to note that the propionate group is rarely found in briarane-type natural products [12,14–18].

Fragilide Q (**2**) was found to have the molecular formula C$_{28}$H$_{38}$O$_{12}$ as determined from its (+)-HRESIMS at *m/z* 589.22562 (calcd. for C$_{28}$H$_{38}$O$_{12}$ + Na, 589.22555) (Ω = 10). Its absorption peaks in the IR spectrum showed ester carbonyl, γ-lactone, and broad OH stretching at 1740, 1778, and 3273 cm^{-1}, respectively. It was found that the ^{1}H and ^{13}C-NMR spectra of **2** resembled those of a known analogue, juncin X (**5**) (Figure 1), isolated from gorgonian coral *Junceella juncea* collected off the South China Sea [11], except that the signals corresponding to the acetoxy group at C-4 in **5** were replaced by a proton in **2**. The locations of the functional groups were further confirmed by HMBC and COSY correlations (Figure 2); hence, fragilide Q was assigned the structure of **2**, with the same stereochemistry as that of **1**, and the configurations of the stereogenic carbons were elucidated as 1*S*, 2*S*, 7*S*, 8*R*, 9*S*, 10*S*, 11*S*, 14*S*, and 17*R* (Figure 3) (see Figures S11–S20). Due to the chemical shifts for C-11 and C-20 which appeared at δ_C 62.4 and 59.0 ppm, respectively, the epoxy group was β-oriented and the cyclohexane ring should exist in a twisted boat conformation [12].

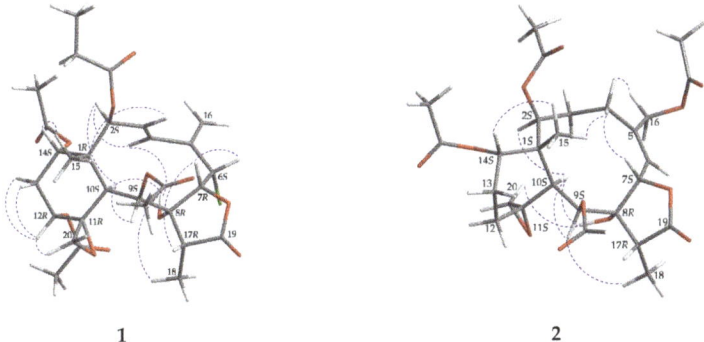

Figure 3. Selected protons with key NOESY ( ) correlations of **1** and **2**.

Two known briaranes were isolated and identified as robustolide F (**3**) [9,10] and juncin Z (**4**) [11] by way of comparison with the spectroscopic and physical data reported in the literature.

In an in vitro anti-inflammatory activity assay, it was found that briarane **4** (juncin Z) showed a 25.56% inhibitory effect on the generation of superoxide anions by human neutrophils at a concentration of 10 µM, and briaranes **1–3** were inactive.

3. Materials and Methods

3.1. General Experimental Procedures

The optical rotations were recored using a Jasco P-1010 digital polarimeter (Japan Spectroscopic, Tokyo, Japan). IR spectra were measured on a Thermo Scientific Nicolet iS5 FT-IR spectrophotometer (Waltham, MA, USA). NMR spectra were taken on a Jeol Resonance ECZ 400S (Tokyo, Japan) or on a Varian Inova (Palo, Alto, CA, USA) 500 NMR spectrometer using the residual CHCl$_3$ signal (δ_H 7.26 ppm) and CDCl$_3$ (δ_C 77.1 ppm) as the internal standard for ^{1}H and ^{13}C-NMR, respectively; coupling constants (J) are presented in Hz. Multiplicities of ^{13}C-NMR data were determined by Distortionless Enhancement by Polarization Transfer (DEPT) experiments. ESIMS and HRESIMS mass spectra were measured on a Bruker mass spectrometer with 7 tesla magnets (model: SolariX FTMS system; Bruker, Bremen, Germany). HPLC separations were carried out on a Hitachi L-2130 pump (Tokyo, Japan) equipped with a Hitachi L-2455 photodiode array detector. The column used for HPLC was reversed-phase silica (250 mm × 21.2 mm, 5 µM, Luna RP-18e; Phenomenex Inc., Torrance, CA, USA). Column chromatography was carried out with Kieselgel 60 (230–400 mesh, Merck, Darmstadt, Germany). TLC was performed on precoated Kieselgel 60 F$_{254}$ (0.25 mm thick, Merck), then sprayed with 10% H$_2$SO$_4$ solution, followed by heating to visualize the spots.

3.2. Animal Material

The sea whip gorgonian coral *Junceella fragilis* was collected by hand in April 2017 using self-contained underwater breathing apparatus (SCUBA) gear at depths of 10–15 m off the coast of South Bay, Kenting, Taiwan. The samples were then stored in a −20 °C freezer until extraction. A voucher specimen was deposited in the National Museum of Marine Biology and Aquarium, Taiwan (NMMBA-TW-GC-2017-022). Identification of the species of this organism was performed by comparison as described in previous publications [3–5].

3.3. Extraction and Isolation

The freeze-dried and sliced bodies (wet/dry weight = 795/313 g) of the coral specimen were prepared and extracted with a 1:1 mixture of MeOH and CH$_2$Cl$_2$ to give 19.0 g of crude extract which was partitioned between EtOAc and H$_2$O. The EtOAc extract (8.0 g) was applied on silica gel column chromatography (C.C.) and eluted with gradients of n-hexane/acetone (50:1 to 1:2, stepwise) to furnish eight fractions (fractions A–H). Fraction G was chromatographed on silica gel C.C. and eluted with gradients of n-hexane/EtOAc (4:1 to 1:1, stepwise) to afford 16 subfractions (fractions G1–G16). Afterward, fraction G9 was separated by RP-HPLC using a mixture of MeOH and H_2O (with volume/volume = 60:40; at a flow rate of 4.0 mL/min) to afford fragilide P (**1**, 2.7 mg), fragilide Q (**2**, 1.8 mg), robustolide F (**3**, 1.4 mg), and juncin Z (**4**, 1.2 mg).

Fragilide P (**1**): amorphous powder; $[\alpha]_D^{27}$ −14 (c 0.9, $CHCl_3$); IR (ATR) ν_{max} 3466, 1783, 1735 cm^{-1}; ^1H and ^{13}C-NMR data (see Table 1); ESIMS: m/z 635 [M + Na]$^+$; HRESIMS: m/z 635.18683 (calcd. for $C_{29}H_{37}{}^{35}ClO_{12}$ + Na, 635.18658).

Fragilide Q (**2**): amorphous powder; $[\alpha]_D^{28}$ −59 (c 0.6, $CHCl_3$); IR (ATR) ν_{max} 3273, 1778, 1740 cm^{-1}; ^1H and ^{13}C-NMR data (see Table 1); ESIMS: *m/z* 589 [M + Na]$^+$; HRESIMS: *m/z* 589.22562 (calcd. for $C_{28}H_{38}O_{12}$ + Na, 589.22555).

Robustolide F (**3**): amorphous powder; $[\alpha]_D^{23}$ −37 (c 0.07, $CHCl_3$) (ref. [9] $[\alpha]_D^{26}$ −26.8 (c 1.038, $CHCl_3$)); ref. [10] $[\alpha]_D^{25}$ −28 (c 0.24, $CHCl_3$)); IR (ATR) ν_{max} 3288, 1780, 1735 cm^{-1}; ^1H and ^{13}C-NMR data were found to be in absolute agreement with previous studies [9]; ESIMS: *m/z* 565 [M + Na]$^+$.

Juncin Z (**4**): amorphous powder; $[\alpha]_D^{23}$ +28 (c 0.06, $CHCl_3$) (ref. [11] $[\alpha]D$ +31.57 (c 0.95, $CHCl_3$)); IR (ATR) ν_{max} 3433, 1782, 1738 cm^{-1}; ^1H and ^{13}C-NMR data were found to be in absolute agreement with previous studies [11]; ESIMS: *m/z* 617 [M + Na]$^+$.

3.4. Molecular Mechanics Calculations

The molecular models were generated by implementing the MM2 force field [13] in ChemBio 3D Ultra software (version 12.0) which was created by CambridgeSoft (PerkinElmer, Cambridge, MA, USA).

3.5. Superoxide Anion Generation by Human Neutrophils

Human neutrophils were obtained by means of dextran sedimentation and Ficoll centrifugation. Measurements of elastase release and superoxide anion generation were carried out according to previously described procedures [19]. Briefly, superoxide anion production was assayed by monitoring the superoxide-dismutase-inhibitable reduction of ferricytochrome c. Elastase release experiments were performed using MeO-Suc-Ala-Ala-Pro-Valp-nitroanilide as the elastase substrate.

4. Conclusions

The sea whip gorgonian coral *Junceella fragilis*, a zooxanthella-containing species [20], has been demonstrated to have a wide structural diversity of interesting marine-origin briarane-type diterpenoids [7], and the compounds of this type were suggested originally to be produced by the host corals and not by its zooxanthellae [21]. In our continued study of *Junceella fragilis* collected in the waters of Taiwan, two previously unreported briaranes, fragilides P (**1**) and Q (**2**), were isolated along with two previously described analogues, robustolide F (**3**) and juncin Z (**4**). The structures, including the absolute configurations of **1** and **2**, were determined by using spectroscopic methods and comparing the spectroscopic and rotation values with those of a known related analogue, robustolide F (**3**) [9,10]. Juncin Z (**4**) was found to display an inhibitory effect on the generation of superoxide anions by human neutrophils.

Supplementary Materials: The Supplementary Materials are available online. ESIMS, HRESIMS, IR, 1D (^1H, ^{13}C-NMR, and DEPT spectra) and 2D (HSQC, COSY, HMBC, and NOESY) spectra of new compounds **1** and **2** and ESIMS, ^1H, ^{13}C-NMR, and DEPT spectra of **3** and **4**.

Author Contributions: C.-C.L., L.-C.H., T.-L.H. and P.-J.S. designed the whole experiment and contributed to manuscript preparation. J.-H.S., W.-F.C., Z.-H.W. and B.-R.P. analyzed the data.

Funding: This research was supported by grants from the National Museum of Marine Biology and Aquarium; the National Dong Hwa University; and the Ministry of Science and Technology, Taiwan (Grant Nos: MOST 104-2320-B-291-001-MY3 and 107-2320-B-291-001-MY3) awarded to Ping-Jyun Sung.

Conflicts of Interest: The authors declare no conflicts of interest.

References

1. Burks, J.E.; van der Helm, D.; Chang, C.Y.; Ciereszko, L.S. The crystal and molecular structure of briarein A, a diterpenoid from the gorgonian *Briareum asbestinum*. *Acta Cryst.* **1977**, *33*, 704–709. [CrossRef]
2. Samimi-Namin, K.; van Ofwegen, L.P. Overview of the genus *Briareum* (Cnidaria, Octocorallia, Briareidae) in the Indo-Pacific, with the description of a new species. *ZooKeys* **2016**, *557*, 1–44. [CrossRef] [PubMed]
3. Bayer, F.M. Key to the genera of octocorallia of Pennatulacea (Coelenterata: Anthozoa), with diagnoses of new taxa. *Proc. Biol. Soc. Wash.* **1981**, *94*, 902–947.
4. Bayer, F.M.; Grasshoff, M. The genus group taxa of the family Ellisellidae, with clarification of the genera established by J.E. Gary (Cnidaria: Octocorallia). *Senckenberg. Biol.* **1994**, *74*, 21–45.
5. Chen, C.-C.; Chang, K.-H. Gorgonacea (Coelenterata: Octocorallia) of Southern Taiwan. *Bull. Inst. Zool. Acad. Sin.* **1991**, *30*, 149–181.
6. Su, Y.-M.; Fan, T.-Y.; Sung, P.-J. 11,20-Epoxybriaranes from the gorgonian coral *Ellisella robusta* (Ellisellidae). *Nat. Prod. Res.* **2007**, *21*, 1085–1090. [CrossRef]
7. Chung, H.-M.; Wang, Y.-C.; Tseng, C.-C.; Chen, N.-F.; Wen, Z.-H.; Fang, L.-S.; Hwang, T.-L.; Wu, Y.-C.; Sung, P.-J. Natural product chemistry of gorgonian corals of genus *Junceella*–Part III. *Mar. Drugs* **2018**, *16*, 339. [CrossRef]
8. Su, Y.-D.; Su, J.-H.; Hwang, T.-L.; Wen, Z.-H.; Sheu, J.-H.; Wu, Y.-C.; Sung, P.-J. Briarane diterpenoids isolated from octocorals between 2014 and 2016. *Mar. Drugs* **2017**, *15*, 44. [CrossRef]
9. Tanaka, C.; Yamamoto, Y.; Otsuka, M.; Tanaka, J.; Ichiba, T.; Marriott, G.; Rachmat, R.; Higa, T. Briarane diterpenes from two species of octocorals, *Ellisella* sp. and *Pteroeides* sp. *J. Nat. Prod.* **2004**, *67*, 1368–1373. [CrossRef]
10. Sung, P.-J.; Chiang, M.Y.; Tsai, W.-T.; Su, J.-H.; Su, Y.-M.; Wu, Y.-C. Chlorinated briarane-type diterpenoids from the gorgonian coral *Ellisella robusta* (Ellisellidae). *Tetrahedron* **2007**, *63*, 12860–12865. [CrossRef]
11. Qi, S.-H.; Zhang, S.; Qian, P.-Y.; Xiao, Z.-H.; Li, M.-Y. Ten new antifouling briarane diterpenoids from the South China Sea gorgonian *Junceella juncea*. *Tetrahedron* **2006**, *62*, 9123–9130. [CrossRef]
12. Sheu, J.-H.; Chen, Y.-P.; Hwang, T.-L.; Chiang, M.Y.; Fang, L.-S.; Sung, P.-J. Junceellolides J–L, 11,20-epoxybriaranes from the gorgonian coral *Junceella fragilis*. *J. Nat. Prod.* **2006**, *69*, 269–273. [CrossRef] [PubMed]
13. Allinger, N.L. Conformational analysis. 130. MM2. A hydrocarbon force field utilizing V_1 and V_2 torsional terms. *J. Am. Chem. Soc.* **1977**, *99*, 8127–8134. [CrossRef]
14. Guerriero, A.; D'Ambrosio, M.; Pietra, F. Bis-allylic reactivity of the funicolides, 5,8(17)-diunsaturated briarane diterpenes of the sea pen *Funiculina quadrangularis* from the Tuscan archipelago, leading to 16-nortaxane derivatives. *Helv. Chim. Acta* **1995**, *78*, 1465–1478. [CrossRef]
15. Chiasera, G.; Guerriero, A.; D'Ambrosio, M.; Pietra, F. On the funicolides, briaranes of the Pennatulacean coral *Funiculina quadrangularis* from the Tuscan archipelago: Conformational preferences in this class of diterpenes. *Helv. Chim. Acta* **1995**, *78*, 1479–1489. [CrossRef]
16. Sheu, J.-H.; Sung, P.-J.; Su, J.-H.; Wang, G.-H.; Duh, C.-Y.; Shen, Y.-C.; Chiang, M.Y.; Chen, I.-T. Excavatolides U–Z, new briarane diterpenes from the gorgonian *Briareum excavatum*. *J. Nat. Prod.* **1999**, *62*, 1415–1420. [CrossRef]
17. Sung, P.-J.; Chen, Y.-P.; Su, Y.-M.; Hwang, T.-L.; Hu, W.-P.; Fan, T.-Y.; Wang, W.-H. Fragilide B: A novel briarane-type diterpenoid with a s-cis diene moiety. *Bull. Chem. Soc. Jpn.* **2007**, *80*, 1205–1207. [CrossRef]
18. Cheng, W.; Ji, M.; Li, X.; Ren, J.; Yin, F.; van Ofwegen, L.; Yu, S.; Chen, X.; Lin, W. Fragilolides A–Q, norditerpenoid and briarane diterpenoids from the gorgonian coral *Junceella fragilis*. *Tetrahedron* **2017**, *73*, 2518–2528. [CrossRef]
19. Yu, H.-P.; Hsieh, P.-W.; Chang, Y.-J.; Chung, P.-J.; Kuo, L.-M.; Hwang, T.-L. 2-(2-Fluorobenzamido) benzoate ethyl ester (EFB-1) inhibits superoxide production by human neutrophils and attenuates hemorrhagic shock-induced organ dysfunction in rats. *Free Radic. Biol. Med.* **2011**, *50*, 1737–1748. [CrossRef]
20. Walker, T.A.; Bull, G.D. A newly discovered method of reproduction in gorgonian coral. *Mar. Ecol. Prog. Ser.* **1983**, *12*, 137–143. [CrossRef]
21. Kokke, W.C.M.C.; Epstein, S.; Look, S.A.; Rau, G.H.; Fenical, W.; Djerassi, C. On the origin of terpenes in symbiotic associations between marine invertebrates and algae (zooxanthellae). *J. Biol. Chem.* **1984**, *259*, 8168–8173. [PubMed]

Sample Availability: Samples of the compounds **1–4** are not available from the authors.

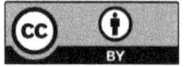 © 2019 by the authors. Licensee MDPI, Basel, Switzerland. This article is an open access article distributed under the terms and conditions of the Creative Commons Attribution (CC BY) license (http://creativecommons.org/licenses/by/4.0/).

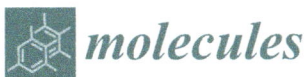

Review

Topical Administration of Terpenes Encapsulated in Nanostructured Lipid-Based Systems

Elwira Lasoń

Faculty of Chemical Engineering and Technology, Cracow University of Technology, Warszawska St 24, 31-155 Kraków, Poland; elwira.lason@pk.edu.pl; Tel.: +48-12-628-2761

Academic Editors: Pavel B. Drasar and Vladimir A. Khripach
Received: 25 October 2020; Accepted: 3 December 2020; Published: 7 December 2020

Abstract: Terpenes are a group of phytocompounds that have been used in medicine for decades owing to their significant role in human health. So far, they have been examined for therapeutic purposes as antibacterial, anti-inflammatory, antitumoral agents, and the clinical potential of this class of compounds has been increasing continuously as a source of pharmacologically interesting agents also in relation to topical administration. Major difficulties in achieving sustained delivery of terpenes to the skin are connected with their low solubility and stability, as well as poor cell penetration. In order to overcome these disadvantages, new delivery technologies based on nanostructures are proposed to improve bioavailability and allow controlled release. This review highlights the potential properties of terpenes loaded in several types of lipid-based nanocarriers (liposomes, solid lipid nanoparticles, and nanostructured lipid carriers) used to overcome free terpenes' form limitations and potentiate their therapeutic properties for topical administration.

Keywords: terpenes; terpenoids; lipid nanoparticles; nanostructured lipid carriers; topical administration; lipid-based systems

1. Introduction

Terpenes and their oxygenated derivatives terpenoids are the largest and most common class of secondary metabolites. Terpenoids are modified terpenes where methyl groups are moved or removed, or additional functional groups (usually oxygen-containing) are added. The two terms are often used interchangeably. They are found in higher plants, as representing the majority of molecules in essential oils, mosses, liverworts, and algae lichens, as well as insects, microbes, and marine organisms [1–3]. These compounds are a very diverse group of molecules with an extremely varied structure and function [4]. The basic chemical structure of terpenes and terpenoids contains several repeated isoprene units (C_5H_8) used to classify them. Thus, e.g., hemiterpenes (hemiterpenoids) are formed by one isoprene unit, monoterpenes (monoterpenoids) have two isoprene units (C10), sesquiterpenes (sesquiterpenoids) have three (C15), and diterpenes (diterpenoids) have four (C20) isoprene units. Terpenes may also be classified as linear, monocyclic, and bicyclic [3,5]. The volatility of these compounds decreases with an increased number of isoprene units [6]. Smaller terpenes are not only highly volatile but also susceptible to degradation mainly by oxidation and isomerization and usually thermolabile [5,7].

Targeted delivery of typically hydrophobic terpenoids has been the subject of much research, finding applications in a wide variety of fields. As naturally occurring compounds, they have been applied in transdermal research since the 1960s and are reported to be a safe and effective class of penetration enhancers [8,9]. Plenty of them have been used as antispasmodics, carminatives, flavoring agents, or perfumes [3]. Several studies also indicated that terpenoids can suppress nuclear factor-κB (NF-κB) signaling, the major regulator in the pathogenesis of inflammatory diseases and cancer [10], thus confirming anti-inflammatory [11] and antineoplastic applications [12,13]. Additionally, terpenes were also found as cutaneous wound healing accelerators [14]. Because that class of compounds appears to offer great benefits for therapeutic purposes, it is understood that the proper carriers play an important role in their administration. Therefore, efficient, safe, and natural delivery systems are of great interest.

Lipid-based nanocarriers are novel drug delivery systems that have been widely explored for topical and transdermal delivery of pharmaceuticals. Encapsulation of terpenoids in such a system is an interesting strategy to provide better stability and protection against environmental factors that may cause chemical degradation. In addition, nanoencapsulation can decrease the toxicity, solubilize poorly soluble terpenes, improve bioavailability, and achieve controlled and sustained delivery, in addition to drug targeting at the site of action [15,16].

In the present review, the topical administration of selected terpenoids is discussed with special emphasis on nanostructured delivery systems applied as carriers for these groups of bioactive compounds.

2. Topical Route of Terpenes Administration

The topical administration of bioactive compounds acting as drugs relies on the localized administration of formulations to a body through dermal and mucosal (e.g., ocular, vaginal, nasal, and rectal) routes. Skin is one of the most easily accessible organs in the human body for topical administration and is the major route of localized drug delivery [5,17]. The drug delivery system can be considered dermal when the targeting site of the drug is the skin or transdermal when the drug has to pass through skin layers to reach the target and, by analogy, for mucosal tissue administration, delivery can be mucosal and transmucosal [18].

The intact skin is much less permeable than other tissues and penetration of the active compounds depends on the physicochemical properties of the penetrant, the condition of the skin, and the nature of the carrier [17]. Topically applied drugs may diffuse through the skin by hair follicles, sweat glands, or sebaceous glands, but the predominant and very slow route is through multiple lipid bilayers of the stratum corneum (Figure 1). Terpenes can be applied topically mainly for local action, e.g., as wound healing, antiseptic, anti-fungal, or anti-inflammatory agents but at the same time, this route can be used to reach the deeper layer of the skin or even for systemic drug delivery like in case of anesthetic or antihypertensive acting terpenes.

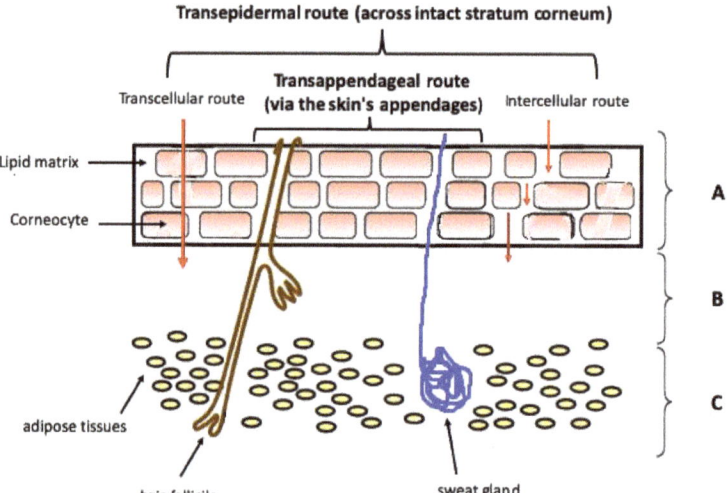

Figure 1. Diagrammatic illustration of the skin's structure and routes of permeation through the skin. A—Epidermis (SC), B—Dermis, C—Subcutaneous layer.

Drug administration through mucosal and transmucosal routes like oral, nasal, and ocular is still a challenge for scientists mainly because of the presence of mucus, saliva, and lacrimal fluids, which can restrict the access of bacteria or virus to the deeper layers but can also affect the bioavailability of bioactive compounds like terpenes [18,19].

Topical terpenoids application can be an attractive route of administration as it allows the reduction of side effects, avoids the injectable route, the first-pass metabolism, and pre-systemic elimination within the gastrointestinal tract. Moreover, it is a safe route with the easiness of application and fast action [20].

2.1. Terpenes as Skin Permeation Enhancers

The effectiveness of transdermal drug delivery depends on the sufficient capability of drugs to penetrate through the skin to reach the therapeutic level. An important barrier of the skin for drug absorption is the stratum corneum (SC) [21,22]. The stratum corneum consists of keratin-enriched dead cells, surrounded by crystalline intercellular lipid lamellar structures. These are continuous structures in the SC and are required for competent skin barrier function [3]. To facilitate drug delivery through the skin and increase percutaneous absorption, penetration enhancers are extensively used, as they ideally cause a temporary reversible reduction in the barrier function of the SC [9].

Terpenes and terpenoids have attracted great interest as effective enhancers from natural products [3,23–26]. They are commonly considered to be less toxic with low irritancy potential compared to other synthetic skin penetration enhancers or surfactants. Moreover, this class of penetration enhancers has been classified by the Food and Drug Administration (FDA) as generally recognized as safe (GRAS) agents [8,24]. Terpenes can increase skin permeation by one or more mechanisms, including interaction with SC lipids and/or keratin and increasing the solubility of a drug into SC lipids. Nevertheless, the interaction of terpenes with SC in the presence of various solvents may not be similar due to differences in the physicochemical properties of these solvents and their interactions with SC, but there are some instrumental methods (e.g., differential scanning calorimetry (DSC) and Fourier transform infrared spectroscopy (FTIR)), which can help to determine these interactions [24].

Terpenes acting as permeation enhancers are usually used as excipients in formulations (Table 1) and are capable of facilitating the passage of the main drug through the skin. The nanostructured lipid-based systems in which terpenes are used as enhancers are mainly invasomes, liposomes, nanoemulsions, and SLN (Solid Lipid Nanoparticles)/NLC (Nanostructured Lipid Carriers) [5]. Invasomes are composed of phosphatidylcholine, ethanol, and a mixture of terpenes and are most popular in recent years among the formulations of nanosystems using terpenes as excipients [27,28]. They present elasticity and deformability, which favors penetration across skin layers, and thus they work as penetration-enhancing vesicles [29]. Terpenes applied in the formulations of invasomes or other lipid-based carriers are mainly representatives of monoterpenes and monoterpenoids (Figure 2) [27–38].

Table 1. Terpenes as skin permeation enhancers encapsulated in nanostructured lipid systems.

Terpenes	Nanosystem	Administration Route	Experimental Model	Reference
Limonene, citral, cineole	Invasomes	Transdermal	In vitro (abdominal human skin)	[27,28]
β-citronellene	Invasomes	Transdermal	In vivo (rat skin)	[30,31]
Limonene, cineole, fenchone, citral	Invasomes	Cutaneous	In vivo (rat skin)	[32]
Limonene	Liposomes	Transdermal	In vitro (porcine skin)	[33]
Limonene	PEGylated liposomes	Transdermal	In vitro (porcine skin)	[34,35]
Limonene	Nanoemulsion	Transdermal	In vitro (abdominal human skin)	[36]
Eucalyptol	Nanoemulsion	Transfollicular		[37]
Eucalyptol and pinene	Nanoemulsion	Transdermal	In vivo	[38]
Limonene and 1,8-cineole	SLN, NLC, Nanoemulsion	Cutaneous	In vitro	[9]

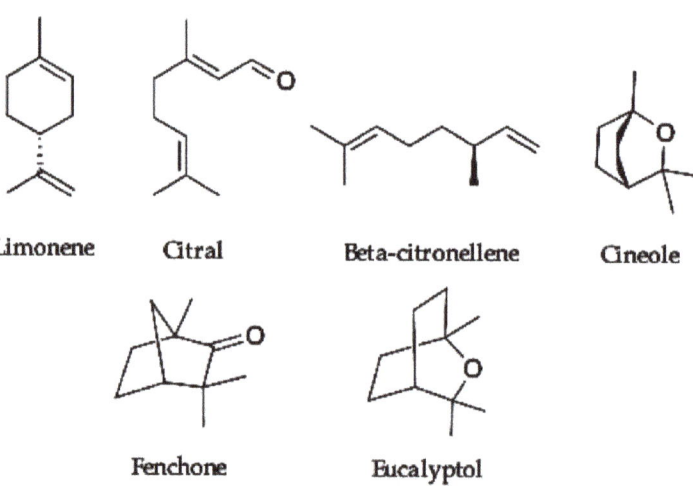

Figure 2. Representatives of monoterpenes and monoterpenoids applied as skin permeation enhancers.

2.2. Terpenes as Bioactive Compounds

The most widely investigated therapeutic potential of terpenes and terpenoids for topical administration is the anti-inflammatory activity, including burns or wounds healing [10–14].

Inflammation is the physiological response of the body to tissue injury (e.g., stress, irritants, radiations), microbial and viral infections, or genetic changes and may have an acute or chronic state [39]. The most common signs of acute inflammation are swelling, pain, erythema, and increased heat. Some chronic diseases can be developed due to inflammation and if the condition causing the damage is not resolved, the inflammatory process evolves toward subacute or chronic inflammation [11]. The chronic state of inflammation has important roles at the beginning of various diseases, including cardiovascular disease, diabetes, cancer, obesity, and asthma, as well as classic inflammatory diseases like arthritis or psoriasis [40–42]. Some chronic diseases may involve the use of anti-inflammatory agents such as steroidal and non-steroidal drugs, but some of them can cause undesirable side effects [11]. Therefore, there is a need to find new therapeutic alternatives that are less toxic, and the perfect candidates seem to be terpenes (Table 2).

Table 2. Terpenes as bioactive compounds encapsulated in lipid-based nanosystems for anti-inflammatory treatment.

Terpenes/Terpenoids	Nanosystem	Administration Route	Activity	Reference
Thymol	SLN	Cutaneous	Anti-inflammatory	[11]
Astragaloside IV	SLN	Cutaneous	Wound healing	[43]
Triptolide	SLN	Cutaneous	Anti-inflammatory	[44]
Ursolic acid	NLC	Cutaneous	Antiarthritic	[45]
Forskolin	NLC	Transdermal	Photoprotector	[46]
Hurpezine A	SLN, NLC, Microemulsion	Transdermal	Alzheimer's treatment	[47]
Triptolide	Nanoemulsion	Percutaneous	Anti-inflammatory, analgesic	[48]
Safranal	Nanoemulsion	Nasal	Cerebral ischemia treatment	[49]
Madecassoside	Liposomes	Cutaneous	Wound healing, psoriasis	[50]
Citral	Liposomes	Transdermal	Anti-inflammatory, antifungal	[51]
Thymol, menthol, camphor and cineol	Invasomes	Transdermal	Anti-inflammatory, bacterial infections e.g., MRSA	[52]

An equally important therapeutic aspect of terpenes is their activity against skin cancer. The number of skin cancer cases has increased rapidly worldwide. Skin cancer, including melanoma and non-melanoma skin cancer (NMSC), represents the most common type of malignancy in the white population [53,54]. The major risk factor of developing cutaneous cancers is chronic exposure of the skin to UV radiation, both natural and artificial [55]. Potential risks for cancer are also genetic predisposition, depressed immune system, or exposure to viral infections (human papillomavirus), or chemicals like aromatic hydrocarbons and arsenic [54]. The huge impact on the prognosis of any type of skin cancer is its early diagnosis and immediate treatment. When it comes to melanoma skin cancer, it has a high propensity for metastasis; therefore, it is more of a systemic disease as far as treatment options are considered. For NMSC, the treatment mainly depends on the number, thickness, and distribution of lesions, then patient preferences like convenience, tolerance, and treatment cost are also taken into consideration [56]. Topical therapies are mainly applied when there are multiple lesions, the affected area is large, or for lesions that take time to cure. They are also used for patients who are not candidates for surgery [54]. Nanostructured systems hold great promise as carriers for skin cancer treatment in topical application. Numerous nanomaterials can be applied as drug vesicles from those based on lipids to polymer micelles, silicone dioxide, carbon nanotubes, gold, silver, and other metal or metal oxides [57,58]. As drug carriers, nanoparticles must have low toxicity and deliver drugs precisely into target tissues in order to achieve the maximum benefit with minimum side effects [59]. The nanocarriers' ability to treat tumors has been extensively investigated by many research groups [54,59–61]. For decades, lipid-based nanoparticle systems have been tested in vitro and in vivo for the topical treatment of skin cancer mainly because of their ability to improve skin and tumor penetration of bioactive compounds. The therapeutic potential of terpenoids and terpenes as antineoplastic drugs is also well known as that which gives promising perspectives in topical skin cancer treatment (Table 3).

Table 3. Terpenes as anticancer bioactive compounds encapsulated in lipid based nanosystems.

Terpenes/Terpenoids	Nanosystem	Administration Route	Activity	Reference
Paclitaxel	SLN	Cutaneous	Antineoplastic	[13]
Tripterine	NLC	Cutaneous	Antimelanoma	[62]
Betulin	Nanoemulsion	Cutaneous	Anti-carcinogenic	[63]
Ursolic acid	Nano lipid vesicles	Nasal	Antineoplastic	[64]
Tripterine	Phytosomes	Oral/Buccal	Antineoplastic	[65]

3. Lipid-Based Nanoparticles for Topical Applications of Terpenes

The choice of vehicle or delivery system in the case of skin diseases has a significant influence on the outcome of topical dermatological drug treatment. Nanoparticulate systems can improve the stability of actives in front of possible degradation by light, heat, and other environmental factors. Moreover, they provide better bioavailability, improve permeation through the skin and other biological barriers, and reach the controlled delivery of drugs [16,66]. These systems can be divided according to their composition on polymer and lipid-based carriers. The lipid-based systems are formed by lipids and include nanoemulsions (NE), liposomes (LS), solid lipid nanoparticles (SLN), nanostructured lipid carriers (NLC), and vesicular systems (VS), which comprehend ethosomes, phytosomes, niosomes, glycerosomes, and invasomes (IV) (Figure 3) [66]. The examples of using different types of the vesicles mentioned above to incorporate and deliver terpenes to the skin are presented in Tables 1–3. A brief overview of some of the most commonly tested lipid systems in topical delivery is introduced below.

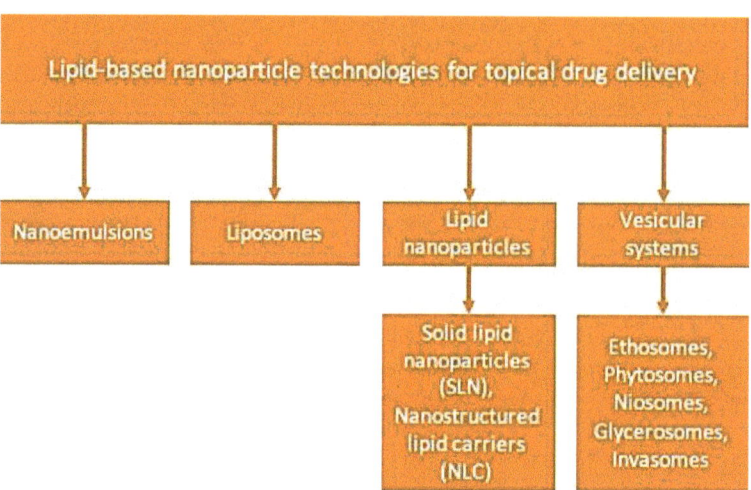

Figure 3. Nanoparticle based on lipids technologies for topical drug delivery.

Nanoemulsions (NE) are thermodynamically stable oil in water (o/w) or water in oil (w/o) dispersions stabilized by surfactant molecules. The mean droplet size, ranging from 20 to 200 nm, and the low percentage of surfactant make them ideal for topical drug delivery with reduced skin irritation [67]. NEs are able to solubilize lipophilic drugs at high loading capacity. Their large surface area makes it possible to create close occlusive contact with the stratum corneum that helps to permeate and deliver drugs (both, lipo- and hydrophilic) deep inside the skin. NE skin permeation is also enhanced by the presence of oil and surfactants in the composition that may change the lipid structure of the stratum corneum [67,68].

Liposomes are vesicles built by amphiphilic lipids, mainly cholesterol and phospholipids. The lipids arrange themselves in bilayers surrounding an aqueous core, where hydrophilic compounds can be entrapped while hydrophobic drugs can be encapsulated on the bilayer. Liposomes are very versatile drug delivery systems since they can incorporate either hydrophilic, hydrophobic, or amphiphilic drugs [66,69]. Liposomes have the ability to improve the pharmacokinetics, specificity, and efficacy of a drug with reduced toxicity [70]. The idea of using liposomes for skin diseases was first proposed by Mezei and Gulasekharam in 1980 [71]. The composition of the liposomes enables their adsorption on the skin surface and fusion with SC lipids, hence initiating the release of the drug into the tissue [72]. It has been shown that liposomes can accumulate in various layers of the skin compared to the free drug, so they can be engineered to achieve a desirable layer. Larger particles remain adsorbed on the surface while liposomes with a mean diameter of less than 50 nm have been shown to accumulate within the deeper layers of the tissue [73].

Lipid nanoparticles are innovative nanocarriers known as solid lipid nanoparticles (SLN) and nanostructured lipid carriers (NLC) and represent a revolution in the efficient encapsulation of hydrophobic drugs and long-term physicochemical stability of lipid-based drug delivery systems [18]. They are highly tolerable and protect drugs from degradation while maintaining a steady release for extended periods [54]. SLNs are colloidal systems consisting of a blend of biodegradable and biocompatible solid lipids, emulsifiers, and water and range from less than 50 to 1000 nm in size. Typically used lipids include triglycerides, glycerides, fatty acids, and waxes [74]. SLNs adhere to the skin to form a monolayer that creates an occlusive effect to increase the water retention of the skin. This helps to increase the penetration of drug-loaded particles into the skin [75]. Unfortunately, these systems possess some disadvantages associated with poor drug loading due to a compact lipid matrix and possible active expulsion during storage connected with matrix polymorphic transition. Nevertheless, as a result of the solid nature of SLN, they have enhanced physical stability over nanoemulsions [76]. NLCs were introduced to overcome some drawbacks represent by SLNs. They are composed of a blend of solid and liquid lipids that do not possess the ideal crystalline structure. The lipid is either enclosed within the solid lipid matrix or localized on the surfactant layer [77], which allows it to increase drug loading capacity and improve bioavailability.

Vesicular systems have been among the most studied for topical therapies during recent years [54]. The physicochemical properties of these systems allow the creation of easy-to-produce nano-scaled drug transporters. It is possible to encapsulate either polar compounds, in the inner aqueous compartment of the vesicle, or non-polar molecules, embedded in the membrane [78]. Depending on its membrane composition, vesicular systems are often classified as ethosomes, phytosomes, niosomes, glycerosomes, and invasomes [5]. Many researchers have also classified liposomes into this group due to the resemblance to the structure and composition.

Niosomes are a form of liposomes composed of nonionic surfactants that produce more stable, less toxic, and more flexible vesicles. They are also less expensive and more economical to manufacture [79]. Niosomes can modify the SC barrier by blending with the lipids. They can also increase the smoothness of the SC by recovering the lost lipids and reducing the transepidermal water loss. All these depend on the physicochemical properties of the drug, the vesicle, and the lipids used to produce the niosomes [79,80].

Ethosomes are elastic vesicles composed of phospholipids, cholesterol, water, and large amounts of ethanol that help to improve the solubility of lipophilic drugs and aid in disrupting the SC. Therefore, the delivery of drugs into the deep dermal layers or even into the systemic circulation is possible [81,82]. When compared to classic liposomes, ethosomes are more stable and achieved superior antifungal activity [83].

Invasomes represent vesicular carriers for enhanced skin delivery. They are composed of unsaturated phospholipids, small amounts of ethanol, terpenes, and water. Different penetration studies performed in vitro in human skin were represented in order to show the penetration-enhancing ability of invasomes. They are characterized by elasticity and deformability, which favors penetration across skin layers [27–29,84].

4. Conclusions

Nowadays, phytochemicals like terpenes and terpenoids have promising potential to prevent and treat different types of diseases. Although several terpenes are considered GRAS, few studies investigated the safety of these compounds in direct topical application. Their poor water solubility, stability, and bioavailability, as well as other side effects (e.g., irritant index), have limited their clinical application. New drug delivery systems based on lipids represent an encouraging approach for topical applications of terpenes. These systems are attractive, non-invasive, and especially beneficial for patients that are not viable for surgery or highly intensive non-specific systemic therapies. Encapsulation of terpenes in lipid-based nanocarriers is widely described in the literature as an approach providing protection against environmental factors that can cause chemical degradation and volatilization of these compounds. Moreover, nanostructured lipid systems allow controlled drug release and enable the passage of the bioactive compounds through biological barriers making them ideal candidates for topical applications. Finally, terpenes and lipid-based nanosystems represent a sustainable alternative in pharmaceuticals, giving increasing importance to greener chemistry.

Funding: This research received no external funding.

Conflicts of Interest: The author declares no conflict of interest.

References

1. Heras, B.D.L.; Hortelano, S. Molecular Basis of the Anti-Inflammatory Effects of Terpenoids. *Inflamm. Allergy Drug Targets* **2009**, *8*, 28–39. [CrossRef] [PubMed]
2. Bilia, A.R.; Guccione, C.; Isacchi, B.; Righeschi, C.; Firenzuoli, F.; Bergonzi, M.C. Essential Oils Loaded in Nanosystems: A Developing Strategy for a Successful Therapeutic Approach. *Evidence-Based Complement. Altern. Med.* **2014**, *2014*. [CrossRef] [PubMed]
3. Sapra, B.; Jain, S.; Tiwary, A.K. Percutaneous Permeation Enhancement by Terpenes: Mechanistic View. *AAPS J.* **2008**, *10*, 120–132. [CrossRef] [PubMed]
4. Reddy, L.H.; Couvreur, P. Squalene: A natural triterpene for use in disease management and therapy. *Adv. Drug Deliv. Rev.* **2009**, *61*, 1412–1426. [CrossRef]
5. De Matos, S.P.; Teixeira, H.F.; De Lima Ádley, A.N.; Veiga-Junior, V.F.; Koester, L.S. Essential Oils and Isolated Terpenes in Nanosystems Designed for Topical Administration: A Review. *Biomolecules* **2019**, *9*, 138. [CrossRef]
6. Hamm, S.; Bleton, J.; Connan, J.; Tchapla, A. A chemical investigation by headspace SPME and GC–MS of volatile and semi-volatile terpenes in various olibanum samples. *Phytochemistry* **2005**, *66*, 1499–1514. [CrossRef]
7. Turek, C.; Stintzing, F.C. Stability of Essential Oils: A Review. *Compr. Rev. Food Sci. Food Saf.* **2013**, *12*, 40–53. [CrossRef]
8. Vikas, S.; Seema, S.; Gurpreet, S.; Rana, A.C.; Baibhav, J. Penetration enhancers: A novel strategy for enhancing transdermal drug delivery. *Int. Res. J. Pharm.* **2011**, *2*, 32–36.
9. Charoenputtakun, P.; Pamornpathomkul, B.; Opanasopit, P.; Rojanarata, T.; Ngawhirunpat, T. Terpene Composited Lipid Nanoparticles for Enhanced Dermal Delivery of All-trans-Retinoic Acids. *Biol. Pharm. Bull.* **2014**, *37*, 1139–1148. [CrossRef]
10. Salminen, A.; Lehtonen, M.; Suuronen, T.; Kaarniranta, K.; Huuskonen, J. Terpenoids: Natural inhibitors of NF-κB signaling with anti-inflammatory and anticancer potential. *Cell. Mol. Life Sci.* **2008**, *65*, 2979–2999. [CrossRef]

11. Pivetta, T.P.; Simões, S.; Araújo, M.M.; Carvalho, T.; Arruda, C.; Marcato, P.D. Development of nanoparticles from natural lipids for topical delivery of thymol: Investigation of its anti-inflammatory properties. *Colloids Surf. B Biointerfaces* **2018**, *164*, 281–290. [CrossRef] [PubMed]
12. Tosta, F.V.; Andrade, L.M.; Mendes, L.P.; Anjos, J.L.V.; Alonso, A.; Marreto, R.N.; Lima, E.M.; Taveira, S.F. Paclitaxel-loaded lipid nanoparticles for topical application: The influence of oil content on lipid dynamic behavior, stability, and drug skin penetration. *J. Nanopart. Res.* **2014**, *16*, 1–12. [CrossRef]
13. Bharadwaj, R.; Das, P.J.; Pal, P.; Mazumder, B. Topical delivery of paclitaxel for treatment of skin cancer. *Drug Dev. Ind. Pharm.* **2016**, *42*, 1482–1494. [CrossRef]
14. Takada, H.; Yonekawa, J.; Matsumoto, M.; Furuya, K.; Sokabe, M. Hyperforin/HP-β-Cyclodextrin Enhances Mechanosensitive Ca^{2+} Signaling in HaCaT Keratinocytes and in Atopic Skin Ex Vivo Which Accelerates Wound Healing. *BioMed Res. Int.* **2017**, *2017*. [CrossRef] [PubMed]
15. Kumar, M.N.V.R. Nano and microparticles as controlled drug delivery devices. *J. Pharm. Pharm. Sci.* **2000**, *3*, 234–258.
16. Bilia, A.R.; Piazzini, V.; Guccione, C.; Risaliti, L.; Asprea, M.; Capecchi, G.; Bergonzi, M.C. Improving on Nature: The Role of Nanomedicine in the Development of Clinical Natural Drugs. *Planta Med.* **2017**, *83*, 366–381. [CrossRef]
17. Bhowmik, D.; Gopinath, H.; Kumar, B.P.; Duraivel, S.; Kumar, K.S. Recent advances in novel topical drug delivery system. *Pharma Innov.* **2012**, *1*, 12.
18. Guilherme, V.A.; Ribeiro, L.N.D.M.; Tofoli, G.R.; Franz-Montan, M.; De Paula, E.; De Jesus, M.B. Current Challenges and Future of Lipid Nanoparticles Formulations for Topical Drug Application to Oral Mucosa, Skin, and Eye. *Curr. Pharm. Des.* **2018**, *23*, 6659–6675. [CrossRef]
19. Lesch, C.; Squier, C.; Cruchley, A.; Speight, P.; Williams, D. The Permeability of Human Oral Mucosa and Skin to Water. *J. Dent. Res.* **1989**, *68*, 1345–1349. [CrossRef]
20. Sanz, R.; Calpena, A.C.; Mallandrich, M.; Clares, B. Enhancing topical analgesic administration: Review and prospect for transdermal and transbuccal drug delivery systems. *Curr. Pharm. Des.* **2015**, *21*, 2867–2882. [CrossRef]
21. Pathan, I.; Setty, C. Chemical Penetration Enhancers for Transdermal Drug Delivery Systems. *Trop. J. Pharm. Res.* **2009**, *8*, 173–180. [CrossRef]
22. Morgan, C.; Renwick, A.; Friedmann, P.S. The role of stratum corneum and dermal microvascular perfusion in penetration and tissue levels of water-soluble drugs investigated by microdialysis. *Br. J. Dermatol.* **2003**, *148*, 434–443. [CrossRef] [PubMed]
23. Michniak, B.; Thakur, R.; Wang, Y. Essential Oils and Terpenes. In *Percutaneous Penetration Enhancers*, 2nd ed.; Informa UK Limited: Bocca Raton, FL, USA, 2005; pp. 159–173.
24. Williams, A.C.; Barry, B.W. Terpenes and the lipid–protein-partitioning theory of skin penetration enhancement. *Pharm. Res.* **1991**, *8*, 17–24. [CrossRef] [PubMed]
25. Monti, D.; Najarro, M.; Chetoni, P.; Burgalassi, S.; Saettone, M.; Boldrini, E. Niaouli oil as enhancer for transdermal permeation of estradiol Evaluation of gel formulations on hairless rats in vivo. *J. Drug Deliv. Sci. Technol.* **2006**, *16*, 473–476. [CrossRef]
26. Monti, D.; Tampucci, S.; Chetoni, P.; Burgalassi, S.; Bertoli, A.; Pistelli, L. Niaouli oils from different sources: Analysis and influence on cutaneous permeation of estradiol in vitro. *Drug Deliv.* **2009**, *16*, 237–242. [CrossRef]
27. Dragicevic, N.; Scheglmann, D.; Albrecht, V.; Fahr, A. Temoporfin-loaded invasomes: Development, characterization and in vitro skin penetration studies. *J. Control. Release* **2008**, *127*, 59–69. [CrossRef]
28. Dragicevic-Curic, N.; Scheglmann, D.; Albrecht, V.; Fahr, A. Development of different temoporfin-loaded invasomes—Novel nanocarriers of temoporfin: Characterization, stability and in vitro skin penetration studies. *Colloids Surf. B Biointerfaces* **2009**, *70*, 198–206. [CrossRef]
29. Sinico, C.; Fadda, A.M. Vesicular carriers for dermal drug delivery. *Expert Opin. Drug Deliv.* **2009**, *6*, 813–825. [CrossRef]
30. Qadri, G.R.; Ahad, A.; Aqil, M.; Imam, S.S.; Ali, A. Invasomes of isradipine for enhanced transdermal delivery against hypertension: Formulation, characterization, and in vivo pharmacodynamic study. *Artif. Cells Nanomed. Biotechnol.* **2016**, *45*, 139–145. [CrossRef]

31. Kamran, M.; Ahad, A.; Aqil, M.; Imam, S.S.; Sultana, Y.; Ali, A. Design, formulation and optimization of novel soft nano-carriers for transdermal olmesartan medoxomil delivery: In vitro characterization and in vivo pharmacokinetic assessment. *Int. J. Pharm.* **2016**, *505*, 147–158. [CrossRef]
32. El-Nabarawi, M.A.; Shamma, R.N.; Farouk, F.; Nasralla, S.M. Dapsone-Loaded Invasomes as a Potential Treatment of Acne: Preparation, Characterization, and In Vivo Skin Deposition Assay. *AAPS PharmSciTech* **2018**, *19*, 2174–2184. [CrossRef] [PubMed]
33. Subongkot, T.; Wonglertnirant, N.; Songprakhon, P.; Rojanarata, T.; Opanasopit, P.; Ngawhirunpat, T. Visualization of ultradeformable liposomes penetration pathways and their skin interaction by confocal laser scanning microscopy. *Int. J. Pharm.* **2013**, *441*, 151–161. [CrossRef] [PubMed]
34. Rangsimawong, W.; Obata, Y.; Opanasopit, P.; Ngawhirunpat, T.; Takayama, K. Enhancement of Galantamine HBr Skin Permeation Using Sonophoresis and Limonene-Containing PEGylated Liposomes. *AAPS PharmSciTech* **2017**, *19*, 1093–1104. [CrossRef] [PubMed]
35. Ngawhirunpat, T.; Rangsimawong, W.; Opanasopit, P.; Rojanarata, T. Mechanistic study of decreased skin penetration using a combination of sonophoresis with sodium fluorescein-loaded PEGylated liposomes with D-limonene. *Int. J. Nanomed.* **2015**, *10*, 7413–7423. [CrossRef]
36. Sandig, A.G.; Campmany, A.C.; Fernandez-Campos, F.; Villena, M.M.; Clares, B. Transdermal delivery of imipramine and doxepin from newly oil-in-water nanoemulsions for an analgesic and anti-allodynic activity: Development, characterization and in vivo evaluation. *Colloids Surf. B Biointerfaces* **2013**, *103*, 558–565. [CrossRef]
37. Abd, E.; Benson, H.A.E.; Roberts, M.S.; Grice, J.E. Follicular Penetration of Caffeine from Topically Applied Nanoemulsion Formulations Containing Penetration Enhancers: In vitro Human Skin Studies. *Skin Pharmacol. Physiol.* **2018**, *31*, 252–260. [CrossRef]
38. Nikolic, I.; Mitsou, E.; Pantelic, I.; Randjelovic, D.; Markovic, B.; Papadimitriou, V.; Xenakis, A.; Lunter, D.J.; Žugic, A.; Savic, S. Microstructure and biopharmaceutical performances of curcumin-loaded low-energy nanoemulsions containing eucalyptol and pinene: Terpenes' role overcome penetration enhancement effect? *Eur. J. Pharm. Sci.* **2020**, *142*, 105135. [CrossRef]
39. Conte, R.; Marturano, V.; Peluso, G.; Calarco, A.; Cerruti, P. Recent Advances in Nanoparticle-Mediated Delivery of Anti-Inflammatory Phytocompounds. *Int. J. Mol. Sci.* **2017**, *18*, 709. [CrossRef]
40. Montecucco, F.; Liberale, L.; Bonaventura, A.; Vecchiè, A.; Dallegri, F.; Carbone, F. The Role of Inflammation in Cardiovascular Outcome. *Curr. Atheroscler. Rep.* **2017**, *19*, 11. [CrossRef]
41. Chen, W.-W.; Zhang, X.; Huang, W.-J. Role of neuroinflammation in neurodegenerative diseases (Review). *Mol. Med. Rep.* **2016**, *13*, 3391–3396. [CrossRef]
42. Perretti, M.; Cooper, D.; Dalli, J.; Norling, M.P.D.C.J.D.L.V. Immune resolution mechanisms in inflammatory arthritis. *Nat. Rev. Rheumatol.* **2017**, *13*, 87–99. [CrossRef] [PubMed]
43. Chen, X.; Peng, L.-H.; Shan, Y.-H.; Li, N.; Wei, W.; Yu, L.; Li, Q.-M.; Liang, W.-Q.; Gao, J.-Q. Astragaloside IV-loaded nanoparticle-enriched hydrogel induces wound healing and anti-scar activity through topical delivery. *Int. J. Pharm.* **2013**, *447*, 171–181. [CrossRef] [PubMed]
44. Mei, Z.-N.; Wu, Q.; Hu, S.; Lib, X.; Yang, X. Triptolide Loaded Solid Lipid Nanoparticle Hydrogel for Topical Application. *Drug Dev. Ind. Pharm.* **2005**, *31*, 161–168. [CrossRef] [PubMed]
45. Ahmada, A.; Abuzinadah, M.F.; Alkreathy, H.M.; Banaganapalli, B.; Mujeeb, M. Ursolic acid rich *Ocimum sanctum* L leaf extract loaded nanostructured lipid carriers ameliorate adjuvant induced arthritis in rats by inhibition of COX-1, COX-2, TNF-α and IL-1: Pharmacological and docking studies. *PLoS ONE* **2018**, *13*, e0193451. [CrossRef]
46. Lason, E.; Sikora, E.; Miastkowska, M.; Escribano, E.; Garcia-Celma, M.J.; Solans, C.; Llinas, M.; Ogonowski, J. NLCs as a potential carrier system for transdermal delivery of forskolin. *Acta Biochim. Pol.* **2018**, *65*, 437–442. [CrossRef]
47. Patel, P.A.; Patil, S.C.; Kalaria, D.R.; Kalia, Y.N.; Patravale, V. Comparative in vitro and in vivo evaluation of lipid based nanocarriers of Huperzine A. *Int. J. Pharm.* **2013**, *446*, 16–23. [CrossRef]
48. Yang, M.; Gu, Y.; Yang, D.; Tang, X.; Liu, J. Development of triptolide-nanoemulsion gels for percutaneous administration: Physicochemical, transport, pharmacokinetic and pharmacodynamic characteristics. *J. Nanobiotechnol.* **2017**, *15*, 88. [CrossRef]

49. Ahmad, N.; Ahmad, R.; Naqvi, A.A.; Ashafaq, M.; Alam, A.; Ahmad, F.J.; Al-Ghamdi, M.S. The effect of safranal loaded mucoadhesive nanoemulsion on oxidative stress markers in cerebral ischemia. *Artif. Cells Nanomed. Biotechnol.* **2017**, *45*, 775–787. [CrossRef]
50. Liu, M.; Li, Z.; Wang, H.; Du, S. Increased cutaneous wound healing effect of biodegradable liposomes containing madecassoside: Preparation optimization, in vitro dermal permeation, and in vivo bioevaluation. *Int. J. Nanomed.* **2016**, *11*, 2995–3007. [CrossRef]
51. Usach, I.; Margarucci, E.; Manca, M.L.; Caddeo, C.; Aroffu, M.; Petretto, G.L.; Manconi, M.; Peris, J.E. Comparison between Citral and Pompia Essential Oil Loaded in Phospholipid Vesicles for the Treatment of Skin and Mucosal Infections. *Nanomaterials* **2020**, *10*, 286. [CrossRef]
52. Kaltschmidt, B.P.; Ennen, I.; Greiner, J.; Dietsch, R.; Patel, A.V.; Kaltschmidt, B.; Kaltschmidt, C.; Hütten, A. Preparation of Terpenoid-Invasomes with Selective Activity against S. aureus and Characterization by Cryo Transmission Electron Microscopy. *Biomedicines* **2020**, *8*, 105. [CrossRef] [PubMed]
53. Apalla, Z.; Lallas, A.; Sotiriou, E.; Lazaridou, E.; Ioannides, D. Epidemiological trends in skin cancer. *Dermatol. Pract. Concept.* **2017**, *7*, 1–6. [CrossRef] [PubMed]
54. Krishnan, V.; Mitragotri, S. Nanoparticles for topical drug delivery: Potential for skin cancer treatment. *Adv. Drug Deliv. Rev.* **2020**, *153*, 87–108. [CrossRef] [PubMed]
55. Zhang, M.; Qureshi, A.A.; Geller, A.C.; Frazier, L.; Hunter, D.J.; Han, J. Use of Tanning Beds and Incidence of Skin Cancer. *J. Clin. Oncol.* **2012**, *30*, 1588–1593. [CrossRef]
56. Goldenberg, G.; Perl, M. Actinic keratosis: Update on field therapy. *J. Clin. Aesth. Dermatol.* **2014**, *7*, 28–31.
57. Tang, J.-Q.; Hou, X.-Y.; Yang, C.-S.; Li, Y.-X.; Xin, Y.; Guo, W.-W.; Wei, Z.-P.; Liu, Y.-Q.; Jiang, G. Recent developments in nanomedicine for melanoma treatment. *Int. J. Cancer* **2017**, *141*, 646–653. [CrossRef]
58. Kang, L.; Gao, Z.; Huang, W.; Jin, M.; Wang, Q. Nanocarrier-mediated co-delivery of chemotherapeutic drugs and gene agents for cancer treatment. *Acta Pharm. Sin. B* **2015**, *5*, 169–175. [CrossRef]
59. Khallaf, R.A.; Salem, H.F.; Abdelbary, A. 5-Fluorouracil shell-enriched solid lipid nanoparticles (SLN) for effective skin carcinoma treatment. *Drug Deliv.* **2016**, *23*, 3452–3460. [CrossRef]
60. Chen, D.; Lian, S.; Sun, J.; Liu, Z.; Zhao, F.; Jiang, Y.; Gao, M.; Sun, K.; Liu, W.; Fu, F. Design of novel multifunctional targeting nano-carrier drug delivery system based on CD44 receptor and tumor microenvironment pH condition. *Drug Deliv.* **2014**, *23*, 798–803. [CrossRef]
61. Csanyi, E.; Bakonyi, M.; Kovács, A.; Budai-Szűcs, M.; Csóka, I.; Berkó, S. Development of Topical Nanocarriers for Skin Cancer Treatment Using Quality by Design Approach. *Curr. Med. Chem.* **2019**, *26*, 6440–6458. [CrossRef]
62. Zhou, L.; Chen, Y.; Zhang, Z.-H.; Liu, X.; Wu, Q.; Yuan, L. Formulation, characterization, and evaluation of in vitro skin permeation and in vivo pharmacodynamics of surface-charged tripterine-loaded nanostructured lipid carriers. *Int. J. Nanomed.* **2012**, *7*, 3023–3033. [CrossRef] [PubMed]
63. Dehelean, C.A.; Feflea, S.; Gheorgheosu, D.; Ganta, S.; Cimpean, A.M.; Muntean, D.; Amiji, M. Anti-angiogenic and anti-cancer evaluation of betulin nanoemulsion in chicken chorioallantoic membrane and skin carcinoma in Balb/c mice. *J. Biomed. Nanotechnol.* **2013**, *9*, 577–589. [CrossRef] [PubMed]
64. Khan, K.; Aqil, M.; Imam, S.S.; Ahad, A.; Moolakkadath, T.; Sultana, Y.; Mujeeb, M. Ursolic acid loaded intra nasal nano lipid vesicles for brain tumour: Formulation, optimization, in vivo brain/plasma distribution study and histopathological assessment. *Biomed. Pharmacother.* **2018**, *106*, 1578–1585. [CrossRef] [PubMed]
65. Freag, M.S.; Saleh, W.M.; Abdallah, O.Y. Laminated chitosan-based composite sponges for transmucosal delivery of novel protamine-decorated tripterine phytosomes: Ex vivo mucopenetration and in vivo pharmacokinetic assessments. *Carbohydr. Polym.* **2018**, *188*, 108–120. [CrossRef]
66. De Matos, S.P.; Lucca, L.G.; Koester, L.S. Essential oils in nanostructured systems: Challenges in preparation and analytical methods. *Talanta* **2019**, *195*, 204–214. [CrossRef]
67. Solans, C.; Izquierdo, P.; Nolla, J.; Azemar, N.; Garcia-Celma, M.J. Nano-emulsions. *Curr. Opin. Colloid Interface Sci.* **2005**, *10*, 102–110. [CrossRef]
68. Bouchemal, K.; Briançon, S.; Perrier, E.; Fessi, H. Nano-emulsion formulation using spontaneous emulsification: Solvent, oil and surfactant optimisation. *Int. J. Pharm.* **2004**, *280*, 241–251. [CrossRef]
69. Laouini, A.; Jaafar-Maalej, C.; Limayem-Blouza, I.; Sfar, S.; Charcosset, C.; Fessi, H. Preparation, Characterization and Applications of Liposomes: State of the Art. *J. Colloid Sci. Biotechnol.* **2012**, *1*, 147–168. [CrossRef]
70. Anselmo, A.C.; Mitragotri, S. Nanoparticles in the clinic. *Bioeng. Transl. Med.* **2016**, *1*, 10–29. [CrossRef]

71. Mezei, M.; Gulasekharam, V. Liposomes—A selective drug delivery system for the topical route of administration I. Lotion dosage form. *Life Sci.* **1980**, *26*, 1473–1477. [CrossRef]
72. El Maghraby, G.M.; Barry, B.W.; Williams, A.C. Liposomes and skin: From drug delivery to model membranes. *Eur. J. Pharm. Sci.* **2008**, *34*, 203–222. [CrossRef] [PubMed]
73. Hood, R.R.; Kendall, E.L.; Junqueira, M.; Vreeland, W.N.; Quezado, Z.; Finkel, J.C.; DeVoe, D.L. Microfluidc—Enabled liposomes elucidate size-dependent transdermal transport. *PLoS ONE* **2014**, *9*, e92978. [CrossRef] [PubMed]
74. Muller, R.H.; Shegokar, R.; Keck, C.M. 20 years of lipid nanoparticles (SLN and NLC): Present state of development and industrial applications. *Curr. Drug Discov. Technol.* **2011**, *8*, 207–227. [CrossRef] [PubMed]
75. Jain, S.; Patel, N.; Shah, M.K.; Khatri, P.; Vora, N. Recent Advances in Lipid-Based Vesicles and Particulate Carriers for Topical and Transdermal Application. *J. Pharm. Sci.* **2017**, *106*, 423–445. [CrossRef] [PubMed]
76. Mukherjee, S.; Ray, S.; Thakur, R.S. Solid lipid nanoparticles: A modern formulation approach in drug delivery system. *Indian J. Pharm. Sci.* **2009**, *71*, 349–358. [CrossRef] [PubMed]
77. Desai, P.; Patlolla, R.R.; Singh, M. Interaction of nanoparticles and cell-penetrating peptides with skin for transdermal drug delivery. *Mol. Membr. Biol.* **2010**, *27*, 247–259. [CrossRef]
78. Estupiñan, O.R.; Garcia-Manrique, P.; Blanco-Lopez, M.D.C.; Matos, M.; Gutiérrez, G. Vitamin D3 Loaded Niosomes and Transfersomes Produced by Ethanol Injection Method: Identification of the Critical Preparation Step for Size Control. *Foods* **2020**, *9*, 1367. [CrossRef]
79. Kazi, K.M.; Mandal, A.S.; Biswas, N.; Guha, A.; Chatterjee, S.; Behera, M.; Kuotsu, K. Niosome: A future of targeted drug delivery systems. *J. Adv. Pharm. Technol. Res.* **2010**, *1*, 374–380.
80. Gupta, M.; Vaidya, B.; Mishra, N.; Vyas, S.P. Effect of Surfactants on the Characteristics of Fluconazole Niosomes for Enhanced Cutaneous Delivery. *Artif. Cells Blood Sub. Biotechnol.* **2011**, *39*, 376–384. [CrossRef]
81. Godin, B.; Touitou, E. Ethosomes: New prospects in transdermal delivery. *Crit. Rev. Ther. Drug Carr. Syst.* **2003**, *20*, 63–102. [CrossRef]
82. Hua, S. Lipid-based nano-delivery systems for skin delivery of drugs and bioactives. *Front. Pharmacol.* **2015**, *6*, 219. [CrossRef] [PubMed]
83. Bhalaria, M.K.; Naik, S.; Misra, A.N. Ethosomes: A novel delivery system for antifungal drugs in the treatment of topical fungal diseases. *Indian J. Exp. Boil.* **2009**, *47*, 368–375.
84. Dragicevic-Curic, N.; Verma, D.D.; Fahr, A. Invasomes: Vesicles for Enhanced Skin Delivery of Drugs. In *Percutaneous Penetration Enhancers Chemical Methods in Penetration Enhancement*; Springer Science and Business Media LLC: Berlin, Germany, 2016; pp. 77–92.

Publisher's Note: MDPI stays neutral with regard to jurisdictional claims in published maps and institutional affiliations.

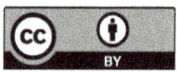

© 2020 by the author. Licensee MDPI, Basel, Switzerland. This article is an open access article distributed under the terms and conditions of the Creative Commons Attribution (CC BY) license (http://creativecommons.org/licenses/by/4.0/).

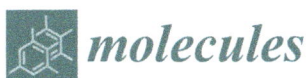

Review

Synthesis, Modification and Biological Activity of Diosgenyl β-D-Glycosaminosides: An Overview

Daria Grzywacz *, Beata Liberek[ID] and Henryk Myszka

Laboratory of Glycochemistry, Faculty of Chemistry, University of Gdańsk, Wita Stwosza 63, 80-308 Gdańsk, Poland; beata.liberek@ug.edu.pl (B.L.); henryk.myszka@ug.edu.pl (H.M.)
* Correspondence: daria.grzywacz@ug.edu.pl; Tel.: +48-58-523-50-70

Academic Editors: Pavel B. Drasar, Vladimir A. Khripach and Valeria Patricia Sülsen
Received: 9 September 2020; Accepted: 17 November 2020; Published: 20 November 2020

Abstract: Saponins are a structurally diverse class of natural glycosides that possess a broad spectrum of biological activities. They are composed of hydrophilic carbohydrate moiety and hydrophobic triterpenoid or steroid aglycon. Naturally occurring diosgenyl glycosides are the most abundant steroid saponins, and many of them exhibit various pharmacological properties. Herein, we present an overview of semisynthetic saponins syntheses–diosgenyl β-D-glycosaminosides (D-gluco and D-galacto). These glycosides possess a 2-amino group, which creates great possibilities for further modifications. A wide group of glycosyl donors, different N-protecting groups and various reaction conditions used for their synthesis are presented. In addition, this paper demonstrates the possibilities of chemical modifications of diosgenyl β-D-glycosaminosides, associated with functionalisation of the amino group. These provide N-acyl, N-alkyl, N,N-dialkyl, N-cinnamoyl, 2-ureido and 2-thiosemicarbazonyl derivatives of diosgenyl β-D-glycosaminosides, for which the results of biological activity tests (antifungal, antibacterial, anti-cancer and hemolytic) are presented.

Keywords: steroid saponin; diosgenin glycosides; diosgenyl β-D-glucosaminoside; diosgenyl β-D-galactosaminoside; amine group modifications; antimicrobial activity; anti-cancer activity; hemolytic activity

---

1. Introduction

The aim of this review is to provide information on the methods of synthesis and biological activity of diosgenyl β-D-glycosaminosides and their derivatives. These are semisynthetic saponins with proven antimicrobial and antitumor activity. This makes them very promising candidates for use as an antifungal or antibacterial drug. A significant advantage of these compounds is that they are not toxic. The toxicity of saponins is a particular limitation in the clinical application of this group of compounds.

2. Saponins, Their Occurrence, Properties and Structure

Saponins are a structurally diverse group of glycosides and are widely distributed in nature. Although these compounds are typical for plants [1,2], they have also been isolated from animals [3,4].

Saponins have the characteristic ability to reduce the surface tension of aqueous solutions and maintain a stable foam [5]. Therefore, they are useful in the production of emulsions and cleaning agents [5]. Most of them have been extracted from herbal preparations used in folk medicine, especially in Asian countries. In the form of herbal extracts, ointments, and various types of infusions, they are used as anti-malarial drugs, antidotes against snake and insect venoms, and as antiseptics, bactericides and antivirals [6]. Saponins also present interesting pharmacological properties, such as anti-diabetic [7–9], anti-cancer [10–12] and anti-inflammatory [13–16], and specific physiological properties—they change the structure of cell membranes, making them more permeable to compounds [17]. Saponins can also impair the digestion of intestinal proteins and the absorption of vitamins and minerals [18].

Saponins are composed of hydrophilic carbohydrate moiety and hydrophobic sapogenin. Due to their structure classic methods of saponin isolation, such as: solvent extraction, column chromatography and preparative TLC, are in many cases insufficient to isolate single saponins from plant material. Therefore, various, more modern, often combined separation techniques are used. Depending on the type of plant material, the following methods of extracting saponins can be distinguished: microwave-assisted solvent extraction (MAE); ultrasound-assisted solvent extraction (UAE); solid phase extraction (SPE); preparative column chromatography (CC); high-performance liquid chromatography (HPLC) coupled with other techniques [19,20].

The division of saponins depends mainly on the type of sapogenin. Triterpenoid and steroid saponins are one of the most important families of these plant secondary metabolites. Triterpenoid aglycones have the most varied structures among all types of sapogenins and dominate in the plant kingdom [21]. Their aglycon usually contains 30 carbon atoms and comprises five six-carbon rings (oleanane and ursane type; Figure 1) or four six- and one five-carbon ring (lupane type, Figure 1). A common feature of this type of sapogenins is the arrangement of the methyl substituents. Groups at the C-4, C-8 and C-10 atoms occupy the β position, whereas groups at the C-4 and C-14 atoms occupy the α position. The presence of a hydroxyl group at the secondary carbon atom (C-3) is also typical for triterpenoid sapogenins.

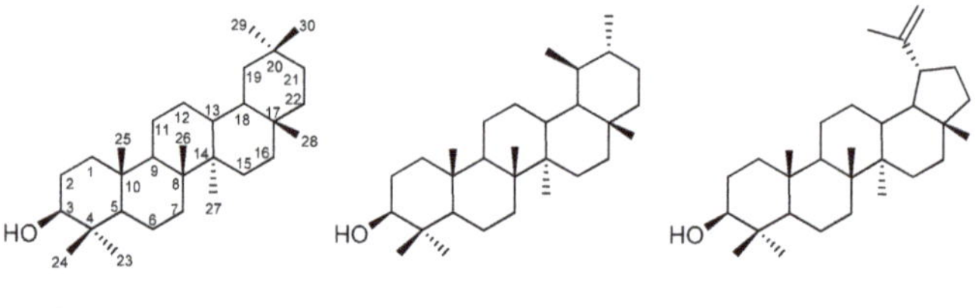

Figure 1. Chemical structures of triterpenoid sapogenins and the numbering system of carbon atoms.

The basic aglycone of steroid saponins contains 17 carbon atoms and is based on the sterane skeleton (1,2-cyclopentanoperhydrophenantrene), which comprises three six- and one five-carbon ring (Figure 2). Steroid sapogenins differ in the structure of the substituent located at the C-17 atom, which could be an additional heterocyclic ring or an aliphatic chain. Due to the nature of this substituent, steroid saponins are divided into three types: spirostane, furostane and cholestane (Figure 2) [22]. A common feature in the structure of steroid sapogenins is the arrangement of the methyl substituents located at the C-10 and C-13 atoms, which occupy the β position, whereas these occupy the α position at the C-21 atom. The presence of a hydroxyl group at the C-3 atom is also typical for steroidal saponins. Individual sapogenins differ in the presence of double bonds (e.g., C5 = C6), the configuration of the methyl group at the C-25 atom in spirostane saponins (25R or 25S) and sometimes the presence of additional functional groups (e.g., -OH).

The structural diversity of saponins lies also in the hydrophilic fragment, which usually comprises one or more sugar units. Analysis of the structure–activity relationship (SAR) has proven that the sugar portion plays an important role in the biological activity and might be the key pharmacophore for saponins' anti-cancer activities [23]. The most common saccharides found in saponins are: β-D-glucopyranose, β-D-galactopyranose, α-L-rhamnopyranose and β-D-xylopyra- nose; di-tri- and tetrasaccharides also occur. N-Acetyl-D-glucosamine residue sometimes is attached as the first sugar to the triterpenoid sapogenin [24]; however, in spirostane saponins D-glucose, and less frequently,

D-galactose, are usually directly attached to sapogenin. Natural steroidal saponins that contain an amino sugar fragment are very rare.

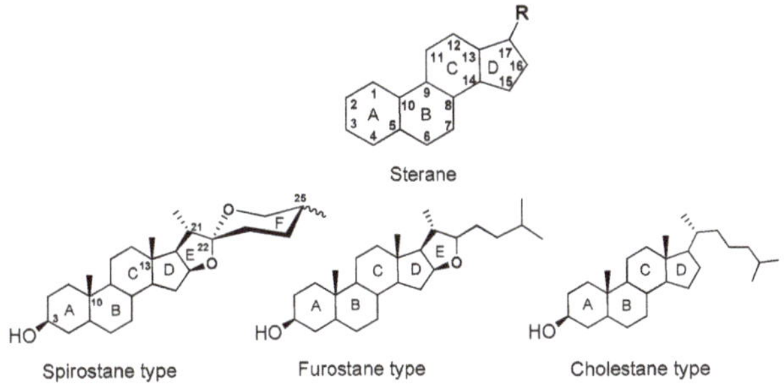

Figure 2. Chemical structures of steroidal sapogenins and the numbering system of carbon atoms.

3. Diosgenyl Saponins

Diosgenin ((25R)-spirost-5-en-3β-ol; DsOH; Figure 3) is a spirostane, and it has a very high structural similarity to steroid hormones. Therefore, it is a valuable and often used precursor in the synthesis of hormones and corticosteroids, including cortisone, pregnenolone and progesterone, on an industrial scale [25]. It is known for its anti-inflammatory and antioxidant properties and can also be used in the treatment of allergic and metabolic diseases (hypercholesterolemia, dyslipidaemia, diabetes and obesity), as well as for menopause symptoms and skin aging [26].

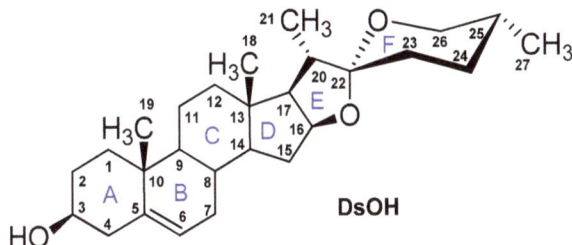

Figure 3. The structure of diosgenin (DsOH) with the numbering system of carbon atoms.

Diosgenin in combination with carbohydrate forms diosgenyl glycosides. In these natural compounds, D-glucose is usually the saccharide directly attached to sapogenin. However, combinations of diosgenin with other sugars have also been found: D-galactose (e.g., smilacinoside A, funcioside B or indioside E) and L-arabinose (e.g., conwallasaponin E and polyphilin F). Diosgenyl glycosides are the most abundant and, from the pharmaceutical point of view, the most explored natural steroid saponins. They occur mainly in the family of fungus plants (*Dioscoreaceae*), as well as in some species of solanaceae (*Solanaceae*), bean plants (*Fabaceae*) and fenugreek (*Trigonella*) [26]. Many of them exhibit antifungal [27], anti-thrombotic [28], antivirial, antioxidative and tissue-protective properties [29]. Diosgenyl glycosides also exerted an antitumor effect by inducing apoptosis in cancer cells and have great potential to be explored for cancer treatment [30–32].

Diosgenin saponins are commonly present in Chinese herbal preparations used in traditional folk medicine. The turning point in the research on this saponin was the discovery of the anti-cancer properties of the Chinese preparation 'Yunnan Baiyao' in the 1960s and the isolation of active substances with it [33]. Since then, research on methods of diosgenin saponins synthesis and their activity has been intensified. In the following years, numerous studies of representatives this class of compounds were carried out to find compounds useful in the fight against cancer cells and in therapies of diverse clinical disorders.

Among the most explored compounds are dioscin (^3O-{α-L-Rha-(1→4)-[α-L-Rha-(1→2)]-β-D-Glc}-diosgenin), gracillin (^3O-{α-D-Glc-(1→3)-[α-L-Rha-(1→2)]-β-D-Glc}-diosgenin) and their analogs [34–36].

4. D-Glycosaminosides of Diosgenin

Given that steroid–carbohydrate conjugates exhibit a broad spectrum of biological properties, research is ongoing not only to isolate these compounds from plant materials but also to improve the methods of their synthesis. The latter endeavour offers enormous opportunities to obtain non-naturally occurring compounds. Their design is based on the leading structure of a biologically active substance with confirmed activity. After finding that the compound exhibits biological activity, it is often chemically modified to improve its properties (physicochemical or biological) or to eliminate undesirable properties, such as high toxicity or poor solubility.

Diosgenyl D-glycosaminosides, which contain 2-amino-2-deoxy sugar residue in the carbohydrate moiety, have not yet been isolated from natural sources. Typically, D-glucose is linked to diosgenin in naturally occurring saponins. Replacing D-glucose with D-glucosamine or D-galactosamine is a promising modification; the presence of an amino group creates great opportunities for further modifications of these compounds. Amino sugars are of great biological importance and are commonly found as a component of natural oligo- and polysaccharides, glycoproteins, and can significantly increase the bioactivity of compounds. The formation of a glycosidic bond with them presents many problems, and much effort has been put into developing the most convenient conditions for such synthesis [37]. This review presents various synthetic approaches for obtaining diosgenyl β-D-glycosaminosides (different glycosyl donors, different protective groups of the amino function, different solvents used for the reaction, etc.). Moreover, the chemical modifications of the obtained diosgenyl β-D-glycosaminosides that lead to *N*-acyl, *N*-alkyl, *N,N*-dialkyl, *N*-cinnamoyl, 2-ureido and 2-thiosemicarbazyl derivatives, as well as the results of biological activity tests (antifungal, antibacterial, anti-cancer and hemolytic) of these new saponins, are presented.

4.1. Methods of Synthesis

The general strategy for the synthesis of diosgenyl 2-amino-2-deoxy-β-D-glycopyranoside (diosgenyl β-D-glucosaminoside, DsO-β-D-Glc-NH$_2$) relies on the preparation of an appropriately protected glycosyl donor, next, a coupling of the donor with diosgenin and finally, the deprotection of the amine and hydroxyl groups of the obtained diosgenyl glycoside. A properly protected amino group located at the C-2 atom of the glycosyl donor can play a key role in a glycosidic coupling, e.g., amide-type groups participate in the process of bond forming as the *neighbouring group*, which favours the formation of a 1,2-*trans*-glycosidic bond [38]. Therefore, among other things, various *N*-protecting groups were developed for the synthesis of diosgenyl–carbohydrate conjugates.

The first synthesis of diosgenyl 2-amino-2-deoxy-β-D-glucopyranoside was presented by Bednarczyk et al. in 2000 [39]. Two differently *N*-protected bromides (**5,7**) were used as the glycosyl donors (Scheme 1). The first one was 3,4,6-tri-*O*-acetyl-2-deoxy-2-trifluoroacetamido-α-D-glucopyranosyl bromide (**5**), which was syntesised via acetate **3** [40]. A trifluoroacetyl (TFAc) group was introduced on the free NH$_2$ function (**4**), formed by removing the imino group from **2** [41]. The final step was bromination of **4** with TiBr$_4$. The second bromide-3,4,6-tri-*O*-acetyl-2-deoxy-2-(3,4,5,6-tetrachlorophthalimido)-α,β-D-glucopyranosyl bromide (**7**) differs from the former one (**5**) in the amine group protection. In this case, a tetrachlorophthaloyl (TCP)-protecting group was used to block the amine function. From the *N*-TCP-protected acetate **6**, in reaction with TiBr$_4$, bromide **7** was synthesised. This time, the first was acylation of the amine function in hydrochloride **1** with tetrachlorophthalic anhydride (TCPA), followed by acetylation of the *N*-protected product with acetic anhydride in pyridine. This approach afforded compound **6** (α/β), and from this, the mixture of the anomeric bromides **7** was obtained. Furthermore, bromides **5** and **7** were also synthesised with the use of HBr in acetic acid [42]. The yields of both manners of bromination are similar.

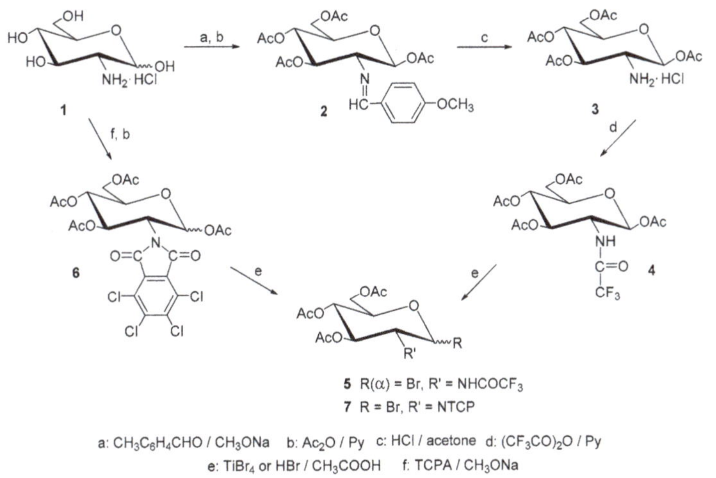

Scheme 1. Preparation of bromides **5** and **7** with the trifluoroacetyl (TFAc) and tetrachlorophthatloyl (TCP), respectively, *N*-protecting groups.

When comparing these approaches, one may see that the overall efficiency of the acetate **4** and **6** synthesis is higher when the acetylation reaction is carried out first, followed by amino function protection. In this approach, only the β-anomer of **4** (81%) is obtained. However, when the amine function is first protected and followed by acetylation, the acetate **6** (62%) is a mixture of α- and β-anomers, with clear dominance of the latter. This observation depends on the protecting groups used and has also been confirmed for different types of amino protecting groups (e.g., 2,2,2-trichoroetoxycarbonyl or phthaloyl groups) [43].

Condensations of the obtained glycosyl donors (bromides **5** and **7**) with diosgenin were carried out according to the modified Koenigs–Knorr method [44] that employed silver triflate (AgOTf) as the reaction promoter, in combination with powdered 4 Å molecular sieves in anhydrous dichloromethane (CH_2Cl_2) under an inert gas, namely nitrogen (Scheme 2) [39,41]. In this way, saponins **8** and **9** were obtained. The reaction of **8** with 1 M sodium methoxide in methanol yielded the partially deprotected diosgenyl 2-deoxy-2-trifluoroacetamido-β-D-glucopyranoside (**10**). The treatment of **10** with 1 M aqueous sodium hydroxide in acetone, followed by neutralisation, yielded the fully deprotected diosgenyl 2-amino-2-deoxy-β-D-glucopyranoside (**11**), which was isolated as the hydrochloride (**11**·HCl). In turn, the full *O*- and *N*-deprotection of **9**, in the presence of hydrazine hydrate in ethanol, was described [43]. This also led to the fully deprotected **11**. Under such conditions, glycosylations were efficient (~65%) and stereoselective, resulting only in β-glycosides. Importantly, this configuration also occurs in the natural diosgenyl glycosides.

In 2007, Yu and co-workers described another way of synthesis protected diosgenyl β-D-glucosaminoside using a different group of the glycosyl donors—trichloroacetimidate (TCAI), namely 3,4,6-tri-*O*-acetyl-2-deoxy-2-*N*-dimethylphosphoryl-α-D-glucopyranosyl trichloroacetimidate (**12**, Figure 4) [45]. Synthesis of **12** involves treatment of acetate **3** with diphenyl chlorophosphate in the presence of 4-dimethylaminopyridine (DMAP) and Et_3N, which gave *N*-diphenylphosphoryl (DPP)-glucosamine derivative. Transesterification of DPP into a dimethylphosphoryl group (DMP) and removal of the anomeric *O*-acetyl group, followed by reaction with trichloroacetonitrile (CCl_3CN), resulted in a new glycosyl donor (**12**). Its reaction with diosgenin in the presence of trimethylsilyl trifluoromethanesulfonate (TMSOTf) gave saponin **17**, with a 92% yield. From glycoside **17**, *O*-acetyl groups and DMP were finally removed in the presence of NaOH or hydrazine [45].

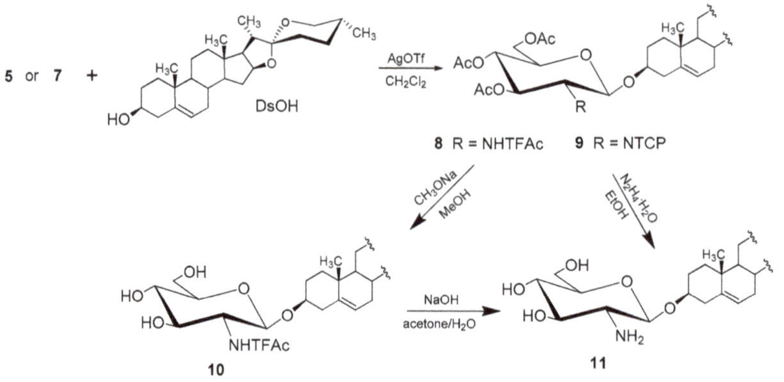

Scheme 2. Glycosylation of diosgenin with bromides **5** and **7**.

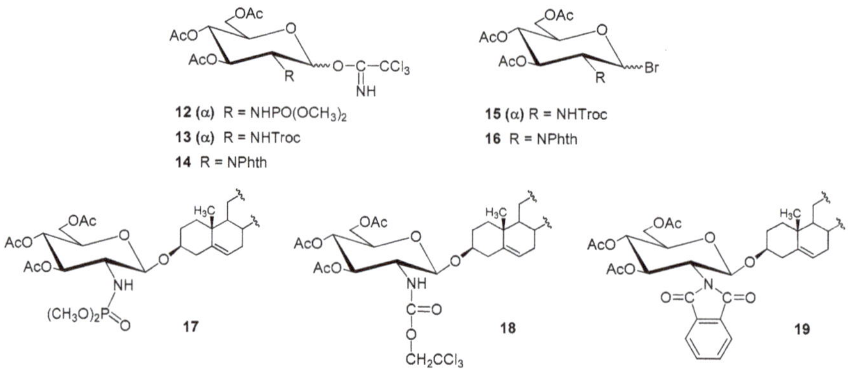

Figure 4. Glycosyl donors: trichloroacetimidates (**12–14**) and bromides (**15,16**) with different protecting groups at the amine function and examples of diosgenyl β-D-glucosaminosides synthesised with them (**17–19**).

In the subsequent years, other glycosyl donors were tested for the synthesis of diosgenyl glucosaminosides. Kaskiw et al. used 3,4,6-tri-O-acetyl-2-deoxy-2-(2′,2′,2′-trichloroethoxycarbonyl-amino)-α-D-glucopyranosyl trichloroacetimidate (**13**) [46]. The 2,2,2-trichoroetoxycarbonyl group (Troc) is stable under a wide range of standard conditions used in the synthesis of glucosamine derivatives. Additionally, it belongs to potential participating groups, which promote the formation of 1,2-*trans*-glycosides. The authors obtained saponin **18** (98%) in the reaction of **13** with diosgenin in the presence of TMSOTf as the catalyst (Figure 4).

The Kaskiw's group also used the glycosyl trichloroacetimidate donor with the Troc-protecting group on an amine function in the synthesis of protected diosgenyl amino disaccharide (**23**) [47]. The attached disaccharide comprises benzoylated D-glucoaminopyranose with a Troc-protecting group (**20**) and acetylated L-rhamnopyranose (**21**) (Scheme 3). The glycosylation of diosgenin was performed with the respective trichloroacetimidate (**22**) in the presence of TMSOTf in an 80% yield. The resulting glycoside was further transformed, and the protecting groups were subsequently removed by treatment with sodium methoxide in methanol.

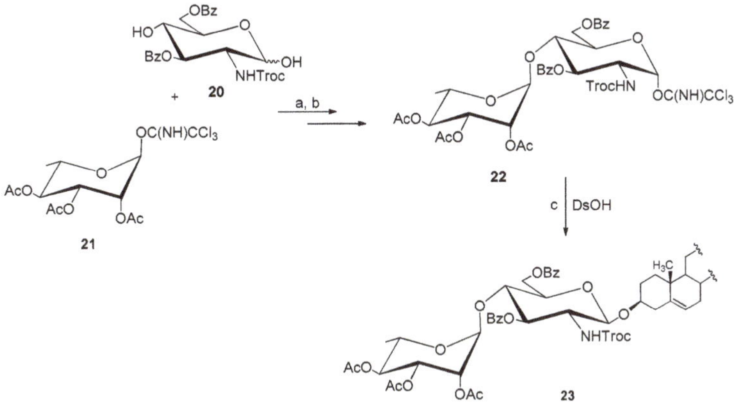

Scheme 3. Glycosylation of diosgenin with *N*-Troc-amino disaccharide (**22**).

In turn, Fernandez-Herrera et al. proposed per-*O*-acetylated 1-*O*-trichloroacetimidate, with phthaloyl protection (Phth) of the amine function (**14**), as a suitable donor for diosgenin glycosylation (Figure 4). They obtained only β-anomer of saponin **19** in a glycosylation reaction promoted by TMSOTf; the yield was 96% [48]. Tan's research group also used a similar procedure to obtain **19**, but with a slightly worse yield (80%) [49]. Saponins **18** and **19** were also synthesised in the reactions of diosgenin with bromides **15** and **16**, respectively (Figure 4) [50]. The authors obtained only the α anomer of **15** and a mixture of anomers α + β in a case of **16**. These bromides were later used without further purification in the coupling reaction with diosgenin in the presence of AgOTf. The reaction yields were 98% and 90%, respectively.

In addition to the above-described and commonly used D-glucosaminosyl donors, the less frequently used D-glucosaminosyl chlorides (**24–27**) and (*N*-phenyl)trifluoroacetimidates (PTFAI, **28–31**) are also noteworthy (Figure 5) [43]. Although glycosyl chlorides are less reactive than corresponding bromides, they are more stable and were used for the synthesis of diosgenyl glycosides.

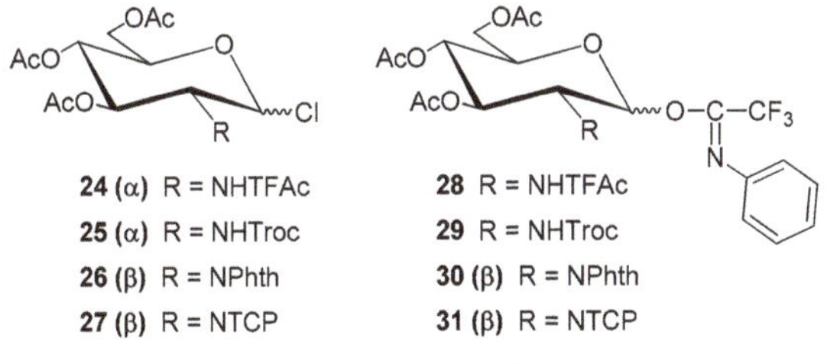

Figure 5. Glycosyl chlorides (**24–27**) and (*N*-phenyl)trifluoroacetimidates (**28–31**) with different protecting groups at the 2-amino function.

There are several ways that a chlorine atom can be introduced on an anomeric carbon atom in *N*-protected and per-*O*-acetylated D-glucosamine. One of the often-used chlorinating agents is 1,1-dichloromethyl methyl ether in the presence of $ZnCl_2$ or $BF_3 \cdot H_2O$ [51]. This reagent was successfully used by Bednarczyk et al. to synthesise chlorides **24–27** [43]. Chlorides with the 2-NHTFAc (**24**) or 2-NHTroc (**25**) groups were solely α anomers, whereas those with imide-type moieties (2-NPhth **26** and 2-NTCP **27**) have the β configuration on the anomeric carbon atom. Glycosyl chlorides (**24–27**) were used in coupling reactions with diosgenin, carried out in CH_2Cl_2 or in its mixture with Et_2O, in the presence of AgOTf as a reaction promoter. The fully protected diosgenyl β-D-glucosaminosides (**8,9,18,19**) were obtained with a yield of 69–99% [43].

The use of (*N*-phenyl) trifluoroacetimidates (PTFAI) instead of trichloroacetimidates (TCAI) as glycosyl donors is an alternative method for the synthesis of glycosides [52,53], including diosgenyl saponins. The synthesis of 1-*O*-(*N*-phenyl)trifluoroacetimidates (**28–31**, Figure 5) from the respective sugar acetates with four different 2-*N*-protecting groups (TFAc, Troc, Phth and TCP) requires the selective removal of the acetyl group from the anomeric carbon, typically with ethylenediamine in a mixture of acetic acid in THF, followed by reaction with (*N*-phenyl)trifluoroacetate imidoyl chloride. This approach was ineffective in the case of D-glucosaminopyranose acetate with the TCP-protecting group (**6**); therefore, its bromide or chloride was hydrolysed in reaction with Ag_2CO_3 in the acetone and H_2O mixture. It was then reacted with freshly prepared (*N*-phenyl)trifluoroacetate imidoyl chloride [43]. Such synthesised glycosyl donors in the reaction with diosgenin in the presence of TMSOTf led to the expected fully protected β-glycosides (**8,9,18,19**) obtained in yields of 52–85%.

In addition to D-glucosamine, 2-amino-2-deoxy-D-galactopyranose (D-galactosamine) was glycosidically attached to diosgenin [54]. Natural diosgenyl D-galactosides have been much less isolated from plants than the corresponding D-glucosides. Similarly to diosgenyl glucosaminosides, spirostane saponins that contain a D-galactosamine in carbohydrate portion are not found in nature. To synthesise diosgenyl β-D-galactosaminosides (**35**), analogous reactions were performed, such as those described for the D-glucosamine series (Scheme 4). Thus, to obtain bromide **33**, D-galactosamine hydrochloride (**32**) was used. It was first acylated with tetrachlorophthalic anhydride (TCPA), followed by acetylation with acetic anhydride in pyridine. Then, the obtained anomeric mixture of the product was brominated with $TiBr_4$, which led to an anomeric mixture of bromides (**33**), with a clear predominance of the β anomer (α:β = 1:4). Due to the high reactivity of bromides, this donor was immediately used in the condensation reaction with diosgenin in CH_2Cl_2, in the presence of AgOTf as the reaction promoter. There was an 80% yield of synthetic protected diosgenyl β-D-galactosaminoside (**34**) [54]. Deprotection of the *O*-acetyl groups and NTCP group of **34** was achieved by using 98% hydrazine hydrate in EtOH and yielded diosgenyl 2-amino-2-deoxy-β-D-galactopyranoside (**35**), which was converted into hydrochloride **35·HCl**.

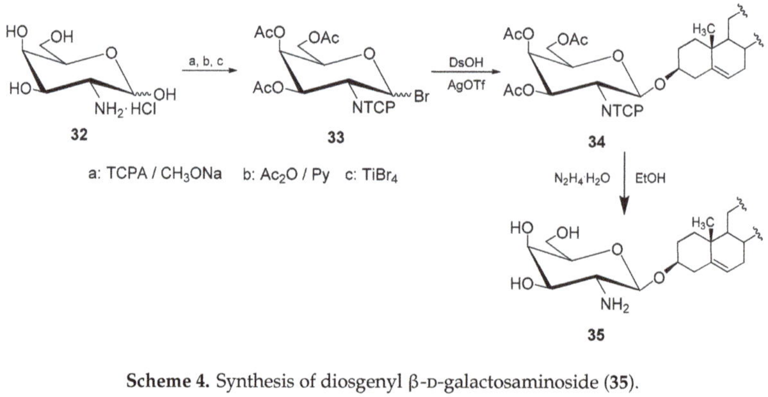

Scheme 4. Synthesis of diosgenyl β-D-galactosaminoside (**35**).

Glycosylation of diosgenin with D-glycosamine derivatives mainly proceeds according to the S_N1 and/or S_N2, mechanism, usually with the contribution of protected 2-amino groups (NHTFAc, NHTroc, NPhth and NTCP). The presence of these groups promotes the formation of 1,2-*trans* glycosides, which in the case of D-glucosamine and D-galactosamine means formation of β-configurated glycosides.

The type of promoter used (heavy metal salt or TMSOTf), as well as the solvent and temperature, are also significant. Table 1 summarizes the most useful procedures of providing diosgenyl β-D-glycosaminosides. The type of glycosyl donor (bromides, chlorides and imidates) and the order of reagent addition has a noticeable influence on the efficiency of the reaction. For the glycosidation reaction, two procedures are recognized: *normal* and *reverse*. In the *normal* procedure, the promoter (AgOTf or TMSOTf) is added as the last to the solution containing the glycosyl donor and acceptor, whereas in the *reverse* procedure, the glycosyl donor is added to the mixture of the promoter and glycosyl acceptor [55].

Table 1. Most commonly used procedures for glycosylation of diosgenin.

Entry	Procedure	Glycosyl Donor			Solvent	Promotor	Product	Yield (%)	Lit.
1	normal	5 (α)	Bromide	NHTFAc	CH_2Cl_2	AgOTf	8	65	[39]
2	normal	5 (α)	Bromide	NHTFAc	CH_2Cl_2/Et_2O	AgOTf	8	69	[41]
3	reverse	5 (α)	Bromide	NHTFAc	CH_2Cl_2/Et_2O	AgOTf	8	77	[50]
4	normal	7 (α + β)	Bromide	NTCP	CH_2Cl_2	AgOTf	9	65	[39]
5	normal	7 (α + β)	Bromide	NTCP	CH_2Cl_2/Et_2O	AgOTf	9	73	[41]
6	reverse	7 (α + β)	Bromide	NTCP	CH_2Cl_2	AgOTf	9	93	[50]
7	normal	10 (α)	TCAI	NDMP	CH_2Cl_2	TMSOTf	15	92	[45]
8	normal	11 (α)	TCAI	NHTroc	CH_2Cl_2	TMSOTf	16	98; 84	[47,56]
9	normal	12 (α + β)	TCAI	NPhth	CH_2Cl_2	TMSOTf	17	96; 80	[48,49]
10	reverse	13 (α)	Bromide	NHTroc	CH_2Cl_2/Et_2O	AgOTf	16	98	[50]
11	normal	14 (α + β)	Bromide	NPhth	CH_2Cl_2/Et_2O	AgOTf	17	51	[50]
12	reverse	14 (α + β)	Bromide	NPhth	CH_2Cl_2/Et_2O	AgOTf	17	55	[50]
13	reverse	14 (α + β)	Bromide	NPhth	CH_2Cl_2	AgOTf	17	90	[50]
14	reverse	18 (α)	Chloride	NHTFAc	CH_2Cl_2/Et_2O	AgOTf	8	69	[43]
15	reverse	19 (α)	Choride	NHTroc	CH_2Cl_2/Et_2O	AgOTf	16	86	[43]
16	reverse	20 (β)	Chloride	NPhth	CH_2Cl_2	AgOTf	17	99	[43]
17	reverse	21 (β)	Chloride	NTCP	CH_2Cl_2	AgOTf	9	87	[43]
18	normal	22 (α + β)	PTFAI	NHTFAc	CH_2Cl_2	TMSOTf	8	85	[50]
19	normal	23 (α + β)	PTFAI	NHTroc	CH_2Cl_2	TMSOTf	16	81	[50]
20	normal	24 (β)	PTFAI	NPhth	CH_2Cl_2	TMSOTf	17	83	[50]
21	normal	25 (β)	PTFAI	NTCP	CH_2Cl_2	TMSOTf	9	52	[50]
22	reverse	27 (α + β)	Bromide	NTCP	CH_2Cl_2	AgOTf	28	80	[54]

The choice of glycosylation procedure should also consider the orthogonality of the protecting groups, and thus the possibility of removing them independently. This factor is especially important when there is a planned modification of the obtained glycoside, e.g., by attaching further saccharide units or functionalising the amino group.

O-Acetyl groups used in the above presented syntheses could be easily removed under basic conditions (typically with sodium methoxide in methanol). It is possible to remove only *O*-acetyl groups while the amino-protecting groups remain intact (8→10, Scheme 2). This approach is important if further attachment of the sugar units to such saponin is planned. To remove the TFAc amino-protecting group, a solution of NaOH in an acetone–water mixture is typically used (10→11, Scheme 2). Under these conditions, the *O*-acetyl groups could be also removed [57]. Likewise, the *O*-acetyl groups, the TCP- and TFAc-protecting groups can be removed simultaneously under weakly basic conditions, e.g., with hydrazine hydrate in EtOH, at the reflux temperature (9→11 and 34→35). If diethylamine is used instead of hydrazine hydrate, an *N*-acetyl derivative of saponin is often formed as a by-product [57]. Removal of the phthaloyl group requires a high temperature and quite a long reaction time. This reaction usually uses hydrazine hydrate or *n*-butylamine in ethanol (19→11) [58]. It is worth adding that the order in which the protecting groups are removed must be taken into account. Generally, *O*-deacetylation should be done first, otherwise *O*→*N* acetyl migration may occur.

Sometimes, to functionalise an amino group, it is necessary to remove only the protecting group from the amine function, leaving the acetyl groups on the hydroxyl functions. In that case, it is preferable to use a trichloroethoxycarbonyl group, which could be selectively removed under reductive β-elimination with zinc dust or zinc-copper powder in acetic acid (18 → 36, Scheme 5) [43,46].

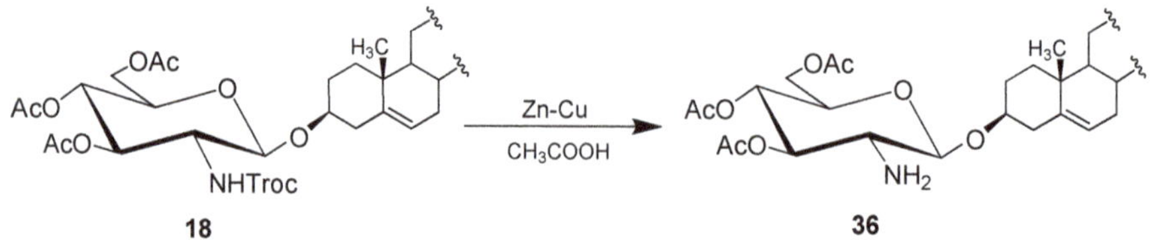

Scheme 5. Removal of Troc protecting group from amino function.

4.2. Chemical Modification

Difficulties associated with the isolation and purification of saponins from natural sources force its synthesis. In addition, chemical modifications create opportunities to obtain new compounds, often with more favourable therapeutic properties compared to naturally occurring or reference substances. Saponins, especially diosgenyl glycosides, are attractive candidates for new drug design and development due to their valuable properties: anti-inflammatory [13,14], antimicrobial [27], anti-coagulant [28], anti-cancer [30–32] and gelling [59].

Chemical modifications of diosgenyl saponins mainly concern the sugar part. The changes most often involve attachment of other sugar residues or extension of the sugar chain and introduction of various functional groups or substituents. Modifications of aglycon have also been described in the literature [60].

Research related to the chemical modification of diosgenyl β-D-glycosaminosides is mainly associated with the functionalisation of the amino group. Thus, the following sections present the procedures for modifying the -NH_2 group and the results of studies on the biological activity of the most interesting derivatives of diosgenyl glycosaminosides.

4.2.1. N-alkyl and N,N-dialkyl Derivatives

A series of *N*-alkyl and *N,N*-dialkyl derivatives of diosgenyl 2-amino-2-deoxy-β-D-gluco- and D-galactopyranosides have been synthesised [50,54]. The synthesis of these compounds used a method of reductive alkylation of amines [61]. *N*-Monoalkyl derivatives were obtained by treatment of the primary amine group in diosgenyl β-D-glycosaminoside with an appropriate aldehyde (*R*-CHO), followed by reduction in the resulting imine with sodium cyanoborohydride (NaBH$_3$CN).

The *N*-alkyl derivatives, as the secondary amines, can react under the same conditions with another aldehyde molecule to form an enamine, from which the *N,N*-dialkyl derivative is obtained after reduction. Such alkylation reactions are not selective and usually provide mixtures of mono- and dialkylated products, which should be separated by column chromatography.

Using reductive alkylation of diosgenyl β-D-glucosaminoside (**11**) with respective aldehyde, four *N*-alkyl (**37–40**) and six *N,N*-dialkyl derivatives (**41–46**) were obtained, whereas using alkylation of diosgenyl β-D-galactosaminoside (**35**) one *N*-alkyl (**47**) and two *N,N*-dialkyl (**48** and **49**) derivatives were synthesized (Figure 6).

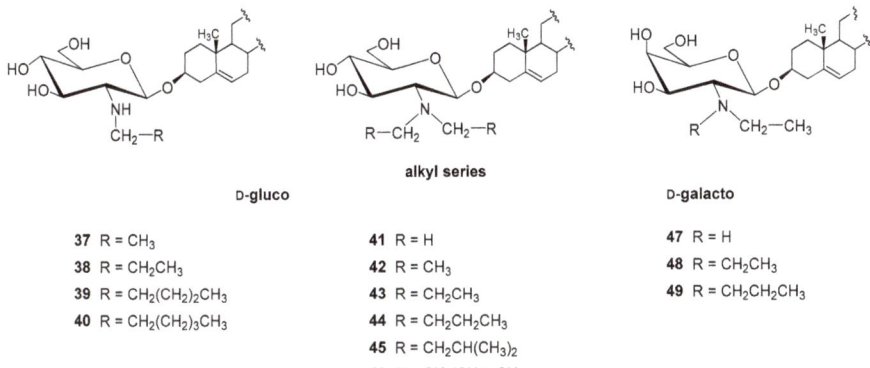

Figure 6. N-Alkyl and N,N-dialkyl derivatives of diosgenyl β-D-gluco-(**37–46**) and β-D-galactosaminosides (**47–49**).

4.2.2. N-acyl Derivatives

N-Acetylation with acetic or trifluoroacetic anhydride, in methanol or pyridine, of the free amino group in diosgenyl β-D-glycosaminosides (**11** and **35**), provided four new saponins (**50**, **51**, **57**, **58**, Figure 7) [41,54].

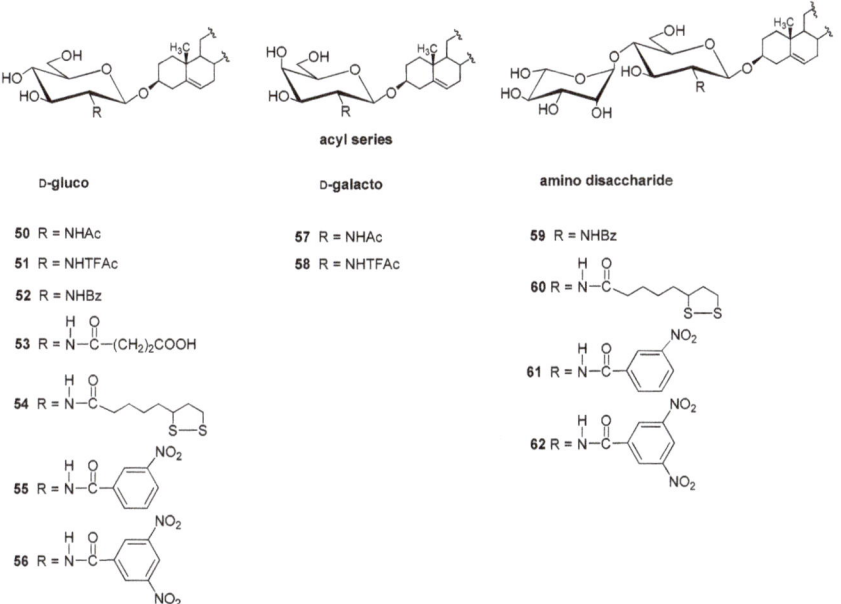

Figure 7. N-acyl derivatives of diosgenyl D-gluco- (**50–56**), D-galactosaminosides (**57**, **58**) and amino disaccharide (**59–62**).

Kaskiw at al. synthesised the other group of diosgenyl β-D-glucosaminosides with different acyl substituents at the amino group. Glycoside **36** was used for the synthesis, and the amino function of this saponin was acetylated with: benzoyl chloride, succinic anhydride in pyridine and (±)-α-lipoic acid, 3-nitrobenzoic acid, 3,5-dinitrobenzoic acid in the presence of 2-(1*H*-benzotriazole-1-yl)-1,1,3,3-tetra-methylaminium hexafluorophosphate (HBTU) and *N,N*-diisopropylethylamine (DIPEA). The final removal of the *O*-acetyl groups from obtained derivatives with sodium methoxide in CH_2Cl_2/MeOH mixture generated the respective diosgenyl glycosides **52–56** with good yields (73–92%; Figure 7) [46,47].

The same approach was used to obtain *N*-acyl derivatives of diosgenyl glycoside containing a disaccharide residue (**59–62**, Figure 7). After removing the Troc protecting group from the saponin **23** by treating it with zinc dust in acetic acid, the free amino group was acylated under the same conditions used for monosaccharide saponins with benzoyl chloride, (±)-α-lipoic acid, 3-nitrobenzoic acid and 3,5-dinitrobenzoic acid (76–83%). Finally, *O*-acetyl and *O*-benzoyl groups from the obtained saponins were removed by treating with sodium methoxide in methanol to yield *N*-acyl diosgenyl disaccharide consisting of glucosaminose (**59–62**).

To search for pharmaceuticals that may be well-delivered to a cell, Grzywacz et al. synthesised the *N*-acyl derivatives of diosgenyl β-D-glucosaminoside (**11**) with a series of amino acids, peptide and hydroxy acids conjugated with saponin (**63–76**, Scheme 6) [62]. The use of amino acids and peptide as drug delivery vectors is growing due to their large structural diversity, biocompatibility as well as low toxicity [63,64]. Hydroxy acids used in these explorations are structural analogs of some amino acids.

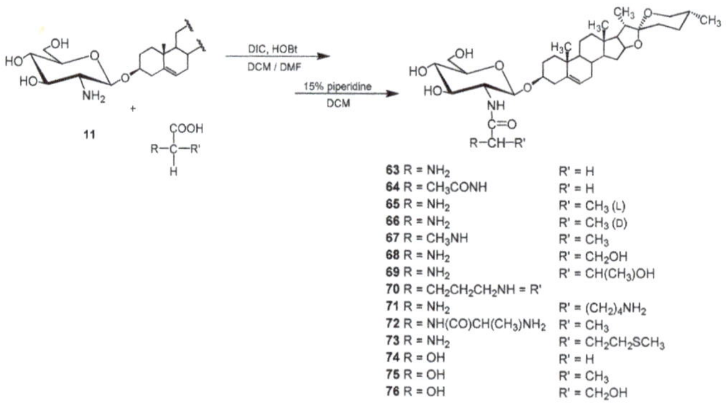

Scheme 6. Synthesis of *N*-aminoacyl (**63–73**) and *N*-hydroxyacyl (**74–76**) derivatives of diosgenyl 2-amino-2-deoxy-β-D-glucopyranoside.

N-Aminoacyl and *N*-hydroxyacyl derivatives of diosgenyl 2-amino-2-deoxy-β-D-glucopyranoside (**63–76**) were obtained using the solution-phase method of peptide synthesis in DCM/DMF mixture. Fmoc-protected amino acids were used for the synthesis, whereas *N,N*'-diisopropylcarbodiimide (DIC) and 1-hydroxybenzotriazole (HOBt) were used as the coupling agents (Scheme 6). Reactions with amino acids and peptide were carried out with and without microwave assistance. In both procedures, the reaction yields were similar, but the duration was markedly reduced (even several fold) in the case of the reactions carried out in microwave reactor. Reactions of hydroxy acids were conducted solely without microwave assistance. For modifications of diosgenyl β-D-glucosaminoside (**11**), the following protected amino acids were selected: glycine, *N*-acetylglycine, sarcosine, L- and D-alanine, L-serine, L-threonine, L-lysine, L-proline, L-methionine and dipeptide (L-Ala-L-Ala). From the obtained diosgenyl *N*-aminoacyl saponins, the Fmoc-protecting group was removed by treatment with a freshly prepared 15% piperidine solution in DCM. Three hydroxy acids, namely glycolic acid, L-lactic acid and L-glyceric acid, were also attached to diosgenyl β-D-glucosaminoside (**11**). The formation of *N*-acyl derivatives of diosgenyl glucosaminoside in the presence of DIC and HOBt from the mentioned amino acids proceeds according to the known mechanism of amide bond formation using HOBt in order to minimize the formation of unreactive *N*-acylurea [65].

4.2.3. Other Derivatives

Urea derivatives—not only of carbohydrates—exhibit a broad spectrum of biological activity. They can be part of antibiotics, enzyme inhibitors or compounds with documented cytotoxicity, such as streptozotocin or chlorozotocin [66,67]. The presence of amino group in diosgenyl glycosaminosides creates the possibility of ureido derivatives' formation. Therefore, such saponins were also synthesised and explored.

The first saponin with a 2-phenylureido moiety, glycoside **77**, was obtained by Myszka et al. in the reaction of diosgenyl β-D-glucosaminoside (**11**) with phenyl isocyanate in a CHCl$_3$/MeOH mixture [34]. In the same way, using isocyanates, three different ureido derivatives of diosgenyl β-D-galactosaminoside (**82–84**) were obtained [54]. Wang et al. proposed a different route for the synthesis of 2-ureido diosgenyl saponins [56]. To obtain several urea derivatives (**78–81**) they used diosgenyl 3,4,6-tri-O-acetyl-N-Troc-2-amino-2-deoxy-β-D-glucopyranoside (**18**) and commercially available amines, including benzyl-, 4-fluoro-benzyl-, 4-methoxy-benzyl-, and *tert*-butyl-amine (Figure 8). Notably, this modification was made without the need for removal of the Troc- and O-acetyl-protecting group from glycoside **18**. The reactions were carried out in dimethyl sulfoxide (DMSO) at 70 °C in the presence of DIPEA. Only after completion of the reaction were the acetyl-protecting groups removed with a solution of NH$_3$ in methanol. The reactions yields were 54–75%.

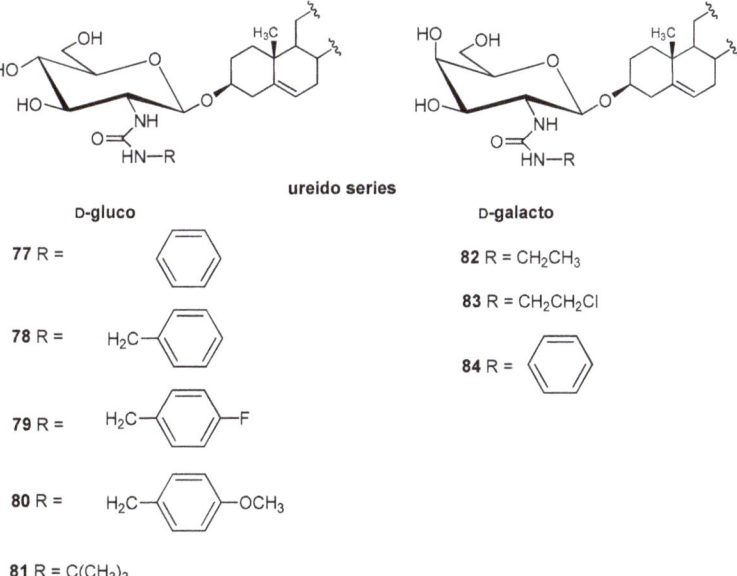

Figure 8. 2-Ureido derivatives of diosgenyl D-gluco-(**77–81**) and D-galactosaminosides (**82–84**).

The same group of researchers synthesised two other series of diosgenyl β-D-glucosaminoside derivatives with a cinnamoyl and thiosemicarbazonyl moiety at the C-2 atom (Figure 9) [56]. Before the introduction of sulfonamides, cinnamic acid and its derivatives performed the function of chemotherapeutics. Derivatives that contained a thiosemicarbazonyl moiety can be valuable bioeffectors with a wide range of pharmaceutical applications. Some of them are antiviral, antibacterial or antifungal drugs [68–70].

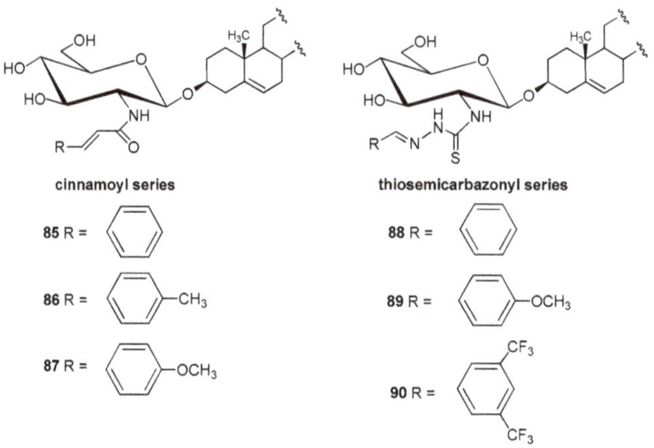

Figure 9. Examples of diosgenyl β-D-glucosaminosides with *N*-cinnamoyl (**85–87**) and 2-thiosemicarbazonyl (**88–90**) functional groups.

For the synthesis of both series, it was necessary to remove the Troc protecting group (zinc dust in acetic acid) from the amine function in **18** and obtain saponin **36** (Scheme 5). The reaction of **36** with cinnamoyl chlorides with differently substituted phenyl rings formed the respective *N*-cinnamoyl derivatives of the *O*-acetylated diosgenyl glucosaminoside. Their *O*-deprotection with NH_3 in MeOH provided a series of new diosgenyl *N*-cinnamoyl-β-D-glucosaminosides (**85–87**, Figure 9). Reaction yields were 55–71%.

To synthesise thiosemicarbazonyl derivatives of diosgenyl glucosaminoside (**88–90**), Wang et al. first converted the free amino group of **36** to isosulfocyanide in reaction of **36** with thiocarbonyl chloride in the presence of $CaCO_3$ in DCM/H_2O mixture [56]. They then treated it with 80% hydrazine hydrate in ethanol, followed by the appropriate benzaldehyde. Finally, the *O*-acetyl groups were removed, which gave saponins **88–90** (total yields were 48–53%).

4.3. Pharmacological Properties

Over the past 30 years, a significant increase in the incidence of fungal infections, multi-drug resistance to bacteria and the number of cases of cancer have been observed. Therefore, alternative therapeutic methods are being sought, in particular, effective therapies with new mechanisms of action against resistant pathogens.

Natural diosgenyl glycosides exhibit a broad spectrum of pharmaceutical properties [27–32]. The diverse biological activity of these compounds is closely connected with their diverse structural construction. Therefore, their synthetic analogs are designed and synthesised to find pharmaceutics with improved activities. This also applies to diosgenyl β-D-glycosaminosides, for which syntheses are presented above.

4.3.1. Antibacterial Activity

Saponins exhibit antibacterial activity by inhibiting the growth of Gram-positive (G+) or Gram-negative (G−) bacteria. However, some of them are not effective against G− bacteria, probably because they cannot penetrate the cell membranes of these microorganisms [71]. The cell wall of G- bacteria has a much more complex structure; it is composed of an additional outer membrane, phospholipids and lipopolysaccharide, which are not present in the cell wall of G+ bacteria. The mechanism of saponins' action is based on their ability to form complexes with the sterols present in the surface membrane of eukaryotic cells/microorganisms (bacteria and fungi). As a consequence, it causes disorders of membrane integration, its perforation and rupture, and loss of intracellular components. Nucleic acids and proteins are key components of pathogens, and the integrity of the cytoplasmic membrane is essential for cell growth [72–74]. Studies on the obtained diosgenyl β-D-glycosaminosides indicate that none of the above-presented saponins exhibit activity against G− bacteria; the minimum inhibitory concentrations (MIC; μg/mL) were over 512 μg/mL [50,54,62].

The bactericidal effect on a large number of Gram-positive cocci were performed, setting MIC_{50}, MIC_{90}, and the minimum bactericidal concentration (MBC_{50} and MBC_{90}; μg/mL) for diosgenyl β-D-glucosaminoside hydrochloride (**11**·HCl) [75]. The studies were conducted for clinical isolates of: methicillin- and vancomycin-resistant strains (MR and VR), as well as methicillin- and vancomycin-sensitive strains (MS and VS) of *S. aureus* and *E. faecalis*, and for *S. pyogenes* and *R. equi*. As control compounds, widely available antibiotics, including imipenem, doxycycline, erythromycin and ciprofloxacin were used (Table 2). The results of studies showed that **11**·HCl is equally and, in many cases, more active against examined strains to the tested antibiotics used to treat patients infected with these bacteria. Interestingly, the values of the MBC against *R. equi* for **11**·HCl (MBC = 4 μg/mL (50%), 16 μg/mL (90%)) were much lower than the MBC for the standard antibiotics. Additionally, when comparing the MIC_{90} and MBC_{90} values for **11**·HCl and for erythromycin, it can be seen that saponin **11**·HCl in each case gives better results, with the exception of *R. equi* bacteria (MIC_{90} = 4 μg/mL).

Further studies assessing antibacterial activity for **11**·HCl showed that its exhibits relative activity against tested reference strains of G+ bacteria: *E. faecalis*, *S. aureus*, *S. epidermidis* and *R. equi* (MIC = 16 μg/mL), whereas analogous hydrochloride of diosgenyl β-D-galactosaminoside (**35**·HCl) is completely inactive against the listed strains [50,54].

Additionally, the synergism of diosgenyl β-D-glucosaminoside hydrochloride (**11**·HCl) and antibiotics was studied [75]. The results were presented as a Fractionated Inhibitory Concentration (FIC index; FIC ≤ 0.5 indicates synergism, 0.5 < FIC ≤ 1.0 additive activity, 1.0–4 neutral effect and FIC > 4 shows an antagonistic effect). It was observed that the use of **11**·HCl with vancomycin or with daptomycin leads to a synergistic effect against methicillin- and vancomycin-sensitive strains, and against *R. equi* and *S. pyogenes*. The FIC index for these bacterial strains ranged from 0.312 to 0.458, whereas, for other antibiotics, the FIC value was 0.917–2.0. In no case was an antagonistic effect observed.

Taking into account the obtained synergistic results, in vivo studies on an albino strain of inbred BALB/c mice were conducted [75]. As reference antibiotics, vancomycin and daptomycin were chosen and tests were performed on infected mice with MS *S. aureus* and vs. *E. faecalis*. In the case of these infections, the number of colony-forming microorganisms, called CFU/mL, was determined. For staphylococcus-infected tissue not treated with any compound, the CFU/ml value was 6.7×10^7 and was significantly higher than when the infected tissue was treated only with hydrochloride of **11** (CFU/ml = 4.4×10^4), daptomycin (CFU/ml = 3.8×10^3), or vancomycin (CFU/ml = 4.0×10^3). However, when this tissue was treated with saponin **11**·HCl (1 mg of compound/kg of mass) plus daptomycin or vancomycin (7 mg antibiotic/kg of mass), CFU/ml values were 17 and 22, respectively, lower than for antibiotics alone. Thus, the highest bacterial inhibition was obtained for a staphylococcus-infected tissue which was treated with a mixture of saponin and antibiotic. Very similar results were obtained for vs. *E. faecalis*-infected tissue.

Table 2. Selected MIC$_{50}$ (MIC$_{90}$) and MBC$_{50}$ (MBC$_{90}$) values for 11·HCl and clinically used antibiotics against clinical isolates of Gram-positive bacteria.

	MIC$_{50}$ (MIC$_{90}$) *						MBC$_{50}$ (MBC$_{90}$) **					
	MR S. aureus (n = 20) ***	MS S. aureus (n = 20)	VR E. faecalis (n = 10)	VS E. faecalis (n = 20)	S. pyogenes (n = 20)	R. equi (n = 20)	MR S. aureus (n = 20)	MS S. aureus (n = 20)	VR E. faecalis (n = 10)	VS E. faecalis (n = 20)	S. pyogenes (n = 20)	R. equi (n = 20)
11·HCl	4 (8)	2 (4)	8 (32)	8 (16)	2 (4)	2 (4)	8 (16)	8 (16)	16 (64)	16 (32)	4 (8)	4 (16)
Imipenem	16 (128)	1 (2)	16 (64)	4 (16)	0,5 (1)	0,25 (1)	64 (256)	4 (8)	64 (128)	16 (64)	1 (4)	8 (32)
Doxycycline	4 (16)	4 (8)	16 (32)	8 (16)	4 (8)	1 (2)	8 (32)	8 (32)	16 (64)	16 (64)	8 (16)	32 (128)
Erythromycin	4 (16)	2 (8)	16 (64)	8 (32)	2 (8)	0,5 (2)	32 (128)	16 (64)	32 (128)	16 (128)	8 (32)	32 (64)
Ciprofloxacin	4 (8)	2 (8)	8 (32)	4 (8)	2 (8)	1 (2)	8 (16)	4 (16)	16 (128)	8 (16)	8 (16)	16 (64)

* MIC$_{50}$ (MIC$_{90}$) = minimum inhibitory concentrations (μg/mL) at which 50% and 90% of the isolates were inhibited, respectively ** MBC$_{50}$ (MBC$_{90}$) = minimum bactericidal concentration (μg/mL) at which 50% and 90% of the isolates were inhibited, respectively *** n is the number of tested isolates of a given bacterium.

In turn, almost all tested mono- and dialkyl diosgenyl glycosaminosides inhibit the growth of G+ bacteria. Saponins with the *N*-ethyl group at the amino function of both D-gluco-(**37**) and D-galactosamine (**47**) are the most active compounds against reference strains of *E. faecalis*, *S. aureus*, *S. epidermidis* and *R. equi* (MIC = 0.5–8 µg/mL) [50,54]. Importantly, the introduction of an additional ethyl group reduces the antimicrobial activity of these derivatives, in particular with respect to *E. faecium* and *S. aureus* (for *N,N*-diethyl diosgenyl galactosaminoside **48** MIC > 1024 µg/mL). Studies have shown that several *N*-alkyl derivatives of **11** exhibit stronger or similar activity than **11**·HCl: saponin **38** with the *N*-propyl group (MIC = 1–8 µg/mL) and saponins **43–45** with *N,N*-dialkyl chains. In turn, two tested saponins with the longest carbons chain, *N*-pentyl (**39**) and *N,N*-diheksyl (**46**) turned out to be completely inactive against to the tested strains of G+ bacteria. These indicate that the extension of the alkyl chain, as well as the addition of another alkyl group, are rather unfavourable from the point of view of antibacterial activity. This is probably related to the lower solubility of saponins with longer alkyl chains or to the ability to form micellar structures [50].

The good activity of the *N*-acetyl derivative of diosgenyl β-D-galactosaminoside (**57**, MIC = 8–32 µg/mL for all tested reference strains of G+ bacteria) is surprising, while the analogous *N*-acetyl derivative of diosgenyl β-D-glucosaminoside (**50**) does not exhibit any microbial activity (MIC > 1024 µg/mL). In the case of *N*-aminoacyl derivatives of **11**, the dependence of saponin structure on its activity is noticeable, and only *N*-aminoacyl analogs with the free α-amino group in the aminoacyl residue are found to be active against tested reference strains of G+ bacteria [62]. Some of them exhibit better antibacterial activity than **11**·HCl: *N*-sarcosyl (**64**), *N*-D-and L-alanyl derivatives (**65,66**, respectively). Any increase or decrease in the amino acid substituent has an unfavourable effect on the biological activity of the compound, and replacing the amino group in amino acid residue by the hydroxyl group also causes a complete lack of the antibacterial activity.

4.3.2. Antifungal Activity

Strains of *Candida albicans* constitute about 60% of the strains isolated from patients suffering from candidiasis, but recent data show the increasing occurrence of strains called non-*albicans Candida*. Species belonging to this group are often characterised by reduced susceptibility to antifungal agents [76].

Based on the conducted tests, the MIC values were determined for diosgenyl glycosides **11**·HCl, **35**·HCl and some of their derivatives (**37–49, 63–76**). Hydrochloride of **11** and *N,N*-dialkyl analogs with short carbon chains (**41–43**), are characterised by the highest antifungal activity against reference strains *C. albicans* and *C. tropicalis* [50]. MIC values for tested fungal pathogens are in the range of 0.5–2 µg/mL. A change in the configuration of the C-4 carbon atom in the carbohydrate residue adversely affected the activity of the diosgenyl galactosaminoside. Hydrochloride of **35** in comparison with its D-gluco counterpart (**11**·HCl) inhibits fungal growth to a lesser extent [54]. In the case of *N*-alkyl derivatives of diosgenyl glysocaminosides, good results against both types of *Candida* were obtained for diosgenyl β-D-galactosaminosides **47–49** with MIC values in the range of 2–8 µg/mL, which is similar to those obtained for analogous *N*-alkyl derivatives of diosgenyl β-D-glucosaminosides (**42,43**). In turn, *Aspergillus niger* turned out to be the least susceptible and the majority of *N*-alkyl derivatives of diosgenyl glucosaminosides are inactive against it, with the exception of *N*-ethyl (**37**) and *N*-propyl (**38**) derivatives; MIC = 8 µg/mL. Surprisingly, *N*-acetyl analog of diosgenyl β-D-galactosaminoside (**57**) inhibits the growth of fungal reference strains, which is opposite to the corresponding D-gluco derivative (**50**).

In the case of *N*-acyl analogs, only *N*-aminoacyl derivatives of **11** with the free α-amino group in the amino acid residue are found to be active against reference strains of human pathogenic fungi (MIC = 2–4 µg/mL) [62]. Replacing this amino group by the hydroxyl function causes the lack of antifungal activities. Although part of the tested *N*-aminoacyl derivatives of **11** (**65–69**) inhibit the growth of *C. albicans* and *C. lypolitica*, their activity is slighter weaker than the activity of reference

11·HCl. Noteworthy, for the tested *N*-acyl analogs the antifungal activity does not depend on the type of the attached amino acid, and usually the MIC values are 4 µg/mL.

In view of a large number of non-*albicans Candida* and their drug resistance, the tests of five derivatives of diosgenyl glucosaminoside (**11·HCl, 41–44**, Figure 6) on clinical isolates were attempted [77]. These compounds were selected because of their promising MIC values against the reference strains of fungi *Candida* species. The tests were carried out on clinical strains: *C. glabrata, C. krusei, C. parapsilosis* and *C. tropicalis*, which were collected from patients suffering from vaginal, skin and mouth mycoses. As reference compounds, generally available conventional antifungal agents, including antibiotics, were used: amphotericin B, clotrimazole, fluconazole, itraconazole, natamycin and nystatin. The results of the tests are presented in Table 3.

Table 3. MIC_{50} * and MIC_{90} * values for hydrochloride of **11**, *N,N*-dialkyl saponins **41–44** and antifungal agents against clinical isolates of fungi of genus *non-albicans Candida*.

Saponin Antibiotic		*C. glabrata* (n = 22) **		*C. krusei* (n = 12)		*C. parapsilosis* (n = 19)		*C. tropicalis* (n = 13)	
	Fungus	50%	90%	50%	90%	50%	90%	50%	90%
11·HCl		2	4	16	1024	2	4	4	1024
41		4	4	16	1024	1	2	4	1024
42		4	4	64	1024	2	4	4	512
43		4	8	1024	1024	4	4	8	1024
44		8	16	1024	1024	8	16	128	1024
Amphotericin B		2	2	2	2	2	4	1	2
Clotrimazole		4	8	0.25	0.25	0.25	0.25	4	16
Fluconazole		128	128	32	64	2	8	128	1024
Itrakonazol		4	32	0.25	0.25	0.25	0.25	256	1024
Natamycin		2	2	1	1	4	4	2	4
Nystatin		8	8	2	4	4	8	2	4

* MIC_{50} (MIC_{90}) = minimum inhibitory concentrations (µg/mL) at which 50% and 90% of the isolates were inhibited, respectively. ** n is the number of tested isolates of a given pathogen.

Tested derivatives of diosgenyl glucosaminoside **11·HCl, 41** and **42** exhibited a high efficacy against *C. glabrata* and *C. parapsilosis* species. They inhibit fungal growth in 90% at a concentration of 4 µg/mL and lower. Among them the most active is derivative **41**, i.e., *N,N*-dimethyl derivative, which inhibits 90% growth of *C. parapsilosis* isolates at a concentration of 2 µg/mL. These results are comparable or even stronger than those of conventional antifungal agents, such as clotrimazole and the other three antibiotics, classified as polyenes.

Two species, *C. krusei* and *C. tropicalis*, showed a certain discrepancy in their sensitivity to the tested saponins. While the MIC_{50} values for most isolates are 4–128 µg/mL, the highest concentration (1024 µg/mL) is required to inhibit the growth of individual strains in 90%. Against these two strains, three antibiotics and most conventional antifungal agents appear to be more effective. It has to be added that *C. tropicalis* species, in this examination, are characterised by significant resistance to fluconazole and itraconazole.

4.3.3. Anti-Cancer Activity

Antiproliferative activity is an important biological property of natural saponins. This activity may result from programmed cell death (apoptosis or autophagy) or nonapoptotic (necrosis) and also applies to cancer cells. It has been shown that saponins have significant potential as anti-cancer agents [78].

Hydrochloride of diosgenyl β-ᴅ-glucosaminoside (**11·HCl**) was the first diosgenyl glycosaminoside which has been tested for cytotoxic activity. Importantly, this compound does not exhibit antiproliferative activity against non-tumoral cells—peripheral lymphocyte blood cells [48]. Further antitumor tests on **11·HCl** determined its independent effect and in combination with 2-chlorodeoxyadenosine (2-CdA, cladribine) on lymphocytes isolated from the patients suffering from chronic B-cell lymphocytic leukemia (B-CLL) [41]. It was found that this saponin is cytotoxic towards B-CLL—it induces apoptosis and necrosis of some leukemic B-cells. Additionally, **11·HCl** enhances the cytostatic effect of 2-CdA, significantly reducing (20–30%) the number of lymphatic cancer cells in some patients. This could indicate that the tested saponin increases B-cell membrane permeability and facilitates the penetration of the drug into the tumor cell. In turn, in in vitro studies on the other tumor cells, including cervical carcinoma cells—HeLa, CaSKi, ViBo—and human leukemia cells—HEL, K562, HL60 and melanoma WM9—were conducted. The hydrochloride of **11** shows only a moderate antiproliferative effect (IC_{50} ranging from 10.7 to 41 μM) [48,49]. However, it is worth adding that **11·HCl** shows better inhibitory activity toward the tested cancer cell lines than the starting material, which is diosgenin (IC_{50} values 63.8–81 μM) [49].

N-Acyl derivatives of diosgenyl glucosaminosides **50, 52–56, 59–62** have been also examined for cytotoxic activity [46,47]. Most of the tested saponins show moderate activity against several human cancer cell lines (including SK-N-SH, MCF-7 and HeLa lines). Compound **54**, containing α-lipoic acid residue, turned out to be the most active against all three cancer cell lines (IC_{50} ranging from 4.8 μM to 7.3 μM; IC_{50} is the concentration of an inhibitor where the response is reduced by half). This cytotoxicity may be related to the redox properties of α-lipoic acid, which is a biogenic antioxidant, physiologically acting as a coenzyme in the oxidative decarboxylation of α-ketonic acids. However, the effect of this substituent on cytotoxicity is definitely smaller in the case of the α-lipoic derivative of diosgenyl amino disaccharide (**60**); the IC_{50} values for this compound increased 2-6 times in comparison to IC_{50} of **54** [47]. Further analysis of data for the other derivatives of diosgenyl amino disaccharide (**59–62**) confirmed that they are, in general, less active than their corresponding monosaccharides analogs with the same N-substitution (**52–56**).

In the case of N-cinnamoyl derivatives (**85–87**), SAR studies have shown that a significant effect on the cytotoxic activity clearly depends on the type of introduced substituent and its position in the benzene ring [56]. Electron-donating and electron-withdrawing substituents were introduced at various positions into the benzene ring of compound **85**. N-cinnamoyl derivatives with electron donating groups such as methyl (**86**) or methoxy (**87**) in the *para* position show excellent activity against HeLa and MCF-7 cell lines (IC_{50} ranging from 0.5–6.3 μM) and are much more active than the starting compound **85** (IC_{50} ranging from 12.8–39.1 μM). In turn, the introduction of such a group (OMe) in the *ortho* or *meta* position led to a significant decrease in the activity of the compound.

4.3.4. Hemolytic Activity

Saponins are known to show a high ability to hemolyse red blood cells. This process causes irreversible destruction of the lipid double-layer of erythrocyte membranes and the release of hemoglobin and other intracellular components into the surrounding plasma. This may constitute a significant limitation in the use of saponins in therapies. Hemolytic activity is closely related to the structure of saponins and depends, among others, on the structure of the aglycon, on the length and number of carbohydrate units and the type of its chemical modification [17,35].

Diosgenyl β-D-glucosaminoside hydrochloride (**11·HCl**) and N-alkyl analogs (**41–44**) have been tested for hemolytic activity by determining the minimum hemolytic concentration (MHC) [77]. The results of tests showed that these saponins are non-toxic to human red blood cells. Hemolysis was not observed even when the erythrocytes were exposed to 256 μg/mL concentration of saponins, which is many times higher than the MIC = 2–4 μg/mL for the majority of isolated *Candida* species.

In the case of N-acyl derivatives of **11**, based on SAR research, it can be concluded that the ability to hemolyse red blood cells is correlated to the structure of glycosaminosides and is somewhat correlated with its antimicrobial activity [62]. N-Acetyl (**50**), glycyl (**63**), glycoyl (**74**) and L-lactyl (**75**) derivatives, which do not show or show very weak antimicrobial activity, also do not exhibit hemolytic activity. In turn, L-seryl (**68**), L-threonyl (**69**) and L-lysyl (**71**) derivatives of diosgenyl β-D-glucosaminoside, which exhibit better antifungal than antibacterial activity, turn out to be toxic toward red blood cells. Importantly, compounds with the highest antimicrobial activity, namely sarcosyl (**64**), L-alanyl (**65**) and D-alanyl (**66**) derivatives of **11**, are not toxic towards human red blood cells.

5. Conclusions

In this mini-review, various approaches to diosgenyl aminoglycosides are presented as well as various possibilities of their chemical modifications based on 2-amine function. Respective bromides, chlorides, trichloroacetimidates and (*N*-phenyl)trifluoroacetimidates are demonstrated to be useful donors for glycosidic bond formation between D-glucosamine or D-galactosamine and diosgenin. Since such a reaction demands protection of the amine function, useful protective groups are presented, such as: tetrachlorophthaloyl (TCP), trifluoroacetyl (TFA), 2,2,2-trichloroetoxycarbonyl (Troc), dimethylphosphoryl (DMP) and phthaloyl (Phth). The presented glycosidation reactions generally run with good yields, although these yields are dependent on used conditions, e.g., on the order in which the reagents are added. Regarding the modifications of the amine function, its alkylations, acylations, including acylations with amino acids and hydroxy acids, transformations into ureids and thiosemicarbazones are shown. We would like to emphasize that the presented reactions of glucosamine or galactosamine are of universal importance. The indicated protection groups and reaction pathways can be used to form a glycosidic bond between glucosamine or galactosamine and any aglycone. This universality also applies to the presented modifications of the amine function.

Presented syntheses were aimed at finding semi-natural diosgenin derivatives with favorable pharmacological properties. A wide range of such derivatives is presented, which makes it difficult to discuss the influence of specific modification on pharmacological properties. However, some conclusions can be made.

None of the tested derivatives of diosgenyl glycosaminosides are effective against G- bacteria. This finding confirms the known fact that saponins do not exhibit such activity.

A basic amino group is necessary for the activity of the diosgenyl glucosaminosides against G+ bacteria. Compounds with such a group, i.e., hydrochloride, some of the *N*-alkyl, *N,N*-dialkyl and *N*-aminoacyl derivatives, exhibit relatively strong activity against G+ bacteria. Depriving the diosgenyl glucosaminosides of the basic amino group by acetylation or replacing it with a hydroxyl group results in a loss of antibacterial activity. Among alkyl derivatives, diosgenyl *N*-ethylglucosaminoside is the most active against G+ bacteria, whereas, among *N*-aminoacyl derivatives, diosgenyl *N*-alanylglucosaminoside is the most active. In both cases, further elongations of the *N*-substituent are ineffective from the standpoint of the inhibitory activity towards the G+ bacteria. These findings are probably due to the lower solubility of the compounds with longer *N*-substituents or to the micelle formation.

Basic amino group is also necessary for the activity of the diosgenyl glucosaminosides against tested *Candida* species. The growth of tested fungi is the most efficiently inhibited by the hydrochloride of diosgenyl glucosaminoside and its alkyl derivatives with short carbon chains (*N*-ethyl and *N,N*-dimethyl). *N*-aminoacyl derivatives of diosgenyl glucosaminoside quite effectively acted against fungi, and this effect is independent of the size of amino acid. Again, replacing the amino group by the amido group (acylation), as well as replacing the α-amino group by the hydroxyl group, causes the antifungal activities to decrease.

Switching of the D-glucosamine into D-galactosamine dramatically changes antimicrobial properties of the respective diosgenyl glycosides. While the hydrochloride of diosgenyl glucosaminoside is active against G+ bacteria and against *Candida*, the hydrochloride of diosgenyl galactosamine is not active at all. Conversely, *N*-acetyl derivative of diosgenyl glucosaminoside does not exhibit any antibacterial nor antifungal activity, whereas its galactosamine analogue acts against G+-bacteria-tested and against *Candida*-tested. This result may suggest that these two diosgenyl glycosaminosides act according to different mechanisms.

With regard to anti-cancer properties, promising results were obtained for the hydrochloride of diosgenyl glucosaminoside and some acyl derivatives, particularly for the α-lipoic acid derivative. No alkyl nor aminoacyl derivatives of diosgenyl glycosaminosides were tested for their anti-tumor activity.

Extremely important is that derivatives of diosgenyl D-glucosaminosides, which are active against antimicrobials and/or cancers (hydrochloride, *N*-alkyl, *N*-aminoacyl active), are non-toxic to human red blood cells.

The conclusions drawn in this work may be helpful in designing further modifications of diosgenyl glycosaminosides as well as in designing modifications of other glycosaminosides aimed at the search for effective pharmaceuticals.

Author Contributions: Writing—original draft preparation, review and editing, D.G., literature search and partial draft preparation, H.M.; further management and supervision, B.L. All authors have read and agreed to the published version of the manuscript.

Funding: This research was funded by the Ministry of Science and Higher Education in Poland–DS/531-T100-D687-20.

Conflicts of Interest: The authors declare no conflict of interest.

References

1. Sparg, S.G.; Light, M.E.; van Staden, J. Biological activities and distribution of plant saponins. *J. Ethnopharmacol.* **2004**, *94*, 219–243. [CrossRef] [PubMed]
2. Vincken, J.P.; Heng, L.; de Groot, A.; Gruppen, H. Saponins, classification and occurrence in the plant kingdom. *Phytochemistry* **2007**, *68*, 275–297. [CrossRef] [PubMed]
3. Malyarenko, T.; Malyarenko, O.; Ivanchina, N.; Kalinovsky, A.; Popov, R.; Kicha, A. Four New Sulfated Polar Steroids from the Far Eastern Starfish *Leptasterias ochotensis*: Structures and Activities. *Mar. Drugs* **2015**, *13*, 4418–4435. [CrossRef] [PubMed]
4. Williams, J.R.; Gong, H. Isolation and synthesis of shark-repelling saponins. *Lipids* **2004**, *39*, 795–799. [CrossRef] [PubMed]
5. Smułek, W.; Zdarta, A.; Łuczak, M.; Krawczyk, P.; Jesionowski, T.; Kaczorek, E. *Sapindus* saponins' impact on hydrocarbon biodegradation by bacteria strains after short- and long-term contact with pollutant. *Colloids Surf. B Biointerfaces* **2016**, *142*, 207–213. [CrossRef]
6. Xu, R.; Zhao, W.; Xu, J.; Shao, B.; Qin, G. Studies on bioactive saponins from Chinese medicinal plants. *Adv. Exp. Med. Biol.* **1996**, *404*, 371–382. [CrossRef]
7. Koh, R.; Tay, I. *Saponins Properties, Applications and Health Benefits*; Nova Science Publishers, Inc.: New York, NY, USA, 2012.
8. Barky, A.; Hussein, S.A.; AlmEldeen, A.; Hafez, Y.A.; Mohamed, T.M. Saponins and their potential role in diabetes mellitus. *Diabetes Manag.* **2017**, *7*, 148–158.
9. Elekofehinti, O.O. Saponins: Anti-diabetic principles from medicinal plants—A review. *Pathophysiology* **2015**, *22*, 95–103. [CrossRef]
10. Man, S.; Gao, W.; Zhang, Y.; Huang, L.; Liu, C. Chemical study and medical application of saponins as anti-cancer agents. *Fitoterapia* **2010**, *81*, 703–714. [CrossRef]
11. Lin, Y.-Y.; Chan, S.-H.; Juang, Y.-P.; Hsiao, H.-M.; Guh, J.-H.; Liang, P.-H. Design, synthesis and cytotoxic activity of *N*-modified oleanolic saponins bearing a glucosamine. *Eur. J. Med. Chem.* **2018**, *143*, 1942–1958. [CrossRef]
12. Thakur, M.; Melzig, M.F.; Fuchs, H.; Weng, A. Chemistry and pharmacology of saponins: Special focus on cytotoxic properties. *Bot. Targets Ther.* **2011**, *1*, 19–29. [CrossRef]
13. Hassan, H.S.; Sule, I.M.; Musa, M.A.; Musa, Y.K.; Abubakar, S.M.; Hassan, S.A. Anti-inflammatory activity of crude saponin extracts from five Nigerian medicinal plants. *Afr. J. Tradit. Complementary Altern. Med.* **2012**, *9*, 250–255. [CrossRef] [PubMed]
14. Jang, K.J.; Kim, H.K.; Han, M.H.; Oh, Y.N.; Yoon, H.M.; Chung, Y.H.; Kim, G.Y.; Hwang, H.J.; Kim, B.W.; Choi, Y.H. CytoAnti-inflammatory effects of saponins derived from the roots of *Platycodon grandiflorus* in lipopolysaccharide-stimulated BV2 microglial cells. *Int. J. Mol. Med.* **2013**, *31*, 1357–1366. [CrossRef] [PubMed]

15. Zou, W.; Gong, L.; Zhou, F.; Long, Y.; Li, Z.; Xiao, Z.; Ouyang, B.; Liu, M. Anti-inflammatory effect of traditional Chinese medicine preparation Penyanling on pelvic inflammatory disease. *J. Ethnopharmacol.* **2020**, *23*, 113405. [CrossRef]
16. Gallelli, L. Escin: A review of its anti-edematous, anti-inflammatory, and venotonic properties. *Drug Des. Dev. Ther.* **2019**, *27*, 3425–3437. [CrossRef]
17. Augustin, J.M.; Kuzina, V.; Andersen, S.B.; Bak, S. Molecular activities, biosynthesis and evolution of triterpenoid saponins. *Phytochem* **2011**, *72*, 435–457. [CrossRef]
18. Moses, T.; Papadopoulou, K.K.; Osbourn, A. Metabolic and functional diversity of saponins, biosynthetic intermediates and semi-synthetic derivatives. *Crit. Rev. Biochem. Mol. Biol.* **2014**, *49*, 439–462. [CrossRef]
19. Weng, A.; Jenett-Siems, K.; Schmieder, P.; Bachran, D.; Bachran, C.; Görick, C.; Thakur, M.; Fuchs, H.; Melzig, M. A convenient method for saponin isolation in tumour therapy. *J. Chromatogr. B Anal. Technol. Biomed. Life Sci.* **2010**, *1*, 713–718. [CrossRef]
20. Uddin, M.S.; Ferdosh, S.; Haque Akanda, M.J.; Ghafoor, K.; Rukshana, A.H.; Ali, M.E.; Kamaruzzaman, B.Y.; Fauzi, M.B.; Shaarani, S.; Islam Sarker, M.Z. Techniques for the extraction of phytosterols and their benefits in human health: A review. *Sep. Sci. Technol.* **2018**, *53*, 2206–2223. [CrossRef]
21. Netala, V.R.; Ghosh, S.B.; Bobbu, P.; Anitha, D.; Tartte, V. Triterpenoid saponins: A review on biosynthesis, applications and mechanism of their action. *Int. J. Pharm. Pharm. Sci.* **2015**, *7*, 24–28.
22. Negi, J.S.; Negi, P.S.; Pant, G.J.; Rawat, M.S.; Negi, S.K. Naturally occurring saponins: Chemistry and biology. *J. Poisonous Med. Plant Res.* **2013**, *1*, 1–6.
23. Yan, L.L.; Zhang, Y.J.; Gao, W.Y.; Man, S.L.; Wang, Y. In vitro and in vivo anticancer activity of steroid saponins of Paris polyphylla var. yunnanensis. *Exp. Oncol.* **2009**, *31*, 27–32. [PubMed]
24. Yan, M.-C.; Liu, Y.; Chen, H.; Ke, Y.; Xua, Q.-C.; Cheng, M.-S. Synthesis and antitumor activity of two natural N-acetylglucosamine-bearing triterpenoid saponins: Lotoidoside D and E. *Bioorg. Med. Chem. Lett.* **2006**, *16*, 4200–4204. [CrossRef] [PubMed]
25. Li, H.; Ni, J. Treatment of wastewater from *Dioscorea zingiberensis* tubers used for producing steroid hormones in a microbial fuel cell. *Bioresour. Technol.* **2011**, *102*, 2731–2735. [CrossRef]
26. Patel, K.; Gadewar, M.; Tahilyani, V.; Kumar, D.P. A review on pharmacological and analytical aspects of diosgenin: A concise report. *Nat. Prod. Bioprospect.* **2012**, *2*, 46–52. [CrossRef]
27. Yang, C.-R.; Zhang, Y.; Jacob, M.R.; Khan, S.I.; Zhang, Y.-J.; Li, X.-C. Antifungal activity of C-27 steroidal saponins. *Antimicrob. Agents Chemother.* **2006**, *50*, 1710–1714. [CrossRef]
28. Zhang, R.; Huang, B.; Du, D.; Guo, X.; Xin, G.; Xing, Z.; Liang, Y.; Chen, Y.; Chen, Q.; He, Y.; et al. Anti-thrombosis effect of diosgenyl saponins in vitro and in vivo. *Steroids* **2013**, *78*, 1064–1070. [CrossRef]
29. Zhao, X.; Cong, X.; Zheng, L.; Xu, L.; Yin, L.; Peng, J. Dioscin, a natural steroid saponin, shows remarkable protective effect against acetaminophen-induced liver damage in vitro and in vivo. *Toxicol. Lett.* **2012**, *214*, 69–80. [CrossRef]
30. Li, M.; Han, X.; Yu, B. Synthesis of monomethylated dioscin derivatives and their antitumor activities. *Carbohydr. Res.* **2003**, *338*, 117–121. [CrossRef]
31. Li, W.; Qiu, Z.; Wang, Y.; Zhang, Y.; Li, M.; Yu, J.; Zhang, L.; Zhu, Z.; Yu, B. Synthesis, cytotoxicity, and hemolytic activity of 6'-O-substituted dioscin derivatives. *Carbohydr. Res.* **2007**, *342*, 2705–2715. [CrossRef]
32. Wang, B.; Chun, J.; Liu, Y.; Wang, Y.-S.; Joo, E.-J.; Kim, Y.S.; Cheng, M.S. Synthesis of novel diosgenyl saponin analogues and apoptosis-inducing activity on A549 human lung adenocarcinoma. *Org. Biomol. Chem.* **2012**, *10*, 8822–8834. [CrossRef] [PubMed]
33. Ravikumar, P.R.; Hammesfahr, P.; Sih, C.J. Cytotoxic saponins form the Chinese herbal drug Yunnan Bai Yao. *J. Pharm. Sci.* **1979**, *68*, 900–903. [CrossRef] [PubMed]
34. Mimaki, Y.; Yokosuka, A.; Kuroda, M.; Sashida, Y. Cytotoxic activities and structure–cytotoxic relationships of steroidal saponins. *Biol. Pharm. Bull.* **2001**, *24*, 1286–1289. [CrossRef] [PubMed]
35. Wang, Y.; Zhang, Y.; Zhu, Z.; Zhu, S.; Li, Y.; Li, M.; Yu, B. Exploration of the correlation between the structure, hemolytic activity, and cytotoxicity of steroid saponins. *Bioorg. Med. Chem.* **2007**, *15*, 2528–2532. [CrossRef]
36. Hernandez, J.C.; Leon, F.; Brouard, I.; Torres, F.; Rubio, S.; Quintana, J.; Estevez, F.; Bermejo, J. Synthesis of novel spirostanic saponins and their cytotoxic activity. *Bioorg. Med. Chem.* **2008**, *16*, 2063–2076. [CrossRef]
37. Banoub, J.; Boullanger, P.; Lafont, D. Synthesis of oligosaccharides of 2-amino-2-deoxy sugars. *Chem. Rev.* **1992**, *92*, 1167–1195. [CrossRef]

38. Demchenko, A.V. Stereoselective Chemical 1,2-cis O-Glycosylation: From 'Sugar Ray' to Modern Techniques of the 21st Century. *Curr. Org. Chem.* **2003**, *7*, 35–79. [CrossRef]
39. Bednarczyk, D.; Kaca, W.; Myszka, H.; Serwecińska, L.; Smiatacz, Z.; Zaborowski, A. The synthesis of diosgenyl 2-amino-2-deoxy-β-D-glucopyranoside hydrochloride. *Carbohydr. Res.* **2000**, *328*, 249–252. [CrossRef]
40. Wolfrom, M.L.; Bhat, H.M. Trichloroacetyl and trifluoroacetyl as N-blocking groups in nucleoside synthesis with 2-amino sugars. *J. Org. Chem.* **1967**, *32*, 1821–1823. [CrossRef]
41. Myszka, H.; Bednarczyk, D.; Najder, M.; Kaca, W. Synthesis and induction of apoptosis in B cell chronic leukemia by diosgenyl 2-amino-2-deoxy-β-D-glucopyranoside hydrochloride and its derivatives. *Carbohydr. Res.* **2003**, *338*, 133–141. [CrossRef]
42. Griffiths, S.L.; Madsen, R.; Fraser-Reid, B. Studies towards lipid A: Synthesis of Differentially Protected Disaccharide Fragments. *J. Org. Chem.* **1997**, *62*, 3654–3658. [CrossRef]
43. Bednarczyk, D.; Walczewska, A.; Grzywacz, D.; Sikorski, A.; Liberek, B.; Myszka, H. Differently N-protected 3,4,6-tri-O-acetyl-2-amino-2-deoxy-D-glucopyranosyl chlorides and their application in the synthesis of diosgenyl 2-amino-2-deoxy-β-D-glucopyranoside. *Carbohydr. Res.* **2013**, *367*, 10–17. [CrossRef] [PubMed]
44. Paulsen, H. Advances in Selective Chemical Syntheses of Complex Oligosaccharides. *Angew. Chem. Int. Ed. Engl.* **1982**, *21*, 155–173. [CrossRef]
45. Yang, Y.; Yu, B. N-Dimethylphosphoryl-protected glucosamine trichloroacetimidate as an effective glycosylation donor. *Tetrahedron Lett.* **2007**, *48*, 4557–4560. [CrossRef]
46. Kaskiw, M.J.; Tassotto, M.L.; Th'ng, J.; Jiang, Z.-H. Synthesis and cytotoxic activity of diosgenyl saponin analogues. *Bioorg. Med. Chem.* **2008**, *16*, 3209–3217. [CrossRef] [PubMed]
47. Kaskiw, M.J.; Tassotto, M.L.; Mok, M.; Tokar, S.L.; Pycko, R.; Th'ng, J.; Jiang, Z.-H. Structural analogues of diosgenyl saponins: Synthesis and anticancer activity. *Bioorg. Med. Chem.* **2009**, *17*, 7670–7679. [CrossRef] [PubMed]
48. Fernandez-Herrera, M.A.; Lopez-Munoz, H.; Hernandez-Vazquez, J.M.V.; Sanchez-Sanchez, L.; Escobar-Sanchez, M.L.; Pinto, B.M.; Sandoval-Ramirez, J. Synthesis and selective anticancer activity of steroidal glycoconjugates. *Eur. J. Med. Chem.* **2012**, *54*, 721–727. [CrossRef]
49. Tan, Y.; Xiao, X.; Yao, J.; Han, F.; Lou, H.; Luo, H.; Liang, G.; Ben-David, Y.; Pan, W. Syntheses and anti-cancer activities of glycosylated derivatives of diosgenin. *Chem. Res. Chin. Univ.* **2017**, *33*, 80–86. [CrossRef]
50. Walczewska, A.; Grzywacz, D.; Bednarczyk, D.; Dawgul, M.; Nowacki, A.; Kamysz, W.; Liberek, B.; Myszka, H. N-Alkyl derivatives of diosgenyl 2-amino-2-deoxy-β-D-glucopyranoside; synthesis and antimicrobial activity. *Beilstein J. Org. Chem.* **2015**, *11*, 869–874. [CrossRef]
51. Nilsson, U.; Ray, A.K.; Magnusson, G. Efficient syntheses of 3,4,6-tri-O-acetyl-2-deoxy-2- phthalimido-β- and -α-D-galactopyranosyl chloride. *Carbohydr. Res.* **1990**, *208*, 260–263. [CrossRef]
52. Yu, B.; Tao, H. Glycosyl trifluoroacetimidates. Part 1: Preparation and application as new glycosyl donors. *Tetrahedron Lett.* **2001**, *42*, 2405–2407. [CrossRef]
53. Yu, B.; Sun, J. Glycosylation with glycosyl N-phenyltrifluoroacetimidates (PTFAI) and a perspective of the future development of new glycosylation methods. *Chem. Commun.* **2010**, *46*, 4668–4679. [CrossRef]
54. Myszka, H.; Sokołowska, P.; Cieślińska, A.; Nowacki, A.; Jaśkiewicz, M.; Kamysz, W.; Liberek, B. Diosgenyl 2-amino-2-deoxy-β-D-galactopyranoside: Synthesis, derivatives and antimicrobial activity. *Beilstein J. Org. Chem.* **2017**, *13*, 2310–2315. [CrossRef]
55. Schmidt, R.R.; Toepfer, A. Glycosylation with highly reactive glycosyl donors: Efficiency of the inverse procedure. *Tetrahedron Lett.* **2001**, *42*, 2405–2407. [CrossRef]
56. Wang, B.; Liu, Y.; Wang, Y.; Liu, X.; Cheng, M.-S. Syntheses and structure–activity relationship studies of N-substituted-β-D-glucosaminides as selective cytotoxic agents. *Bioorg. Med. Chem. Lett.* **2012**, *22*, 7110–7113. [CrossRef] [PubMed]
57. Debenham, J.S.; Rodebaugh, R.; Fraser-Reid, B. Recent Advances in N-Protection for Amino Sugar Synthesis. *Liebigs Ann.* **1997**, 791–802. [CrossRef]

58. Iversen, T.; Josephson, S.; Bundle, D.R. The synthesis of streptococcal groups A, C and variant—A antigenic determinants. *J. Chem. Soc. Perkin I* **1981**, 2379–2385. [CrossRef]
59. Guo, X.; Xin, G.; He, S.; Wang, Y.; Huang, B.; Zhao, H.; Xing, Z.; Chen, Q.; Huang, W.; He, Y. Novel organic gelators based on pentose derivatized diosgenyl saponins. *Org. Biomol. Chem.* **2013**, *11*, 821–827. [CrossRef]
60. Fernandez-Herrera, M.; Lopez-Munoz, H.; Hernandes-Vazquez, J.; Lopez-Davila, M.; Mohan, S.; Escobar-Sanchez, M.; Sanchez-Sanches, L.; Pinto, B.; Sandoval-Ramirez, J. Synthesis and biological evaluation of the glycoside (25R)-3β,16β-diacetoxy-22-oxo-cholest-5-en-26-yl β-D-glucopyranoside: A selective anticancer agent in cervicouterine cell lines. *Eur. J. Med. Chem.* **2011**, *46*, 3877–3886. [CrossRef]
61. Liberek, B.; Melcer, A.; Osuch, A.; Wakieć, R.; Milewski, S.; Wiśniewski, A. N-Alkyl derivatives of 2-amino-2-deoxy-D-glucose. *Carbohydr. Res.* **2005**, *340*, 1876–1884. [CrossRef]
62. Grzywacz, D.; Paduszyńska, M.; Norkowska, M.; Kamysz, W.; Myszka, H.; Liberek, B. N-Aminoacyl and N-hydroxyacyl derivatives of diosgenyl 2-amino-2-deoxy-β-D-glucopyranoside: Synthesis, antimicrobial and hemolytic activities. *Bioorg. Med. Chem.* **2019**, *27*, 114923. [CrossRef] [PubMed]
63. Ibrahim, M.A.; Panda, S.S.; Birs, A.S.; Serrano, J.C.; Gonzalez, C.F. Synthesis and antibacterial evaluation of amino acid-antibiotic conjugates. *Bioorg. Med. Chem. Lett.* **2014**, *24*, 1856–1861. [CrossRef] [PubMed]
64. Panda, S.S.; Ibrahim, M.A.; Kucukbay, H.; Meyers, M.J.; Sverdrup, F.M.; El-Feky, S.A.; Katritzky, A.R. Synthesis and antimalarial bioassay of quinine–peptide conjugates. *Chem. Biol. Drug. Des.* **2013**, *82*, 361–366. [CrossRef] [PubMed]
65. Montalbetti, C.A.; Falque, V. Amide bond formation and peptide coupling. *Tetrahedron* **2005**, *61*, 10827–10852. [CrossRef]
66. McKay, M.J.; Nguyen, H.M. Recent developments in glycosyl urea synthesis. *Carbohydr. Res.* **2014**, *385*, 18–44. [CrossRef]
67. Porwański, S. New ureas containing glycosyl and diphenylphosphinyl scaffolds: Synthesis and the first attempts to use them in asymmetric synthesis. *Carbohydr. Res.* **2014**, *394*, 7–12. [CrossRef]
68. Moharana, A.K.; Dash, R.N.; Subudhi, B.B. Thiosemicarbazides: Updates on antivirals strategy. *Mini Rev. Med. Chem.* **2020**, 32811412. [CrossRef]
69. Gutsanu, V.; Lisa, G. Composites containing metal and thiosemicarbazone: Thermal, antimicrobial and antifungal properties. *Polyhedron* **2020**, *191*, 114800. [CrossRef]
70. Santos, F.R.S.; Andrade, J.T.; Sousa, C.D.F.; Fernandes, J.S.; Carmo, L.F.; Araújo, M.G.F.; Ferreira, J.M.S.; Villar, J.A.F.P. Synthesis and Evaluation of the in vitro Antimicrobial Activity of Triazoles, Morpholines and Thiosemicarbazones. *Med. Chem.* **2019**, *15*, 38–50. [CrossRef]
71. Kharkwal, H.; Panthari, P.; Pant, M.K.; Kharkwal, H.; Kharkwal, A.C.; Joshi, D.D. Foaming glycosides: A Review. *IOSR J. Pharm.* **2012**, *2*, 23–28. [CrossRef]
72. Khan, M.I.; Ahhmed, A.; Shin, J.H.; Baek, J.S.; Kim, M.Y.; Kim, J.D. Green Tea Seed Isolated Saponins Exerts Antibacterial Effects against Various Strains of Gram Positive and Gram Negative Bacteria, a Comprehensive Study In Vitro and In Vivo. *Evid. Based Complementary Altern. Med.* **2018**, 3486106. [CrossRef] [PubMed]
73. Dong, S.; Yang, X.; Zhao, L.; Zhang, F.; Hou, Z.; Xue, P. Antibacterial activity and mechanism of action saponins from *Chenopodium quinoa* Willd. husks against foodborne pathogenic bacteria. *Ind. Crops Prod.* **2020**, 112350. [CrossRef]
74. Trdá, L.; Janda, M.; Macková, D.; Pospíchalová, R.; Dobrev, P.I.; Burketová, L.; Matušinsky, P. Dual Mode of the Saponin Aescin in Plant Protection: Antifungal Agent and Plant Defense Elicitor. *Front. Plant Sci.* **2019**, *10*, 1448. [CrossRef] [PubMed]
75. Cirioni, O.; Myszka, H.; Dawgul, M.; Ghiselli, R.; Orlando, F.; Silvestri, C.; Brescini, L.; Kamysz, W.; Guerrieri, M.; Giacometti, A. In vitro activity and in vivo efficacy of the saponin diosgenyl 2-amino-2-deoxy-β-D-glucopyranoside hydrochloride (HSM1) alone and in combination with daptomycin and vancomycin against Gram-positive cocci. *J. Med. Microbiol.* **2011**, *60*, 1337–1343. [CrossRef] [PubMed]
76. Lewis, R.E. Overview of the changing epidemiology of candidemia. *Curr. Med. Res. Opin.* **2009**, *25*, 1732–1740. [CrossRef]

77. Dawgul, M.A.; Grzywacz, D.; Liberek, B.; Kamysz, W.; Myszka, H. Activity of Diosgenyl 2-amino-2-deoxy-β-D-glucopyranoside, its Hydrochloride, and N,N-dialkyl Derivatives against Non-albicans Candida Isolates. *Med. Chem.* **2018**, *14*, 460–467. [CrossRef]
78. Podolak, I.; Galanty, A.; Sobolewska, D. Saponins as cytotoxic agents; a review. *Phytochem. Rev.* **2010**, *9*, 425–427. [CrossRef] [PubMed]

Publisher's Note: MDPI stays neutral with regard to jurisdictional claims in published maps and institutional affiliations.

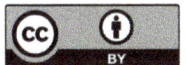
© 2020 by the authors. Licensee MDPI, Basel, Switzerland. This article is an open access article distributed under the terms and conditions of the Creative Commons Attribution (CC BY) license (http://creativecommons.org/licenses/by/4.0/).

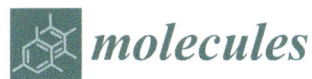

Review

Metabolic Engineering *Escherichia coli* for the Production of Lycopene

Zhaobao Wang [1], JingXin Sun [2], Qun Yang [1,*] and Jianming Yang [1,*]

[1] Energy-Rich Compounds Production by Photosynthetic Carbon Fixation Research Center, Shandong Key Lab of Applied Mycology, College of Life Sciences, Qingdao Agricultural University, Qingdao 266109, China; wangzhaobao123@126.com
[2] College of Food Science and Engineering, Qingdao Agricultural University, Qingdao 266109, China; jxsun20000@163.com
* Correspondence: yqun1001@163.com (Q.Y.); yjming888@126.com (J.Y.); Tel.: +86-131-4543-1413 (Q.Y.); +86-135-8938-5827 (J.Y.); Fax: +86-532-589-57640 (J.Y.)

Academic Editors: Pavel B. Drasar, Vladimir A. Khripach and Derek J. McPhee
Received: 5 June 2020; Accepted: 8 July 2020; Published: 9 July 2020

Abstract: Lycopene, a potent antioxidant, has been widely used in the fields of pharmaceuticals, nutraceuticals, and cosmetics. However, the production of lycopene extracted from natural sources is far from meeting the demand. Consequently, synthetic biology and metabolic engineering have been employed to develop microbial cell factories for lycopene production. Due to the advantages of rapid growth, complete genetic background, and a reliable genetic operation technique, *Escherichia coli* has become the preferred host cell for microbial biochemicals production. In this review, the recent advances in biological lycopene production using engineered *E. coli* strains are summarized: First, modification of the endogenous MEP pathway and introduction of the heterogeneous MVA pathway for lycopene production are outlined. Second, the common challenges and strategies for lycopene biosynthesis are also presented, such as the optimization of other metabolic pathways, modulation of regulatory networks, and optimization of auxiliary carbon sources and the fermentation process. Finally, the future prospects for the improvement of lycopene biosynthesis are also discussed.

Keywords: lycopene; the MEP pathway; the MVA pathway; *Escherichia coli*; metabolic engineering

1. Introduction

Lycopene, a member of the carotenoid family [1], is widely used in food, pharmaceutical, and cosmetic industries because of its potent anti-cancer [2], anti-inflammatory [3], and anti-oxidative activities [4]. Augmentation of lycopene production has become imperative to meet market demand. Currently, lycopene is produced mainly by direct natural extraction, chemical synthesis, and microbial fermentation. Lycopene is also widely found in fruits including tomato, watermelon, guava, and papaya [5–8], with a concentration of as high as 3–14 mg/100 g in tomatoes [9]. However, the purification process is quite complicated due to numerous carotenoids in the raw materials, and also the extraction method cannot match the large market demand. In addition, lycopene production by chemical synthesis is high-cost, low-yielding, and environmentally unfriendly [10]. Notably, lycopene production by chemical synthesis is banned in the European nations [11]. Therefore, metabolic engineering and synthetic biology for producing lycopene using microorganisms is characterized by high efficiency and environmental friendliness and has been applied as a feasible alternative.

Lycopene, a linear carotenoid with a C40 backbone, is composed of seven isopentenyl diphosphates (IPP) and one dimethylallyl diphosphate (DMAPP), both being its biosynthetic precursors [12–15]. The production of IPP and its isomer, DMAPP, in vivo via either the 2-C-methyl-d-erythritol-

4-phosphate (MEP) pathway [16] or the mevalonate (MVA) pathway is reported [17]. The MEP pathway, present in many bacteria, algae, cyanobacteria, plant chloroplasts, and some eukaryotic parasites [18,19], begins with the condensation of pyruvate and glyceraldehyde 3-phosphate derived from glycolysis [16,20]. In contrast, the MVA pathway, present in most eukaryotes, fungi, plants, archaea, and some bacterial species, can produce IPP and DMAPP using acetyl-CoA as the initial substrate [19,21].

Engineered *Escherichia coli* is widely used for the biosynthesis of secondary metabolites and high-value chemicals by metabolic engineering because of its rapid growth and powerful tools to enable genetic manipulation [22]. Moreover, the native MEP pathway present in *E. coli* facilitates the production of terpenoids including lycopene. However, this pathway showed low metabolite flux in metabolic engineering [23], leading to the introduction of the heterogeneous MVA pathway into *E. coli* for lycopene production.

In this review, we summarized the recent advances in lycopene production by the engineered *E. coli* using metabolic engineering strategies. Current investigations on the modification of the two metabolic pathways, MEP and MVA, for lycopene production in *E. coli*, were reviewed. The optimization of other metabolic pathways, modulation of regulatory networks, optimization of auxiliary carbon sources, and the fermentation process were also described. Furthermore, the common challenges, strategies, and prospects for lycopene biosynthesis in metabolically engineered *E. coli* were discussed in this review.

2. Metabolic Engineering of Two Major Pathways in *E. coli* for Lycopene Production

2.1. The Primary Biosynthetic Pathways for Lycopene Production

The MEP and MVA pathways are the major pathways producing the precursors of lycopene, IPP, and DMAPP. As shown in Figure 1, glyceraldehyde 3-phosphate (G3P) and pyruvate are condensed to form 1-deoxy-d-xylulose-5-phosphate (DXP) by DXP synthase (DXS), followed by the conversion into MEP under the catalyzation of DXP reductoisomerase (DXR or IspC) in the MEP pathway. Further, a series of enzymes, including 4-diphosphocytidyl-2C-methyl-d-erythritol (CDP-ME) cytidylyltransferase (IspD), CDP-ME kinase (IspE), 2C-methyl-d-erythritol-2,4-cyclo-diphosphate (MEC) synthase (IspF), 4-hydroxy-3-methyl-2-(E)-butenyl-4-diphosphate (HMBPP) synthase (IspG), and HMBPP reductase (IspH), successively catalyzes the conversion of MEP into IPP, along with the respective intermediates of CDP-ME, 4-diphosphocytidyl-2C-methyl-d-erythritol-2-phosphate (CDP-MEP), MEC, and HMBPP. Subsequently, isopentenyl-diphosphate isomerase (IDI) catalyzes the isomerization of IPP to DMAPP [24,25].

The MVA pathway initiates with acetyl-CoA, which is converted into MVA through three reactions, catalyzed by acetoacetyl-CoA thiolase (ACCT), 3-hydroxy-3-methylglutaryl-CoA (HMG-CoA) synthase (HMGS), and HMG-CoA reductase (HMGR), respectively. Subsequently, MVA is converted to mevalonate-5-phosphate (MVAP) catalyzed by mevalonate kinase (MK). The transformation of MVAP into IPP is reported through different pathways. The one in eukaryotes involves two reactions successively catalyzed by MVAP kinase (PMK) and MVAPP decarboxylase (MDD), while the other pathway in archaea harbors two reactions catalyzed by MVAP decarboxylase (MPD) and isopentenyl phosphate kinase (IPK), respectively [26]. After the production of IPP and DMAPP, the condensation reaction between the two intermediates occurs with the formation of geranyl diphosphate (GPP). Further, farnesyl pyrophosphate (FPP) is formed from GPP catalyzed by FPP synthase (IspA). FPP, in turn, is catalyzed by geranylgeranyl diphosphate (GGPP) synthase (CrtE), phytoene synthase (CrtB), and phytoene desaturase (CrtI) to successively form GGPP, phytoene, and finally lycopene [15,27]. The exogenous genes *crtEBI* from various sources can exhibit differential activities when introduced into the host strains. For instance, when different carotenoid genes *crtEBI* were introduced into *E. coli*, higher lycopene yield and cell growth were reached using the genes derived from *Pantoea agglomerans* compared with those of *Pantoea ananatis*. Furthermore, it was identified that *crtE* was responsible for the difference between the engineered *E. coli* strains harboring the *crtEBI* genes of *P. agglomerans* and *P. ananatis*, respectively [15].

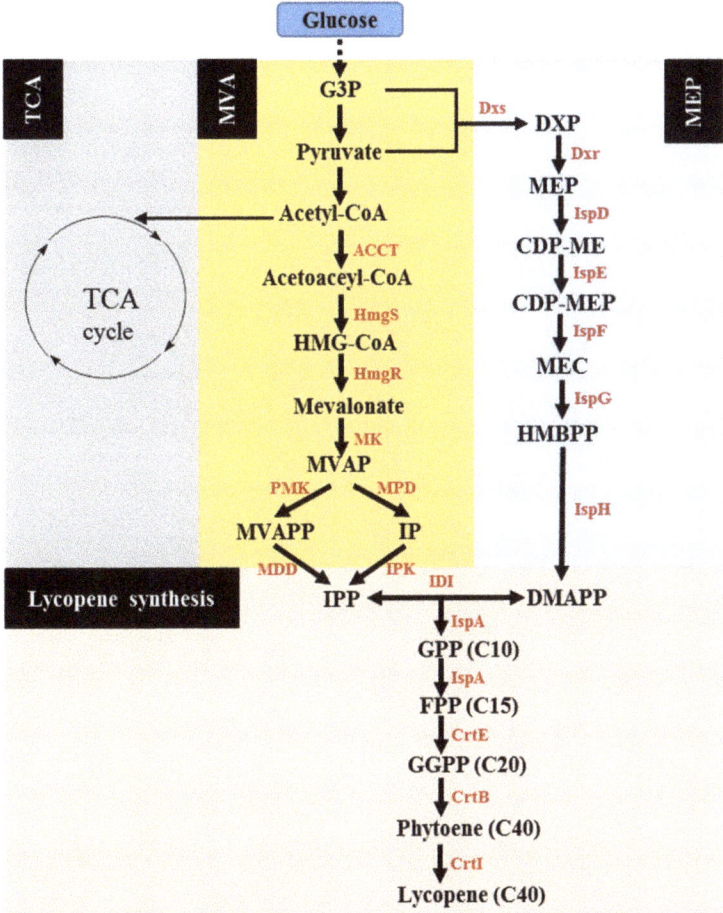

Figure 1. The metabolic pathways for lycopene production. G3P, glyceraldehyde 3-phosphate; DXP, 1-deoxy-d-xylulose-5-phosphate; MEP, methylerythritol phosphate; CDP-ME, 4-diphosphocytidyl-2C-methyl-d-erythritol; CDP-MEP, 4-diphosphocytidyl-2C-methyl-d-erythritol-2-phosphate; MEC, 2C-methyl-d-erythritol-2,4-cyclo-diphosphate; HMBPP, 4-hydroxy- 3-methyl-2-(*E*)-butenyl-4-diphosphate; HMG-CoA, 3-hydroxy-3-methylglutaryl-CoA; MVAP, mevalonate-5-phosphate; MVAPP, mevalonate-5-diphosphate; IP, isopentenyl phosphate; IPP, isopentenyl diphosphate; DMAPP, dimethylallyl diphosphate; GPP, geranyl diphosphate; FPP, farnesyl pyrophosphate; GGPP, geranylgeranyl diphosphate; DXS, DXP synthase; DXR, DXP reductoisomerase; IspD, CDP-ME cytidylyltransferase; IspE, CDP-ME kinase; IspF, MEC synthase; IspG, HMBPP synthase; IspH, HMBPP reductase; ACCT, acetoacetyl-CoA thiolase; HmgS, HMG-CoA synthase; HmgR, HMG-CoA reductase; MK, mevalonate kinase; PMK, MVAP kinase; MDD, MVAPP decarboxylase; MPD, MVAP decarboxylase; IPK, IP kinase; IDI, isopentenyldiphosphate isomerase; IspA, FPP synthase; CrtE, GGPP synthase; CrtB, phytoene synthase; CrtI, phytoene desaturase.

To summarize, the sole utilization of the endogenous MEP pathway or co-expression of the MEP and heterogeneous MVA pathways, and the subsequent expression of three key enzymes, CrtE, CrtB, and CrtI [15,27–30] were the primary biosynthetic route and strategy in the metabolic engineering of *E. coli* for lycopene production. Based on this, further work on the modification of the two major pathways was conducted. Lycopene production via various metabolic engineering optimization strategies in *E. coli* are summarized and listed in Table 1.

Table 1. Summary of the metabolic engineering optimization strategies used for the production of lycopene in *E. coli*.

Major Methods	Optimization Strategies	Yield/Titer	Culture Conditions	References
Overexpression of rate-limiting enzymes	Comparison of *crtEBI* genes from different strains	59 mg/L	-	[15]
	Knockout of *zwf*; overexpression of *idi*, *dxs* and *ispD*, *ispF*	7.55 mg/g DCW	Shake-flask fermentation	[28]
	Overexpression of *crtE*, *crtB*, *crtI*, *ipi*, *dxs*	5.2 mg/g DCW	Shake-flask fermentation	[29]
	Overexpression of *dxs*, *dxr*	22 mg/L	Shake-flask fermentation	[31]
	Overexpression of *dxs*	1.33 mg/g DCW	Shake-flask fermentation	[32]
	The co-expression of *appY*, *crl*, and *rpoS* with *dxs*	4.7 mg/g DCW	-	[29]
Directed evolution	Directed evolution of GGPP synthase	45 mg/g DCW	Shake-flask fermentation	[33]
	Directed co-evolution of *dxs*, *dxr* and *idi*	0.65 mg/L	-	[34]
Whole pathway engineering	Expression of the MVA pathway	4.28 mg/L	Shake-flask fermentation	[35]
	Type 2 IDI; heterologous MVA pathway	198 mg/g DCW	Shake-flask fermentation	[36]
	Heterologous expression of the MVA pathway	-	Shake-flask fermentation	[37]
Removal of competing pathways	Δ*gdhA*, Δ*aceE*, Δ*ytjC* (*gpmB*), Δ*fdhF*	18 mg/g DCW	Batch shake-flask cultivations	[38]
Pathway balancing	Combination of gene knockout and overexpression	2.5 mg/g DCW	-	[20]
	Genome-wide stoichiometric flux balance analysis; genes knockouts	6.6 mg/g DCW	Shake-flask fermentation	[39]
	Gene knockout (Δ*hnr*, Δ*yliE*)	-	Shake-flask fermentation	[40]
Regulatory engineering	Ntr regulon, stimulated by excess glycolytic flux through sensing of ACP	0.16 mg/L/h	Shake-flask fermentation	[41]
	Engineering of the cAMP receptor protein (CRP)	18.49 mg/g DCW	Batch fermentation	[42]
Optimization of carbon sources	Auxiliary carbon source optimization	1050 mg/L	Baffled flask fermentation	[12]
	Supplementing auxiliary carbon sources	40 mg/L/h	Fed-batch culture	[43]
	Fermentation with fatty acids or waste cooking oils	94 mg/g DCW	Fed-batch fermentation	[44]
Optimization of fermentation	High cell density fermentation	220 mg/L	Batch fermentation	[45]
	Different types of plasmid expression; optimization of fermentation conditions	67 mg/g DCW	Shake-flask fermentation	[46]
Targeted engineering	Targeted engineering; targeted proteomic and intermediate analysis	1.23 g/L	Fed-batch fermentation	[47]
	Two-dimensional search for gene targets	16 mg/g DCW	Shake-flask fermentation	[48]
Cofactor engineering	Modulating supply of NADPH and ATP; overexpression of *dxs*, *idi* and the *crt* gene operon	50.6 mg/g DCW	Fed-batch fermentation	[27]
Membrane engineering	Membrane engineering; overexpression of *plsb*, *plsc* and *dgka*	36.4 mg/g DCW	Shake-flask fermentation	[49]
Genome engineering	Synthesis genes were integrated into chromosome	33.43 mg/g DCW	Shake-flask fermentation	[50]
	Large-scale programming used to optimize the MEP pathway	9 mg/g DCW	-	[51]
	A new combinatorial multi-gene pathway assembly scheme	448 mg/g DCW	-	[52]

2.2. Metabolic Engineering of the Endogenous MEP Pathway in E. coli

In the early development stages of lycopene production using engineered *E. coli*, the utilization and modification of the endogenous MEP pathway were extensively investigated. Generally, the overexpression of the key enzymes of the MEP pathway is important in lycopene production, especially the major rate-limiting enzymes (DXS, DXR, and IDI) [19]. When the genes *dxs* and *dxr* were overexpressed solely or jointly on different expression vectors using three different promoters and *E. coli* host strains, the highest lycopene yield (22 mg/L) was reached with the arabinose-inducible promoter on a medium-copy plasmid pBAD24 in the *E. coli* XL1-Blue strain [31].

Several key enzymes involved in the biosynthetic pathway were usually co-overexpressed in metabolic engineering. As described, with the co-overexpression of DXS and exogenous carotenoid biosynthetic enzymes, the engineered *E. coli* strain exhibited lycopene production of 1.3 mg/g dry cell weight (DCW) [32]. Similarly, the combinational overexpression of endogenous DXS and IspA and optimal expression of the four exogenous enzymes of IDI, CrtE, CrtB, and CrtI resulted in lycopene production of 5.2 mg/g DCW [13]. Moreover, the co-overexpression of IDI, DXS, IspD, and IspF in the MEP pathway (Figure 2), showed a 6-fold increase in lycopene production (5.39 mg/g DCW) [28]. Besides the overexpression of the rate-limiting enzymes in the pathway, direct evolution and the optimization of ribosome binding sites (RBS) are conducive for the improvement in lycopene production. RBS libraries were utilized to adjust the expression of *dxs*, *idi*, and the *crt* gene operon, leading to an increase in lycopene yield by 32% [27]. Similarly, directed evolution was applied to modulate both the enzymatic expression and specific activity of CrtE. A combination of this and DXS overexpression reached above 45 mg/g DCW of lycopene production [33]. Lv et al. constructed a lycopene-indicated high-throughput screening method for isoprene production by performing directed co-evolution of the key enzymes (DXS, DXR, and IDI) of the MEP pathway. The result indicated a potential for pathway optimization in lycopene production [34]. In addition, when the expression of *dxs*, *idi*, and *crt* operon genes was modulated using the RBS library, a significant improvement in lycopene yield was observed [27].

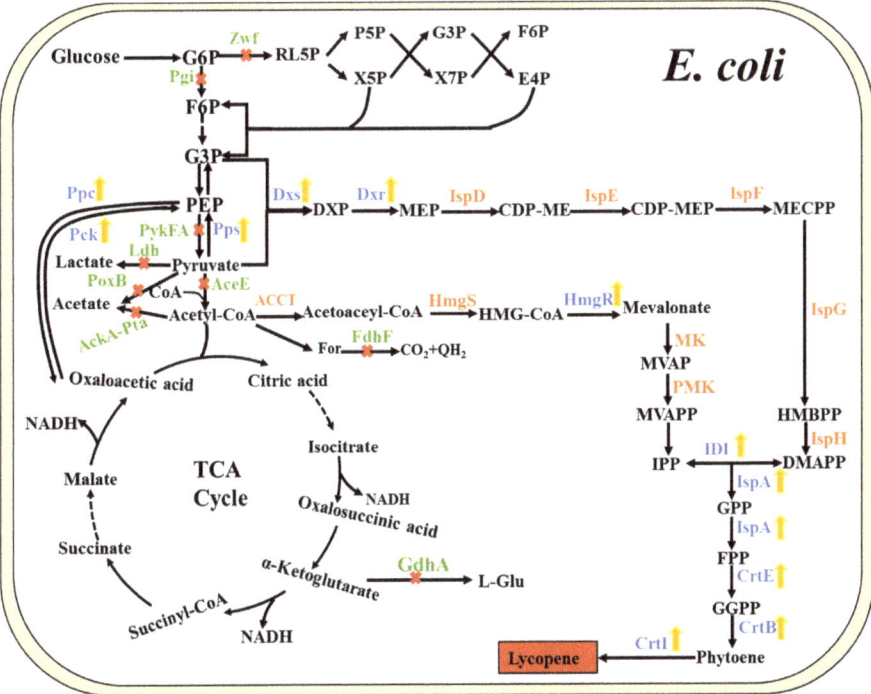

Figure 2. Metabolic engineering strategies of the entire lycopene pathway in *E. coli*. (The yellow arrow represents gene overexpression; the red "×" represents gene knockout or elimination of the pathway). Pps, phosphoenolpyruvate synthase; Pck, PEP carboxykinase; Ppc, PEP carboxylase; Ldh, lactate dehydrogenase; PoxB, pyruvate dehydrogenase; Ack, acetate kinase; Pta, phosphate acetyltransferase; Zwf, glucose-6-phosphate dehydrogenase; Pgi, glucosephosphate isomerase; GdhA, glutamate dehydrogenase; PykFA, pyruvate kinases; AceE, pyruvate dehydrogenase; FdhF, formate dehydrogenase H.

Most research has been focused on improving activities of the desired enzymes via conventional strategies, such as overexpression, direct evolution, and RBS optimization for lycopene production using the MEP pathway. However, fewer studies have been performed to investigate the regulatory mechanisms of the metabolic pathway. Therefore, further understanding of the regulatory mechanism of the MEP pathway and the combination of different strategies for lycopene production in E. coli need to be explored in the future.

2.3. Metabolic Engineering of the Heterogeneous MVA Pathway

Although the MEP pathway is natively present in E. coli [16], the utilization of this pathway has not shown high efficiency and exhibits low metabolite flux [23]. In contrast, the MVA pathway, an alternative pathway for lycopene production, is more energy-saving than the MEP pathway [30], and its introduction paved a new way for the formation of IPP from acetyl-CoA, resulting in a high-efficient lycopene production in E. coli. The MVA pathway is composed of the upper and lower pathway, separate from MVA [53]. When the whole MVA pathway from acetyl-CoA to IPP was engineered into E. coli, lycopene production increased by over 2-fold compared with the control strain [35]. Similarly, when only the lower pathway was employed, and mevalonate was supplied as a substrate, a significant increase in lycopene production was also observed [54]. These results indicated that the introduction of either the complete or the partial MVA pathway could reach an effective lycopene yield when a carbon source or carbon source with mevalonate were supplied, respectively, both through increasing lycopene precursors IPP and DMAPP. The heterologous MVA pathway was transferred into E. coli DH5α, combined with the overexpression of a type 2 IDI from Bacillus licheniformis significantly elevating lycopene production [36]. However, these studies were all implemented at the shake-flask fermentation level, not yet scalable for industrial production. Therefore, Zhu et al. adopted a new, targeted engineering strategy to reconstitute the MVA pathway in E. coli and establish a highly efficient platform which was employed for lycopene production. The fed-batch fermentation process was scaled up to 100 L, reaching 1.23 g/L of lycopene concentration with a maximum productivity of 74.5 mg/L/h [47]. In addition, Miguez et al. had conducted metabolomics analysis to reveal the toxic effects of lycopene production and the metabolic differences caused by induction time variation of the MVA pathway in the engineered E. coli strain. They reported that overnight induction of the MVA pathway was toxic to cells, which could recover if the lycopene pathway was not heterologously expressed simultaneously. Further, they validated that the intermediate homocysteine could contribute to the growth inhibition and the antagonistic effect between the mevalonate and lycopene pathways, resulting in the homocysteine-induced toxicity in lycopene production. This work indicated that metabolomics would be beneficial to reveal the mechanisms of the metabolite toxicity, and subsequently help to improve the metabolic engineering for the biosynthesis of carotenoid [37].

The introduction of the MVA pathway into E. coli caused dramatic improvement in lycopene production and could serve as a platform for the production of carotenoid compounds. This was attributed to the better elucidation of the MVA pathway than the MEP pathway. Moreover, the endogenous MEP pathway could be influenced by native regulation. In contrast, the introduction of the exogenous MVA pathway could play its role without regulation. However, because of the common intermediates (IPP and DMAPP), the two pathways are not totally independent, which provides potential optimization strategies for balancing two different pathways for carotenoid compounds production, including lycopene.

3. Optimization of Other Metabolic Pathways to Enhance Lycopene Production

In metabolic engineering, inhibition or even knockout of the competitive pathway of intermediate products, and elimination of potential bottlenecks in the upstream pathways not only reduces the generation of by-products but also increases the yield of the target products. Meanwhile, the enhancement of some metabolic pathways is also adopted to modulate the metabolite flux in the synthesis of the target products by supplying more precursors or intermediates.

Thus, a rational design strategy of metabolic pathways is of great potential to increase the yield of the target products.

As per the description of the MEP pathway, the initial precursors, G3P and pyruvate, are condensed into DXP in equal amounts. The unbalance between the two precursors can reduce the synthetic efficiency, making it necessary to maintain the balance by modulating the metabolic pathways based on a rational design strategy. As is known, the conversion from phosphoenolpyruvate to pyruvate [55], an essential step in the transformation of G3P to pyruvate, is an irreversible reaction [20] inhibiting the inter-conversion between G3P and pyruvate. Consequently, a new circuit bypassing this irreversible step was reconstructed. This was achieved by deleting pyruvate kinases-I and -II (Pyk-I and-II) to cut off the direct conversion of PEP to pyruvate, and overexpressing Ppc and Pck to introduce the bypass pathway between PEP and pyruvate via the oxaloacetate and TCA cycle (Figure 2). Meanwhile, the PEP synthase (Pps) converting pyruvate to PEP was also overexpressed. Thus, lycopene production was significantly increased with the rational reconstruction of the metabolic pathways from G3P to pyruvate [20].

Similarly, the inactivation of the competing pathways at acetyl-CoA and pyruvate nodes was applied to divert more carbon flux to the precursor IPP, including the deletion of the acetate and lactate production pathways. As a result, the engineered strain with the elimination of the acetate pathway accumulated more lycopene than the control strain [35]. Generally, metabolic engineering of pathways was mainly referred to the manipulation of genes directly connected with the product-synthesizing pathway. At the same time, indirectly related genes could also influence the synthesis of target products. For example, the deletion of the *zwf* gene encoding glucose-6-phosphate dehydrogenase (G6PD) (Figure 2), which controls the entry of carbon into the pentose phosphate pathway, resulted in the increased carbon fluxes in the Embden–Meyerhof–Parnas (EMP) pathway involving G3P and pyruvate, and indirectly led to an increase in lycopene production [28].

Identification of the genes directly or indirectly related to the production of the target products in metabolic engineering is of utmost importance. The elimination or overexpression of these genes can affect metabolic progress, either by redistributing the metabolic precursors or rewiring regulatory networks. Previous research on metabolically engineering *E. coli* for lycopene production employed an artificial phenotypic screening system to identify the genes affecting lycopene formation. As a result, multiple genes, including two unknown genes *elb1* and *elb2*, were identified that might be involved in the early reactions in lycopene synthesis. In more detail, the regulator encoded by *elb2* could regulate the biosynthesis of ubiquinone, including early steps of isoprenoid biosynthesis [56]. Alper et al. performed a genome-wide stoichiometric flux balance analysis to explore potential genes impacting the whole network properties and cellular phenotype. Consequently, seven single and multiple stoichiometric gene deletion mutants were obtained with increased lycopene production compared with the parental strain. Mainly, the triple knockout mutant of *gdhA/aceE/fdhF* (encoding NADP-specific glutamate dehydrogenase, pyruvate dehydrogenase, and formate dehydrogenase, respectively) exhibited a nearly 40% increase in lycopene yield (Figure 2). By exploring the potential reasons, it was found that *gdhA* deletion could increase the availability of NADPH, the knockout of *aceE* would presumably improve carbon flux to pyruvate and formate, and further deletion of *fdhF* might redirect the formate flux back to pyruvate, resulting in the increase of lycopene production [39]. Furthermore, transposon mutagenesis was utilized to identify combinatorial genetic targets for deletion to increase either the cofactor or precursor supply, resulting in the enhancement of lycopene yield. All the validated deletions were directly or indirectly related to cofactor production or metabolic flux [38]. Based on transposon mutagenesis and screening, the Δ*hnr* (aspartokinase/homoserine dehydrogenase) Δ*yliE* (di-GMP phosphodiesterase) mutant was obtained that significantly improved lycopene production. The Hnr protein could function as RpoS degradation, which is important for carotenoid production in *E. coli*. Moreover, the absence of the hypothetical protein YliE could positively influence lycopene production only in the Δ*hnr* background [40]. Subsequently, a two-dimensional gene target search of systematic and combinatorial approaches was developed to identify the overexpression targets and the knockout targets, respectively. More than 40 engineered strains were constructed, and the corresponding lycopene production was detected, combining overexpression with the knockout of the target genes with the highest lycopene yield being 16 mg/g DCW. These mutants involved kinds of genes referring to the synthetic pathway and regulation, and the lycopene of the most mutant strains has been limited by regulatory or metabolic barriers [48]. The adoption of a multi-dimensional search could thus help explore extensive mutant phenotypes. As a result, effective tools and strategies are necessary for identifying potential genes related to product yield in metabolic engineering at a global level. Moreover, the approach used to tune the genetic control of a single gene and modify multiple genes simultaneously also has been developed, including a functional promoter library [57], global transcription machinery engineering [58], engineered global regulators [42], and a functional RBS library [27]. The improvement of these tools and strategies would be beneficial for the optimization of the metabolic landscapes and the construction of effectively engineered strains.

Besides the modulation of the metabolite flux, a specific strategy such as membrane engineering plays a role in improving the lycopene yield. As shown in Figure 3, when Almgs (a membrane-bending protein) and two proteins related to the membrane-synthesis pathway, Plsb (glycerol-3-phosphate acyltransferase) and Plsc (1-acylglycerol-3-phosphate-acyltransferase), were overexpressed, the cells produced sufficient intracellular membrane vesicles and thus provided more space, and the amount of the membrane component, glycerophospholipids, was increased. Finally, 36.4 mg/g DCW of lycopene was accumulated in the cell membranes [49]. This novel membrane engineering strategy could be further explored for the synthesis of a wide range of hydrophobic products.

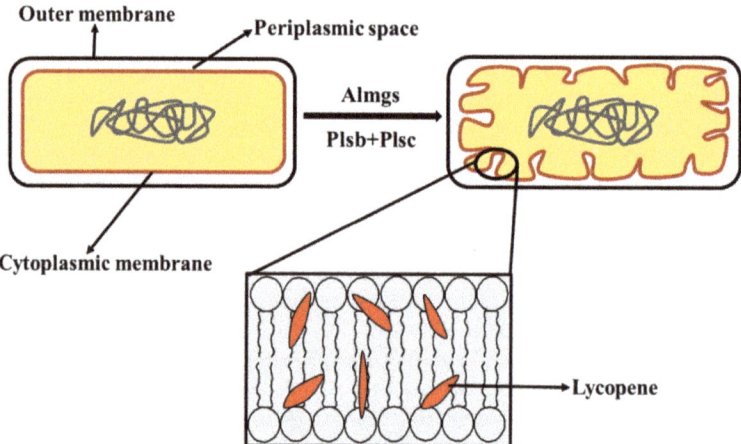

Figure 3. Diagram of membrane engineering strategy to increase the lycopene production in *E. coli*. Almgs, membrane-bending protein; Plsb, glycerol-3-phosphateacyltransferase; Plsc, 1-acylglycerol-3-phosphate-acyltransferase.

In addition, the precursors of lycopene, IPP and DMAPP, were biosynthesized via the MEP or MVA pathway, during which they need NADPH and ATP [19]. Consequently, another critical engineering strategy for enhancing lycopene production is to provide enough NADPH and ATP to the entire metabolic pathway. In another study, the expression of genes encoding a-ketoglutarate dehydrogenase, succinate dehydrogenase, and transaldolase B was modulated to increase NADPH and ATP, resulting in a significant increase in the lycopene yield [27].

4. Engineering Regulatory Networks to Enhance Lycopene Production

As mentioned above, most studies on lycopene production were focused on the overexpression of the key rate-limiting enzymes, and the elimination or inactivation of the competitive branch pathway. The regulation of metabolic pathways could be used to reprogram the metabolic genes to improve the yield of the target products by eliminating metabolic imbalance.

The phosphorylated response regulator NRI (*glnG* product) included in the two-component system Ntr could activate transcription from the *glnAp2* promoter by binding to its cognate binding sites on the DNA. Further, NRI itself is capable of sensing the level of acetyl phosphate (ACP), an indicator of glucose flux. Therefore, an artificially engineered *glnAp2* promoter containing NRI binding sites and the core *glnAp2* promoter was constructed to serve as a control valve that controls gene expression according to the ACP level. Then, this control valve was adopted to regulate the expression of IDI and Pps, which have been identified to control the flux to the final product, and the balance between pyruvate and G3P. The introduction of this regulatory circuit resulted in the full utilization of the excess carbon flux for the enhancement of lycopene production and bypassing the toxic product, acetate [41]. Moreover, transcriptional engineering of the global regulator cAMP receptor protein (CRP) was conducted using an error-prone PCR and site-directed mutagenesis to subtly balance the whole metabolic pathway networks to improve lycopene yield. The mutant strain, MT-1, with the engineered CRP encoded by a mutant gene (mcrp26) showed a higher lycopene production (18.49 mg/g DCW) compared with the original strain. Besides, the differential expression of the global genes between the MT-1 mutant and wild type was also explored, in which the genes of *pfkA*, *fbaA*, and *ispG* involved in the lycopene biosynthetic pathway were up-regulated. Thus, it helped reveal the possible mechanism for the improvement in lycopene production caused by the engineered CRP. As explored, in mcrp26, residue D8 (Asp) had been mutated into V (Val), which belongs to the N-proximal cAMP-binding domain, altering the cAMP-binding capacity. This influenced the CAP-dependent promoters, which raised the differential expression of the above genes related to lycopene production [42]. In addition, the modulation of global regulatory proteins RpoS (Sigma S factor), AppY (transcription activator for genes related to anaerobic energy metabolism), and Crl (transcriptional regulator of *csgBA* for curli surface fiber formation) also enhanced lycopene production by regulating the expression of lycopene synthesis enzymes and energy metabolism operons [59], or the hydrophobic interaction between curli fiber molecules and lycopene [29,48,60]. Another study was performed to disclose the mechanisms involved in the differences in the lycopene production and MEP pathway flux of six *E. coli* host strains through systems analysis including genetic complementation, quantitative sequential windowed acquisition of all theoretical fragment ions (SWATH) proteomics, and biochemical analysis. It revealed that RpoS could help accumulate lycopene by decreasing oxidative stress in the growth stationary phase, which reduced the degradation of lycopene to its colorless oxidation—and cleavage products [61]. These strategies for engineering the regulatory networks to enhance lycopene production in *E. coli* have been summarized in Figure 4. Thus, the engineered regulators controlling the gene expression gave rise to a significant potential for the regulatory design of metabolic pathways in *E. coli* for the production of lycopene and other biochemicals.

Although the biochemistry properties of the MVA pathway have been comprehensively revealed and extensively utilized for the industrial production of isoprenoids, few applications of the regulation of the MVA pathway have been explored in lycopene biosynthesis. Moreover, the regulatory mechanisms of the MEP pathway are also less studied. Thus, the adoption of the regulation of the MVA pathway and the in-depth understanding of the MEP pathway are necessary for further optimization on improving lycopene production in *E. coli*.

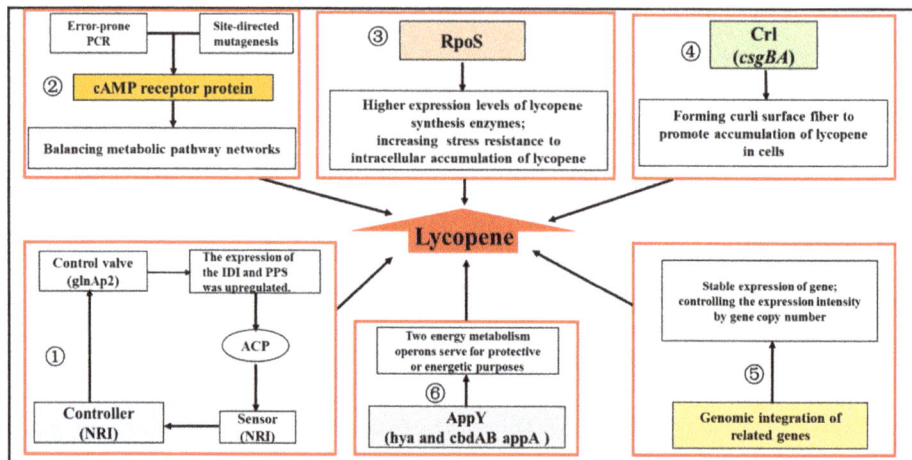

Figure 4. Summary of the strategies for engineering the regulatory networks to enhance lycopene production in *E. coli*. (1) Acetyl phosphate (ACP), as an indicator of glucose flux, was set as a signal of the two-component regulon Ntr, to regulate the expression of *idi* and *pps* for lycopene biosynthesis. (2) Transcriptional engineering on the global regulator cAMP receptor protein (CRP) was conducted by using error-prone PCR and site-directed mutagenesis, to subtly balancing the whole metabolic pathway networks for improving the lycopene yield. (3) RpoS regulates the transcription of genes induced at the stationary phase and energy metabolism. (4) Crl regulated the expression of *csgBA* for curli surface fiber formation to promote the accumulation of lycopene in cells. (5) Genomic integration of related genes made the expression stable and controlled the expression intensity by gene copy number. (6) The AppY transcriptional regulator was relative to anaerobic energy metabolism.

5. Optimization of Auxiliary Carbon Source and Fermentation Modes

Besides the optimization of regulatory networks in a metabolic pathway, the supply of an appropriate carbon source is also an essential factor for improving synthetic efficiency, thereby reducing the production costs at the industrial level. In the biosynthesis of lycopene, glycerol or glucose are usually utilized as the primary carbon source [36,43,45,47,54,62]. Some researchers explored the effect of an auxiliary carbon source on lycopene production in engineered *E. coli*. When glycerol was used as the primary carbon source, the synergistic effect of the auxiliary carbon sources, glucose, and L-arabinose was related to the endogenous metabolism in *E. coli* and the stimulation on the exogenous MVA pathway [43]. When glucose, fructose, glycerol, or arabinose were supplied as an auxiliary carbon source, respectively, to the LB medium for lycopene production, 6 g/L fructose exhibited the highest lycopene yield [12]. Citrate was verified to be a positive auxiliary carbon source for enhancing lycopene production, indicating that the citrate pathway might be responsible for accumulating more isoprenoid in engineered *E. coli* [36]. Similarly, in another study, the MVA lower pathway was introduced into *E. coli*, in which glycerol was supplied as the carbon source with addition of mevalonate, and Tween 80 was added to prevent clump formation, resulting in a significant increase in lycopene production [54]. Moreover, an engineered *E. coli* strain introduced with the fatty acid transport system was capable of utilizing free fatty acids or waste cooking oil to produce lycopene, with the highest yield of 94 mg/g [44].

Optimization of the fermentation process is a traditional and direct strategy for improving lycopene production. Traditional fermentation that includes shake-flask and fed-batch fermentations is usually applied (Table 1). Besides this, various fermentation optimization strategies have been conducted. For instance, high cell density fermentation was performed in two lycopene-producing *E. coli* strains to explore the effect of fermentation parameters on lycopene production. Results demonstrated that high oxygen levels and pH values were critical for increasing the lycopene yield. The importance of oxygen, growth rate, and glutamate flux on lycopene production thus indicated the potential of stoichiometric analysis in optimizing the fermentation strategy [45]. In another study, considering the increased carotenoid yield and productivity at 25 °C in contrast to those at 37 °C [35,63], a temperature-shift culture method (37→25 °C) was adopted to further augment lycopene production [62]. Optimizing the culture conditions of the recombinant *E. coli* 99DH cultivated under exposure to light in 2YT medium (1.6% tryptone, 1% yeast extract, 0.5% NaCl), supplemented with glycine addition, exhibited an increased lycopene production rate by 76% [46].

6. Other Engineering Strategies for Lycopene Production

Besides the conventional engineering approaches adopted to enhance lycopene production in *E. coil*, some novel engineering strategies have been explored. For instance, the enhancement of mRNA stability by varying the mRNA secondary structures was adopted to modulate the metabolic flux to improve lycopene production [64]. Moreover, during the amplification of the fermentation process, it is essential to decrease the requirement of complex media and antibiotics, and the burden caused by exogenous plasmids, as well as to maintain the stability of the engineered strain, based on which chromosomal integration is applied to introduce lycopene synthesis genes into the *E. coli* chromosome [50]. A multiplex automated genome engineering for large-scale programming had been used to optimize the MEP pathway in *E. coli* for lycopene production [51]. Coussement et al. developed a new combinatorial multi-gene pathway assembly scheme based on single-strand assembly (SSA) methods and Golden Gate assembly, and it was adopted to optimize the lycopene biosynthetic pathway, resulting in lycopene production of 448 mg/g DCW [52].

7. Discussion and Future Perspectives

In summary, all these efforts on exploring various engineering strategies have facilitated an increase in lycopene production by metabolically engineering *E. coli*. However, there is still much room for improvement for lycopene yield in engineered *E. coli*. The following perspectives could be focused on in future research. First, the combination of the endogenous MEP pathway and the heterogeneous MVA pathway should be further investigated. The mechanisms of the cross-talk between the two pathways should also be uncovered. Second, the regulatory mechanism of the MEP pathway has not been well understood, giving rise to the potential of exploring regulatory engineering to enhance the biological production of lycopene. Third, the compartmentalization of the lycopene biosynthetic pathway should be paid more attention to, which is beneficial to eliminate the cytotoxicity of IPP and DMAPP as well as enhance the compartmental synthesis efficiency. Accumulation of the target products results in gradual cellular pressure of tolerating the target products, thus requiring the exploration of new strategies to resolve this issue, such as adaptive evolution, membrane engineering and efficient extraction methods. Finally, more concerns are given to the modification of upstream metabolic pathways to increase lycopene production, while the optimization of the downstream fermentation process is ignored. Therefore, more attempts should be made to the process engineering of the fermentation, including optimization of the fermentation mode and process parameters, in situ product recovery (ISPR) processes, and so on. Actually, there are numerous research directions in engineered *E. coli*, showing a promising prospect for lycopene production and other biochemicals.

Funding: This work was supported by grants from the "First class grassland science discipline" program in Shandong Province, the National Natural Science Foundation of China (31860011), the Talents of High Level Scientific Research Foundation (grants 6651117005 and 6651119011) of Qingdao Agricultural University, Key Laboratory of Biofuels, Qingdao Institute of Bioenergy and Bioprocess Technology, Chinese Academy of Sciences (CASKLB201805), and the Shandong Modern Agricultural Technology and Industry System (SDAIT-11-11).

Acknowledgments: The authors would like to thank Caroline S. Harwood for useful suggestions which helped to improve the quality of the manuscript.

Conflicts of Interest: The authors declare no conflict of interest.

References

1. Wang, C.; Zhao, S.; Shao, X.; Park, J.B.; Jeong, S.H.; Park, H.J.; Kwak, W.J.; Wei, G.; Kim, S.W. Challenges and tackles in metabolic engineering for microbial production of carotenoids. *Microb. Cell Fact.* **2019**, *18*, 55. [CrossRef] [PubMed]
2. Giovannucci, E. A review of epidemiologic studies of tomatoes, lycopene, and prostate cancer. *Exp. Biol. Med.* **2002**, *227*, 852–859. [CrossRef]
3. Bignotto, L.; Rocha, J.; Sepodes, B.; Eduardofigueira, M.; Pinto, R.; Chaud, M.V.; De Carvalho, J.; Moreno, H.; Motafilipe, H. Anti-inflammatory effect of lycopene on carrageenan-induced paw oedema and hepatic ischaemia–reperfusion in the rat. *Brit. J. Nutr.* **2009**, *102*, 126–133. [CrossRef] [PubMed]
4. Erdman, J.W.; Ford, N.A.; Lindshield, B.L. Are the health attributes of lycopene related to its antioxidant function. *Arch. Biochem. Biophys.* **2009**, *483*, 229–235. [CrossRef] [PubMed]
5. Choudhari, S.M.; Ananthanarayan, L.; Singhal, R.S. Purification of lycopene by reverse phase chromatography. *Food Bioprocess Tech.* **2009**, *2*, 391–399. [CrossRef]
6. Frengova, G.I.; Beshkova, D.M. Carotenoids from *Rhodotorula* and *Phaffia*: Yeasts of biotechnological importance. *J. Ind. Microbiol. Biot.* **2009**, *36*, 163–180. [CrossRef]
7. Hernández-Almanza, A.; Montañez, J.; Martínez, G.; Aguilar-Jiménez, A.; Contreras-Esquivel, J.C.; Aguilar, C.N. Lycopene: Progress in microbial production. *Trends Food Sci. Tech.* **2016**, *56*, 142–148. [CrossRef]
8. Clinton, S.K. Lycopene: Chemistry, biology, and implications for human health and disease. *Nutr. Rev.* **1998**, *56*, 35–51. [CrossRef] [PubMed]
9. Story, E.N.; Kopec, R.E.; Schwartz, S.J.; Harris, G.K. An update on the health effects of tomato lycopene. *Annu. Rev. Food Sci. Tech.* **2010**, *1*, 189–210. [CrossRef] [PubMed]
10. Liu, X.J.; Liu, R.S.; Li, H.M.; Tang, Y.J. Lycopene production from synthetic medium by *Blakeslea trispora* NRRL 2895 (+) and 2896 (-) in a stirred-tank fermenter. *Bioproc. Biosyst. Eng.* **2012**, *35*, 739–749. [CrossRef]
11. Mantzouridou, F.; Tsimidou, M.Z. Lycopene formation in *Blakeslea trispora*. Chemical aspects of a bioprocess. *Trends Food Sci. Tech.* **2008**, *19*, 363–371. [CrossRef]
12. Zhang, T.C.; Li, W.; Luo, X.G.; Feng, C.X.; Ma, D.Y. Increase of the lycopene production in the recombinant strains of *Escherichia coli* by supplementing with fructose. *Lect. Notes Electr. Eng.* **2015**, *332*, 29–35.
13. Kang, M.J.; Yoon, S.H.; Lee, Y.M.; Lee, S.H.; Kim, S.W. Enhancement of lycopene production in *Escherichia coli* by optimization of the lycopene synthetic pathway. *J. Microbiol. Biotech.* **2005**, *15*, 880–886.
14. Ma, T.; Deng, Z.; Liu, T. Microbial production strategies and applications of lycopene and other terpenoids. *World J. Microb. Biot.* **2016**, *32*, 15. [CrossRef] [PubMed]
15. Yoon, S.-H.; Kim, J.-E.; Lee, S.-H.; Park, H.-M.; Choi, M.-S.; Kim, J.-Y.; Lee, S.-H.; Shin, Y.-C.; Keasling, J.D.; Kim, S.-W. Engineering the lycopene synthetic pathway in *E. coli* by comparison of the carotenoid genes of *Pantoea agglomerans* and *Pantoea ananatis*. *Appl. Microbiol. Biot.* **2007**, *74*, 131–139. [CrossRef] [PubMed]
16. Rohmer, M.; Knani, M.; Simonin, P.; Sutter, B.; Sahm, H. Isoprenoid biosynthesis in bacteria: A novel pathway for the early steps leading to isopentenyl diphosphate. *Biochem. J.* **1993**, *295*, 517. [CrossRef] [PubMed]
17. Yang, J.; Zhao, G.; Sun, Y.; Zheng, Y.; Jiang, X.; Liu, W.; Xian, M. Bio-isoprene production using exogenous MVA pathway and isoprene synthase in *Escherichia coli*. *Bioresource Technol.* **2012**, *104*, 642–647. [CrossRef] [PubMed]
18. Boucher, Y.; Doolittle, W.F. The role of lateral gene transfer in the evolution of isoprenoid biosynthesis pathways. *Mol. Microbiol.* **2000**, *37*, 703–716. [CrossRef]
19. Li, M.; Nian, R.; Xian, M.; Zhang, H. Metabolic engineering for the production of isoprene and isopentenol by *Escherichia coli*. *Appl. Microbiol. Biot.* **2018**, *102*, 7725–7738. [CrossRef]
20. Farmer, W.R.; Liao, J.C. Precursor balancing for metabolic engineering of lycopene production in *Escherichia coli*. *Biotechnol. Progr.* **2001**, *17*, 57–61. [CrossRef]
21. Bloch, K.; Chaykin, S.; Phillips, A.H.; Waard, A.D. Mevalonic acid pyrophosphate and isopentenylpyrophosphate. *J. Biol. Chem.* **1959**, *234*, 2595–2604.
22. Stephanopoulos, G.; Alper, H.; Moxley, J. Exploiting biological complexity for strain improvement through systems biology. *Nat. Biotechnol.* **2004**, *22*, 1261–1267. [CrossRef] [PubMed]

23. Ajikumar, P.K.; Tyo, K.; Carlsen, S.; Mucha, O.; Phon, T.H.; Stephanopoulos, G. Terpenoids: Opportunities for biosynthesis of natural product drugs using engineered microorganisms. *Mol. Pharmaceut.* **2008**, *5*, 167–190. [CrossRef] [PubMed]
24. Grawert, T.; Groll, M.; Rohdich, F.; Bacher, A.; Eisenreich, W. Biochemistry of the non-mevalonate isoprenoid pathway. *Cell Mol. Life. Sci.* **2011**, *68*, 3797–3814. [CrossRef]
25. Hunter, W.N. The non-mevalonate pathway of isoprenoid precursor biosynthesis. *J. Biol. Chem.* **2007**, *282*, 21573–21577. [CrossRef]
26. Dellas, N.; Thomas, S.T.; Manning, G.; Noel, J.P. Discovery of a metabolic alternative to the classical mevalonate pathway. *Elife* **2013**, *2*, e00672. [CrossRef] [PubMed]
27. Sun, T.; Miao, L.; Li, Q.; Dai, G.; Lu, F.; Liu, T.; Zhang, X.; Ma, Y. Production of lycopene by metabolically-engineered *Escherichia coli*. *Biotechnol. Lett.* **2014**, *36*, 1515–1522. [CrossRef] [PubMed]
28. Yan, Z.; Nambou, K.; Wei, L.; Cao, J.; Qiang, H. Lycopene production in recombinant strains of *Escherichia coli* is improved by knockout of the central carbon metabolism gene coding for glucose-6-phosphate dehydrogenase. *Biotechnol. Lett.* **2013**, *35*, 2137–2145.
29. Kang, M.J.; Lee, Y.M.; Yoon, S.H.; Kim, J.H.; Ock, S.W.; Jung, K.H.; Shin, Y.C.; Keasling, J.D.; Kim, S.W. Identification of genes affecting lycopene accumulation in *Escherichia coli* using a shot-gun method. *Biotechnol. Bioeng.* **2005**, *91*, 636–642. [CrossRef]
30. Cunningham, F.X., Jr.; Sun, Z.; Chamovitz, D.; Hirschberg, J.; Gantt, E. Molecular structure and enzymatic function of lycopene cyclase from the cyanobacterium *Synechococcus* sp strain PCC7942. *Plant Cell* **1994**, *6*, 1107–1121.
31. Kim, S.W.; Keasling, J. Metabolic engineering of the nonmevalonate isopentenyl diphosphate synthesis pathway in *Escherichia coli* enhances lycopene production. *Biotechnol. Bioeng.* **2001**, *72*, 408–415. [CrossRef]
32. Matthews, P.D.; Wurtzel, E.T. Metabolic engineering of carotenoid accumulation in *Escherichia coli* by modulation of the isoprenoid precursor pool with expression of deoxyxylulose phosphate synthase. *Appl. Microbiol. Biot.* **2000**, *53*, 396–400. [CrossRef] [PubMed]
33. Wang, C.; Oh, M.K.; Liao, J.C. Directed evolution of metabolically engineered *Escherichia coli* for carotenoid production. *Biotechnol. Prog.* **2000**, *16*, 922–926. [CrossRef] [PubMed]
34. Lv, X.; Gu, J.; Wang, F.; Xie, W.; Liu, M.; Ye, L.; Yu, H. Combinatorial pathway optimization in *Escherichia coli* by directed co-evolution of rate-limiting enzymes and modular pathway engineering. *Biotechnol. Bioeng.* **2016**, *113*, 2661–2669. [CrossRef]
35. Vadali, R.V.; Fu, Y.; Bennett, G.N.; San, K.Y. Enhanced Lycopene Productivity by manipulation of carbon flow to isopentenyl diphosphate in *Escherichia coli*. *Biotechnol. Progr.* **2005**, *21*, 1558–1561. [CrossRef]
36. Rad, S.A.; Zahiri, H.S.; Noghabi, K.A.; Rajaei, S.; Heidari, R.; Mojallali, L. Type 2 IDI performs better than type 1 for improving lycopene production in metabolically engineered *E. coli* strains. *World J. Microbiol. Biot.* **2012**, *28*, 313–321. [CrossRef]
37. Miguez, A.M.; McNerney, M.P.; Styczynski, M.P. Metabolomics analysis of the toxic effects of the production of lycopene and its precursors. *Front. Microbiol.* **2018**, *9*, 760. [CrossRef]
38. Alper, H.; Miyaoku, K.; Stephanopoulos, G. Construction of lycopene-overproducing *E. coli* strains by combining systematic and combinatorial gene knockout targets. *Nat. Biotechnol.* **2005**, *23*, 612–626. [CrossRef]
39. Alper, H.; Jin, Y.S.; Moxley, J.F.; Stephanopoulos, G. Identifying gene targets for the metabolic engineering of lycopene biosynthesis in *Escherichia coli*. *Metab. Eng.* **2005**, *7*, 155–164. [CrossRef]
40. Alper, H.; Stephanopoulos, G. Uncovering the gene knockout landscape for improved lycopene production in *E. coli*. *Appl. Microbiol. Biot.* **2008**, *78*, 801–810. [CrossRef]
41. Farmer, W.R.; Liao, J.C. Improving lycopene production in *Escherichia coli* by engineering metabolic control. *Nat. Biotechnol.* **2000**, *18*, 533–537. [CrossRef] [PubMed]
42. Huang, L.; Pu, Y.; Yang, X.L.; Zhu, X.C.; Cai, J.; Xu, Z.N. Engineering of global regulator cAMP receptor protein (CRP) in *Escherichia coli* for improved lycopene production. *J. Biotechnol.* **2015**, *199*, 55–61. [CrossRef] [PubMed]
43. Kim, Y.; Lee, J.; Kim, N.; Yeom, S.; Kim, S.; Oh, D. Increase of lycopene production by supplementing auxiliary carbon sources in metabolically engineered *Escherichia coli*. *Appl. Microbiol. Biot.* **2011**, *90*, 489–497. [CrossRef] [PubMed]

44. Liu, N.; Liu, B.; Wang, G.; Soong, Y.V.; Tao, Y.; Liu, W.; Xie, D. Lycopene production from glucose, fatty acid and waste cooking oil by metabolically engineered *Escherichia coli*. *Biochem. Eng. J.* **2020**, *155*, 107488. [CrossRef]
45. Alper, H.S.; Miyaoku, K.; Stephanopoulos, G. Characterization of lycopene-overproducing *E. coli* strains in high cell density fermentations. *Appl. Microbiol. Biot.* **2006**, *72*, 968–974. [CrossRef] [PubMed]
46. Xu, J.; Xu, X.; Xu, Q.; Zhang, Z.; Jiang, L.; Huang, H. Efficient production of lycopene by engineered *E. coli* strains harboring different types of plasmids. *Bioproc. Biosyst. Eng.* **2018**, *41*, 489–499. [CrossRef] [PubMed]
47. Zhu, F.; Lu, L.; Fu, S.; Zhong, X.; Hu, M.; Deng, Z.; Liu, T. Targeted engineering and scale up of lycopene overproduction in *Escherichia coli*. *Process Biochem.* **2015**, *50*, 341–346. [CrossRef]
48. Jin, Y.S.; Stephanopoulos, G. Multi-dimensional gene target search for improving lycopene biosynthesis in *Escherichia coli*. *Metab. Eng.* **2007**, *9*, 337–347. [CrossRef]
49. Wu, T.; Ye, L.; Zhao, D.; Li, S.; Li, Q.; Zhang, B.; Bi, C. Engineering membrane morphology and manipulating synthesis for increased lycopene accumulation in *Escherichia coli* cell factories. *3 Biotech.* **2018**, *8*, 269. [CrossRef]
50. Chen, Y.; Shen, H.; Cui, Y.; Chen, S.; Weng, Z.; Zhao, M.; Liu, J. Chromosomal evolution of *Escherichia coli* for the efficient production of lycopene. *BMC Biotechnol.* **2013**, *13*. [CrossRef]
51. Wang, H.H.; Isaacs, F.J.; Carr, P.A.; Sun, Z.Z.; Xu, G.; Forest, C.R.; Church, G.M. Programming cells by multiplex genome engineering and accelerated evolution. *Nature* **2009**, *460*, 894–898. [CrossRef] [PubMed]
52. Coussement, P.; Bauwens, D.; Maertens, J.; De Mey, M. Direct combinatorial pathway optimization. *ACS Synth. Biol.* **2017**, *6*, 224–232. [CrossRef]
53. Yang, J.; Xian, M.; Su, S.; Zhao, G.; Nie, Q.; Jiang, X.; Zheng, Y.; Liu, W. Enhancing production of bio-isoprene using hybrid MVA pathway and isoprene synthase in *E. coli*. *PLoS ONE* **2012**, *7*, e33509. [CrossRef] [PubMed]
54. Yoon, S.H.; Lee, Y.M.; Kim, J.E.; Lee, S.H.; Lee, J.H.; Kim, J.Y.; Jung, K.H.; Shin, Y.C.; Keasling, J.D.; Kim, S.W. Enhanced lycopene production in *Escherichia coli* engineered to synthesize isopentenyl diphosphate and dimethylallyl diphosphate from mevalonate. *Biotechnol. Bioeng.* **2006**, *94*, 1025–1032. [CrossRef] [PubMed]
55. Christian, Q.; Elmar, P.; Pelin, Y.; Jan, G.; Timmy, S.; Pablo, Y.; Jörg, P.; Oliver, G.F. The SILVA ribosomal RNA gene database project: Improved data processing and web-based tools. *Nucleic Acids Res.* **2012**, *41*, 590–596.
56. Hemmi, H.; Ohnuma, S.I.; Nagaoka, K.; Nishino, T. Identification of genes affecting lycopene formation in *Escherichia coli* transformed with carotenoid biosynthetic genes: Candidates for early genes in isoprenoid biosynthesis. *J. Biochem.* **1998**, *123*, 1088–1096. [CrossRef]
57. Alper, H.; Fischer, C.; Nevoigt, E.; Stephanopoulos, G. Tuning genetic control through promoter engineering. *Proc. Natl. Acad. Sci. USA* **2005**, *102*, 12678–12683. [CrossRef]
58. Alper, H.; Moxley, J.; Nevoigt, E.; Fink, G.R.; Stephanopoulos, G. Engineering yeast transcription machinery for improved ethanol tolerance and production. *Science* **2006**, *314*, 1565–1568. [CrossRef]
59. Atlung, T.; Knudsen, K.; Heerfordt, L.; Brondsted, L. Effects of sigmaS and the transcriptional activator AppY on induction of the *Escherichia coli* hya and *cbdAB-appA* operons in response to carbon and phosphate starvation. *J. Bacteriol.* **1997**, *179*, 2141–2146. [CrossRef]
60. Gerhard, S.; Woods, W.S.; Tuveson, R.W. Identification of carotenoids in *Erwinia herbicola* and in a transformed *Escherichia coli* strain. *Fems. Microbiol. Lett.* **1990**, *71*, 77–82.
61. Bongers, M.; Chrysanthopoulos, P.K.; Behrendorff, J.B.; Hodson, M.P.; Vickers, C.E.; Nielsen, L.K. Systems analysis of methylerythritol-phosphate pathway flux in *E. coli*: Insights into the role of oxidative stress and the validity of lycopene as an isoprenoid reporter metabolite. *Microb. Cell Fact.* **2015**, *14*, 193. [CrossRef] [PubMed]
62. Kim, S.W.; Kim, J.B.; Ryu, J.M.; Jung, J.K.; Kim, J.H. High-level production of lycopene in metabolically engineered *E. coli*. *Process. Biochem.* **2009**, *44*, 899–905. [CrossRef]
63. Kim, S.W.; Kim, J.B.; Jung, W.H.; Kim, J.H.; Jung, J.K. Over-production of β-carotene from metabolically engineered *Escherichia coli*. *Biotechnol. Lett.* **2006**, *28*, 897–904. [CrossRef] [PubMed]
64. Smolke, C.D.; Martin, V.J.J.; Keasling, J.D. Controlling the metabolic flux through the carotenoid pathway using directed mRNA processing and stabilization. *Meta. Eng.* **2001**, *3*, 313–321. [CrossRef] [PubMed]

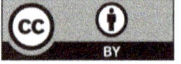 © 2020 by the authors. Licensee MDPI, Basel, Switzerland. This article is an open access article distributed under the terms and conditions of the Creative Commons Attribution (CC BY) license (http://creativecommons.org/licenses/by/4.0/).

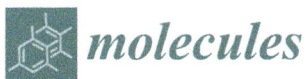

Review

Traps and Pitfalls—Unspecific Reactions in Metabolic Engineering of Sesquiterpenoid Pathways

Maximilian Frey

Institute of Biology, Dept. of Biochemistry of Plant Secondary Metabolism (190b), University of Hohenheim, Garbenstraße 30, 70593 Stuttgart, Germany; maximilian_frey@uni-hohenheim.de

Academic Editors: Pavel B. Drasar and Vladimir A. Khripach
Received: 2 April 2020; Accepted: 21 April 2020; Published: 22 April 2020

Abstract: The characterization of plant enzymes by expression in prokaryotic and eukaryotic (yeast and plants) heterologous hosts has widely been used in recent decades to elucidate metabolic pathways in plant secondary metabolism. Yeast and plant systems provide the cellular environment of a eukaryotic cell and the subcellular compartmentalization necessary to facilitate enzyme function. The expression of candidate genes in these cell systems and the identification of the resulting products guide the way for the identification of enzymes with new functions. However, in many cases, the detected compounds are not the direct enzyme products but are caused by unspecific subsequent reactions. Even if the mechanisms for these unspecific reactions are in many cases widely reported, there is a lack of overview of potential reactions that may occur to provide a guideline for researchers working on the characterization of new enzymes. Here, an across-the-board summary of rearrangement reactions of sesquiterpenes in metabolic pathway engineering is presented. The different kinds of unspecific reactions as well as their chemical and cellular background are explained and strategies how to spot and how to avoid these unspecific reactions are given. Also, a systematic approach of classification of unspecific reactions is introduced. It is hoped that this mini-review will stimulate a discussion on how to systematically classify unspecific reactions in metabolic engineering and to expand this approach to other classes of plant secondary metabolites.

Keywords: rearrangement reactions; sesquiterpenes; sesquiterpene lactones; conjugation; metabolic engineering; enzyme characterization; transannular cyclization; Cope rearrangement

1. Introduction

The sesquiterpenes (ST) are a subgroup of the terpenes with a C15 backbone comprised of three isoprene units; sesquiterpenes with a lactone moiety are called sesquiterpene lactones (STL). The elucidation and metabolic engineering of their biosynthetic pathways have made significant progress in the past decades, as many sesquiterpenes are of commercial interest as fragrances [1], biodiesel [2] or pharmaceuticals [3,4]. The reconstruction of sesquiterpenoid metabolic pathways has been carried out in various prokaryotic and eukaryotic host models such as *Escherichia coli* [5,6], *Saccharomyces cerevisiae* [4,7–12], *Nicotiana benthamiana* [7,8,13–16] and *Physcomitrella patens* [17,18]. The analysis of sesquiterpenes is usually performed by gas or liquid chromatography coupled with mass spectrometry, depending on the volatility of the compound. In the first step of terpene biosynthesis the carbon backbone is formed by a terpene synthase [19]. In a second step, the intermediate is often modified by cytochrome P450 enzymes that introduce oxygen into the core backbone [20,21]. Cytochrome P450 enzymes have been reported to introduce hydroxy-, epoxy-, acid- and estergroups [7–10,13] and the conversion from a germacrene to a guaiane backbone [12]. One of the challenges when expressing biosynthetic enzymes of sesquiterpenoid pathways is the differentiation of the direct enzyme product and artificial products that arise from unspecific subsequent reactions. Here, a concise overview of these unspecific reactions and how to avoid them is presented.

2. Unspecific Reactions

Four categories of unspecific reactions in pathway engineering of sesquiterpenoids can be classified: 1) S-conjugation, 2) O-conjugation, 3) acid-induced rearrangement and 4) heat-induced rearrangement. In each category several unspecific reactions can be observed and several combinations of these can occur. These unspecific reactions are each given a letter from (a) to (k). Irradiation is known to induce rearrangement reactions in germacranolide STL [22–24] as well. So far, there are no reports on unspecific reactions in metabolic engineering of sesquiterpenes caused by light irradiation, yet. However, we know that light does play an important role in the formation of artemisinin in nature [25]. Also, the influence of endogenous enzymes of the host cell system that convert the enzyme product is possible [26].

2.1. S-Conjugation

When expressing the genes of the metabolic pathway to costunolide from various species [7,15,26,27] in *Nicotiana benthamina*, the predominant product found was not free. Instead costunolide had mostly undergone (a) conjugation to cysteine (**1**) to form costunolide-cysteine (**2**) or (b) conjugation to glutathione to form costunolide-glutathione (**3**). The production of costunolide derivatives by expression of the corresponding metabolic pathway in *Nicotiana* such as 3β-costunolide, 14-hydroxycostunolide, eupatolide, parthenolide and 3β-parthenolide resulted in the formation of the cysteine and glutathione conjugates as well [8,13,14]. Also, during *in planta* production of inunolide, the 7,8-*cis* lactone isomer of costunolide resulted in cysteine and glutathione adducts [13]. When the same pathways were expressed in yeast, no cysteine or glutathione conjugates occurred [7,9,14,15].

2.2. O-Conjugation

The production of artemisinic acid (**4**) in *Nicotiana benthamiana* (Figure 1a) has been observed to yield mostly artemisinic acid 12-β-glucoside (**5**), which can be explained by (c) an esterification of the acid moiety of artemisinic acid to diglucose [28]. *In planta* produced epi-kunzeaol (**6**) was linked to two glucose units [29]. This was due to (d) an etherification of the C7-hydroxy moiety of epi-kunzeaol to form epi-kunzeaol-diglucoside (**7**).

2.3. Acid-Induced Rearrangement

Acidic conditions are known to induce transannular cyclization in germacrenes (Figure 1b), which can lead to a great number of rearrangement products, mostly with the C10 ring of a germacrene cyclizing to two C6 rings [22]. In the case of inunolide (**8**) a rearrangement product seems possible with (e) the double bond flipping to the C5-C6 position to form alantolactone (**9**) [13]. One well-observed example is as the rearrangement reaction from a germacrene to a eudesmane backbone. This acid-induced rearrangement converts, for instance, germacrene A acid (**10**) to α-costic acid (**11**), β-costic acid (**12**), and γ-costic acid (**13**) [9,10,30] with the double bond positions Δ3→4 (f), Δ4→15 (g) or Δ4→5 (h). The subsequent introduction of water (i) resulting in ilicic acid (**14**) has also been reported [9,10], likely neutralizing a carbocationic intermediate.

2.4. Heat-Induced Rearrangement

When analyzing the enzyme products of germacrene A synthases from various species in yeast and *Nicotiana* by GC-MS (Figure 1b) the enzyme product germacrene A (**15**) had converted to β-elemene (**16**) by Cope rearrangement [11,30]. Generally, the Cope rearrangement describes the heat-induced cyclization of 1,5-dienes [31].

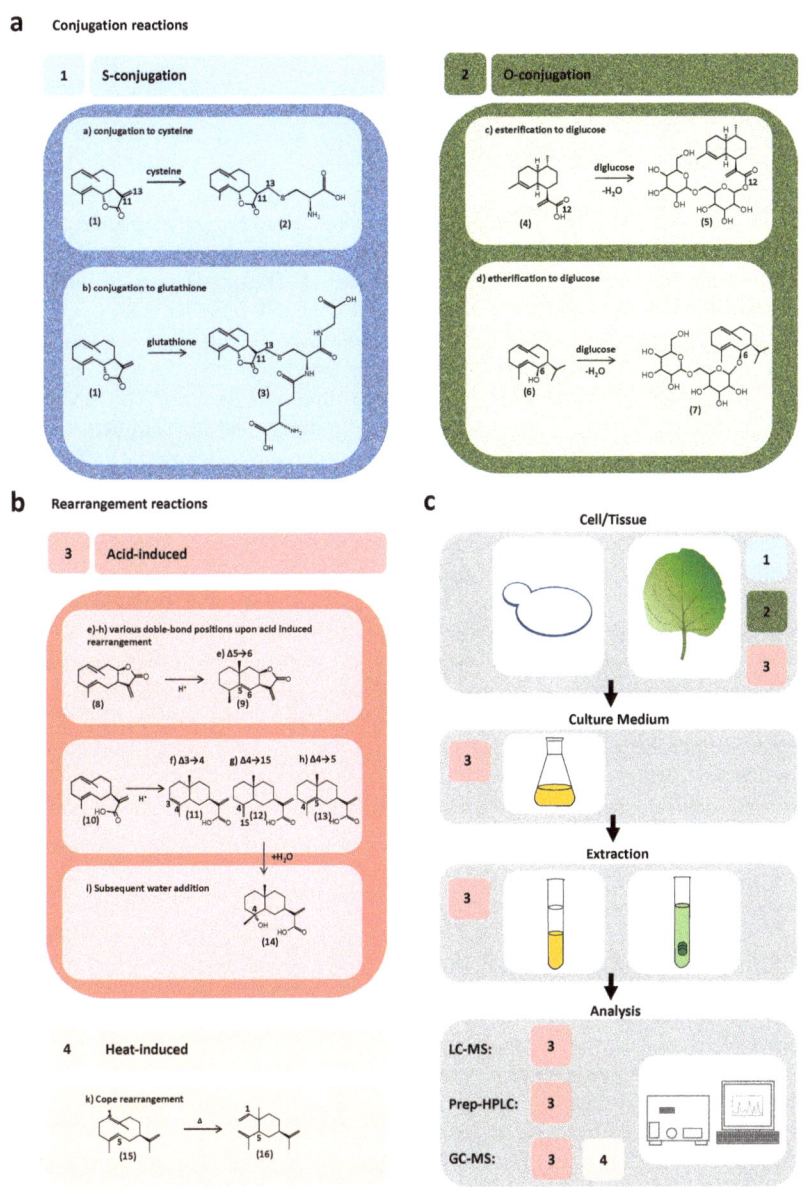

Figure 1. Unspecific rearrangement and conjugation reactions of sesquiterpenoids in heterologous expression systems. (**a**) Conjugation reactions; (**b**) Rearrangement reactions; (**c**) Unspecific reactions in the workflow of enzyme characterization.

3. Where Do the Reactions Happen?

S-conjugation and O-conjugation have so far only been observed in heterologous expression in plant cell systems, where enzyme products accumulate intracellularly (Figure 1c). Acid-induced rearrangement reactions have been observed in plant cell systems [13], during yeast cultivation in unbuffered yeast media and during extraction of yeast cultures [9,10] as well as during liquid and gas chromatography [10,32]. Heat-induced rearrangement has been observed in GC-MS applications [10,11,13,33].

4. What Are the Underlying Mechanisms and Avoiding Strategies?

4.1. S-Conjugation

S-conjugation to the thiol group of cysteine and O-conjugation to the hemiacetal group of glucose are mainly interpreted as a detoxifying mechanism of the host plant cell [7]. Formation of conjugates and transport to the vacuole may allow the plant cells of *Nicotiana benthamiana* to tolerate otherwise toxic cellular concentrations of bioactive metabolites, such as the STL. These conjugates are not observed in yeast expression systems where the enzyme products leave the cells by so far unknown mechanisms and accumulate in the culture medium [20]. The involvement of a glutathione-S-transferase (GST) or a non-enzymatic Michael-type addition have been suggested as an underlying mechanism [7] for cysteine (cys) or glutathione (GSH) conjugates (Table 1). Interestingly, only STL with an exocyclic α-methylene-γ-lactone group have so far been shown to form cys and GSH adducts to the lactone. Examples for this are costunolide (**1**), inunolide (**8**) and its derivatives (exocyclic methylene group: double bond position Δ11→13). On the other hand, the *inplanta* production of epi-dihydrocostunolide (**6**), an STL without an exocyclic methylene group, did not result in cysteine or GSH adducts, which would support a nonenzymatic Michael-type addition [29]. This nucleophilic addition reaction of an α-methylene-γ-lactone with the thiol group of biomolecules such as cysteine has been known for a long time [34] as one of the main reasons for STL bioactivity. It constitutes a special type of Michael addition [35] with an unsaturated lactone in which the nucleophile is a thiol group instead of an enolate [36]. Some STL, such as helenalin can also undergo Michael-type addition via their cyclopentenone moiety with an α,β-unsaturated carbonyl group [37,38]. Consequently, when expression of a metabolic pathway in *Nicotiana* leading to a STL with cyclopentenone moiety is performed, an additional cys or GSH adduct could be expected. GST-tagged STL may be transported into the vacuole by specific transporters and accumulate in the vacuole [7]. The cysteine conjugates are interpreted as breakdown products of the glutathione adducts or result from free cysteine inside the cells that reacts with the STL [7].

4.2. O-Conjugation

Sesquiterpenoids can form di-glucose adducts via esterification of an acid group or, in some cases, etherification of a hydroxy group to the hemiacetal group of glucose. While the formation of S-conjugates could be nonenzymatic due to the spontaneous Michael-type reaction at room temperature the introduction of two glucose units is most likely due to endogenous glycosyl transferases, which lead to the transport of the diglucose-"tagged" sesquiterpene to the vacuole [28]. Interestingly, no glycosylation of artemisinic acid (**4**) was observed when Fuentes et al. (2016) expressed the metabolic pathway to artemisinic acid in the chloroplasts of *Nicotiana tabacum* [16]. This lack of an endogenous glycosyl transferase in this specific subcellular compartment may be the reason why no diglucose-conjugates were formed. Expression of the metabolic pathway to artemisinic acid in *Physcomitrella patens* resulted in the accumulation of nongylcosylated artemisinic acid in the apoplast [18]. Therefore, if glycosylation to an acid-group appears, a promising strategy would be to target a different subcellular localization or to change the expression system.

Table 1. Classification and avoidance of unspecific reactions.

Group	Type	Combinations	Modification	Mass	Functional Group	Reaction Type	Cause	Avoiding Strategies	References
1. S-conjugation	a	f-i	STL-GSH	+307	α-methylene-γ-lactone	Michael-type addition, or GST reaction	Plant cell detoxification	Targeting different subcellular localizations	[7,8,13]
	b	f-i	STL-Cys	+121				Targeting different subcellular localizations	[7,8,13]
2. O-conjugation	c		STLOH-OGlc$_2$	+324	acid-group hydroxy-group	Esterification or etherification	Plant cell detoxification, presumably enzymatic	Targeting different subcellular localizations	[18,28]
	d		STL-OGlc$_2$						[29]
3. Acid	e	a-b	STL**, Δ3→4	±0	1,5-diene (Germacrene)	Acid-induced rearrangement	pH in culture media, cells, chromatography	Buffering of yeast media, pH control of chromatography system, choice of SPME fibers	[9,10,13]
	f	a-b	STL**, Δ4→15						[9,10,13]
	g	a-b	STL**, Δ4→5						[9,10,13]
	h	a-b	STL**, Δ5→6						[13]
	i		STL**-OH	+18					[9,10]
4. Heat	k		STL*	±0	1,5-diene (Germacrene)	Cope rearrangement (heat-induced)	GC-MS Analysis	Reduction of heat in GC-MS inlet	[11,32,33]

4.3. Acid-Induced Rearrangement

Acidic conditions can arise from unbuffered yeast media, as yeast cells rapidly decrease the neutral pH of the culture medium to a pH of ca. 3 [10,20]. Also, acid-induced rearrangement can occur in solid-phase microextraction gas chromatography (SPME-GC) analysis which was shown for the analysis of germacrene D [32] or when acidified solvents are used in high performance liquid chromatography (HPLC) analysis [10]. Recently, it was shown that acid-induced rearrangement may also play a role in plant expression systems and may form rearrangement product combinations with Michael-type adducts [13]. To overcome acid-induced rearrangement in yeast culture, yeast cultures can be buffered [7,39]. The use of MOPS buffer has proven to be better compatible with yeast growth than HEPES buffer [7,39]. If an acidified HPLC system is necessary, run times can be reduced and when preparative HPLC runs are performed, fractions can be collected in neutral buffer [10,39]. The right choice of SPME fibers reduces the acid-induced conversion of enzyme products in SPME-GC-MS analysis [32].

Acidic conditions can induce several other rearrangement reactions. The comparison of kunzeaol production in buffered and unbuffered yeast cultures showed a wide range of murolene and cadinene rearrangement products [40]. Andersen et al. (2015) showed up to 12 acid-induced rearrangement products of germacrene D depending on SPME-GC inlet temperature and fiber material [32].

4.4. Heat-Induced Rearrangement

Enzyme products of sesquiterpene synthases are usually analyzed by GC-MS. A high temperature in the GC inlet causes for instance the backbone of germacrene to rearrange to elemene. Reducing the inlet temperature of the gas chromatography system can overcome the problem with artificial heat-induced rearrangement products [32].

5. How Can Unspecific Enzyme Products Be Identified?

5.1. S-Conjugation

Generally, it is advisable to use nontargeted metabolomics approaches that can lead to the detection of enzyme products and their rearrangement products that were previously not anticipated [7,28]. However, there are several hints that can make the analysis of HPLC, LC-MS or GC-MS runs of putative sesquiterpenoid enzyme products easier. The S-conjugation to cysteine (a) increases the molecular weight from [M(STL)] to [M(STL) + 121], and the conjugation to glutathione increases it from [M(STL)] to [M(STL) + 307] [7,13,14]. This mass shift is a good indication in LC-MS analysis. Cysteine adducts and glutathione adducts elute earlier than the unconjugated STL in reverse-phase HPLC systems. Usually the cysteine and glutathione conjugates of the same STL appear as a peak tandem, with the cysteine adduct being more dominant and eluting slightly earlier [7,13,14]. A good indication for these adducts is also the isotope pattern of the mass peak that indicates the presence of the single sulfur atom from the thiol group of cysteine being introduced into the molecule [13,14]. If the STL is available as a reference compound, synthetic conjugates can easily be produced as reference compounds via Michael-type addition by incubation with cysteine- and glutathione at room temperature [7].

5.2. O-Conjugation

O-conjugation to a sesquiterpene will result in earlier elution from the reversed-phase column and a mass shift from [M(ST)] to [M(ST) + 324] (the mass of two glucose units minus the mass of two water units) [28].

5.3. Acid-Induced Rearrangement

Acid-induced rearrangement reactions can result in many products that are very similar to the enzyme product itself. In the case of a yeast expression system, culture and extraction conditions can be altered to differentiate between specific and unspecific enzyme products. For instance, Nguyen et al. (2010) could show an increase of the specific enzyme product germacrene A acid (**10**) and a decrease of the rearrangement products costic acids and ilicic acid (**11–14**) by comparing extracts from buffered versus unbuffered yeast cultures on a GC-MS and a LC-MS system [10]. Co-elution of acid-induced isomers on GC-MS can be overcome by the use of chiral columns which allow the separation of α-costic acid (**11**) and β-costic acid (**12**) [10].

The acid-induced transannular cyclization of germacranolide ST has been shown to lead to multiple rearrangement products that differ only in the position of one double bond [9,10,13]. These isomers are very difficult to separate from each other as they often co-elute or have very similar retention times on reversed-phase HPLC systems [9,10,13]. Furthermore, they have the same exact mass and strikingly similar MS-MS fragmentation patterns [9,10,13]. The recently reported rearrangement products from the expression of the pathway to germacrene A acid (**10**) in *Nicotiana benthamiana* indicate that acid-induced rearrangement may also appear in the subcellular environment of plant cells used for heterologous expression [13]. The combination of acid-induced rearrangement products with Michael-type reaction can lead to a very complex matrix of rearrangement products, that may be nearly impossible to separate [13]. To disentangle this matrix of products the production of the cysteine and glutathione adducts of reference compounds that match the presumed acid-induced rearrangement products was reported as a solution [13].

If the acid-induced rearrangement is followed by the introduction of a water molecule the resulting rearrangement is easier to spot as the additional hydroxy-group results in an earlier elution from the reversed-phase chromatography system and the molecular weight increases from [M(ST)] to [M(ST) + 18]. This was observed for the rearrangement from germacrene A acid (**10**) to ilicic acid (**14**) and from 8β-hydroxygermacrene A acid to 8β-hydroxyilicic acid [9,10]. Interestingly, costunolide (**1**) and its derivatives, germacranolides with similar structure, appear more stable in acidic conditions and do not show acid-induced rearrangements [9,14].

5.4. Heat-Induced Rearrangement

Similar to acid-induced rearrangements, heat-induced rearrangement does not change the total mass and only slightly changes the MS-MS pattern for the conversion from germacrene A (**15**) to β-elemene (**16**). However, germacrene A (**15**) elutes later (at higher temperatures) from the GC-MS column than its heat-induced rearrangement product β-elemene (**16**) [11].

6. How are Unspecific Reactions Prevented in the Natural Situation?

All the above-mentioned unspecific reactions could theoretically occur in the natural plant except for the heat-induced Cope rearrangement. Why are these reactions rarely observed in nature, where plants can accumulate highly reactive enzyme products in high concentrations in a way that provides protection without poisoning the host plant cell? In the case of STL, several biosynthetic enzymes that have so far been characterized are naturally located in secretory cells of glandular trichomes [8,11,13] or secretory ducts [29]. The upregulation of STL enzyme expression has been shown to be tightly linked to trichome development [8,11,13], which would allow an efficient production of STL before they are transported out of the cell.

7. Outlook

For researchers engaging in the reconstruction of metabolic pathways, it is crucial to have a perception about the unspecific reactions the presumed enzyme product may undergo. Here, a systematic approach to categorize and explain the most frequent unspecific reactions for sesquiterpenes is presented. Expanding this approach to other classes of natural compounds such as mono-, di- and triterpenes as well as polyphenols and alkaloids could create a store of knowledge to better plan and interpret the reconstruction of the metabolic pathways of plant specialized metabolites.

Funding: This research received no external funding.

Acknowledgments: The critical comments of Otmar Spring and Guillermo F. Padilla-Gonzalez are highly appreciated.

Conflicts of Interest: The authors declare no conflict of interest.

References

1. Cankar, K.; van Houwelingen, A.; Bosch, D.; Sonke, T.; Bouwmeester, H.; Beekwilder, J. A chicory cytochrome P450 mono-oxygenase CYP71AV8 for the oxidation of (+)-valencene. *FEBS Lett.* **2011**, *585*, 178–182. [CrossRef]
2. Peralta-Yahya, P.P.; Ouellet, M.; Chan, R.; Mukhopadhyay, A.; Keasling, J.D.; Lee, T.S. Identification and microbial production of a terpene-based advanced biofuel. *Nat. Commun.* **2011**, *2*, 483. [CrossRef] [PubMed]
3. Chang, M.C.Y.; Keasling, J.D. Production of isoprenoid pharmaceuticals by engineered microbes. *Nat. Chem. Biol.* **2006**, *2*, 674–681. [CrossRef] [PubMed]
4. Ro, D.; Paradise, E.M.; Ouellet, M.; Fisher, K.J.; Newman, K.L.; Ndungu, J.M.; Ho, K.A.; Eachus, R.A.; Ham, T.S.; Kirby, J.; et al. Production of the antimalarial drug precursor artemisinic acid in engineered yeast. *Nature* **2006**, *440*, 3–6. [CrossRef] [PubMed]
5. Chang, M.C.Y.; Eachus, R.A.; Trieu, W.; Ro, D.-K.; Keasling, J.D. Engineering Escherichia coli for production of functionalized terpenoids using plant P450s. *Nat. Chem. Biol.* **2007**, *3*, 274–277. [CrossRef]
6. Yu, F.; Okamoto, S.; Harada, H.; Yamasaki, K.; Misawa, N.; Utsumi, R. Zingiber zerumbet CYP71BA1 catalyzes the conversion of α-humulene to 8-hydroxy-α-humulene in zerumbone biosynthesis. *Cell. Mol. Life Sci.* **2011**, *68*, 1033–1040. [CrossRef]
7. Liu, Q.; Majdi, M.; Cankar, K.; Goedbloed, M.; Charnikhova, T.; Verstappen, F.W.A.; de Vos, R.C.H.; Beekwilder, J.; van der Krol, S.; Bouwmeester, H.J. Reconstitution of the costunolide biosynthetic pathway in yeast and Nicotiana benthamiana. *PLoS ONE* **2011**, *6*. [CrossRef]
8. Liu, Q.; Manzano, D.; Tanić, N.; Pesic, M.; Bankovic, J.; Pateraki, I.; Ricard, L.; Ferrer, A.; de Vos, R.; van de Krol, S.; et al. Elucidation and in planta reconstitution of the parthenolide biosynthetic pathway. *Metab. Eng.* **2014**, *23*, 145–153. [CrossRef]
9. Ikezawa, N.; Göpfert, J.C.; Nguyen, D.T.; Kim, S.U.; O'Maille, P.E.; Spring, O.; Ro, D.K. Lettuce costunolide synthase (CYP71BL2) and its homolog (CYP71BL1) from sunflower catalyze distinct regio- and stereoselective hydroxylations in sesquiterpene lactone metabolism. *J. Biol. Chem.* **2011**, *286*, 21601–21611. [CrossRef] [PubMed]
10. Nguyen, D.T.; Göpfert, J.C.; Ikezawa, N.; MacNevin, G.; Kathiresan, M.; Conrad, J.; Spring, O.; Ro, D.K. Biochemical conservation and evolution of germacrene A oxidase in Asteraceae. *J. Biol. Chem.* **2010**, *285*, 16588–16598. [CrossRef]
11. Göpfert, J.C.; Macnevin, G.; Ro, D.-K.; Spring, O. Identification, functional characterization and developmental regulation of sesquiterpene synthases from sunflower capitate glandular trichomes. *BMC Plant Biol.* **2009**, *9*, 86. [CrossRef] [PubMed]
12. Liu, Q.; Beyraghdar Kashkooli, A.; Manzano, D.; Pateraki, I.; Richard, L.; Kolkman, P.; Lucas, M.F.; Guallar, V.; de Vos, R.C.H.; Franssen, M.C.R.; et al. Kauniolide synthase is a P450 with unusual hydroxylation and cyclization-elimination activity. *Nat. Commun.* **2018**, *9*, 4657. [CrossRef] [PubMed]
13. Frey, M.; Schmauder, K.; Pateraki, I.; Spring, O. Biosynthesis of Eupatolide-A Metabolic Route for Sesquiterpene Lactone Formation Involving the P450 Enzyme CYP71DD6. *ACS Chem. Biol.* **2018**, *13*, 1536–1543. [CrossRef] [PubMed]
14. Frey, M.; Klaiber, I.; Conrad, J.; Bersch, A.; Pateraki, I.; Ro, D.-K.; Spring, O. Characterization of CYP71AX36 from Sunflower (Helianthus annuus L., Asteraceae). *Sci. Rep.* **2019**, *9*, 1–8. [CrossRef] [PubMed]
15. Eljounaidi, K.; Cankar, K.; Comino, C.; Moglia, A.; Hehn, A.; Bourgaud, F.; Bouwmeester, H.; Menin, B.; Lanteri, S.; Beekwilder, J. Cytochrome P450s from Cynara cardunculus L. CYP71AV9 and CYP71BL5, catalyze distinct hydroxylations in the sesquiterpene lactone biosynthetic pathway. *Plant Sci.* **2014**, *223*, 59–68. [CrossRef] [PubMed]
16. Fuentes, P.; Zhou, F.; Erban, A.; Karcher, D.; Kopka, J.; Bock, R. A new synthetic biology approach allows transfer of an entire metabolic pathway from a medicinal plant to a biomass crop. *Elife* **2016**, *5*, e13664. [CrossRef]

17. King, B.C.; Vavitsas, K.; Ikram, N.K.B.K.; Schrøder, J.; Scharff, L.B.; Hamberger, B.; Jensen, P.E.; Simonsen, H.T. In vivo assembly of DNA-fragments in the moss, Physcomitrella patens. *Sci. Rep.* **2016**, *6*, 25030. [CrossRef]
18. Khairul Ikram, N.K.B.; Beyraghdar Kashkooli, A.; Peramuna, A.V.; van der Krol, A.R.; Bouwmeester, H.; Simonsen, H.T. Stable Production of the Antimalarial Drug Artemisinin in the Moss Physcomitrella patens. *Front. Bioeng. Biotechnol.* **2017**, *5*, 47. [CrossRef]
19. Chen, F.; Tholl, D.; Bohlmann, J.; Pichersky, E. The family of terpene synthases in plants: A mid-size family of genes for specialized metabolism that is highly diversified throughout the kingdom. *Plant J.* **2011**, *66*, 212–229. [CrossRef]
20. Nguyen, T.D.; MacNevin, G.; Ro, D.K. De novo synthesis of high-value plant sesquiterpenoids in yeast. In *Methods in Enzymology*; Elsevier Inc.: San Diego, CA, USA, 2012; Volume 517, ISBN 9780124046344.
21. Pateraki, I.; Heskes, A.M.; Hamberger, B. Cytochromes p450 for terpene functionalisation and metabolic engineering. *Adv. Biochem. Eng. Biotechnol.* **2015**, *148*, 107–139. [CrossRef]
22. Adio, A. Germacrenes A–E and related compounds: Thermal, photochemical and acid induced transannular cyclizations. *Tetrahedron* **2009**, *65*, 1533–1552. [CrossRef]
23. Reijnders, P.J.M.; van Putten, R.G.; de Haan, J.W.; Koning, H.N.; Buck, H.M. Conformational dependence in the photochemistry of (E,E)-germacra-1(10),4,7(11)-triene. *Recl. des Trav. Chim. des Pays-Bas* **1980**, *99*, 67–69. [CrossRef]
24. Peijnenburg, W.J.G.M.; Dormans, G.J.M.; Buck, H.M. Quantumchemical calculations on the photochemistry of germacrene and germacrol. The exclusive role of the exocyclic double bond isomerization. *Tetrahedron* **1988**, *44*, 2339–2350. [CrossRef]
25. Sy, L.-K.; Brown, G.D. The mechanism of the spontaneous autoxidation of dihydroartemisinic acid. *Tetrahedron* **2002**, *58*, 897–908. [CrossRef]
26. Frey, M.; Klaiber, I.; Conrad, J.; Spring, O. CYP71BL9, the missing link in costunolide synthesis of sunflower. *Phytochemistry* **2020**. submitted.
27. Ramirez, A.M.; Saillard, N.; Yang, T.; Franssen, M.C.R.; Bouwmeester, H.J.; Jongsma, M.A. Biosynthesis of Sesquiterpene Lactones in Pyrethrum (Tanacetum cinerariifolium). *PLoS ONE* **2013**, *8*. [CrossRef]
28. van Herpen, T.W.J.M.; Cankar, K.; Nogueira, M.; Bosch, D.; Bouwmeester, H.J.; Beekwilder, J. Nicotiana benthamiana as a production platform for artemisinin precursors. *PLoS ONE* **2010**, *5*. [CrossRef]
29. Andersen, T.B.; Martinez-Swatson, K.A.; Rasmussen, S.A.; Boughton, B.A.; Jørgensen, K.; Andersen-Ranberg, J.; Nyberg, N.; Christensen, S.B.; Simonsen, H.T. Localization and in-Vivo Characterization of Thapsia garganica CYP76AE2 Indicates a Role in Thapsigargin Biosynthesis. *Plant Physiol.* **2017**, *174*, 56–72. [CrossRef]
30. De Kraker, J.-W.; Franssen, M.C.R.; De Groot, A.; Konig, W.A.; Bouwmeester, H.J. (+)-Germacrene A biosynthesis: The committed step in the biosynthesis of bitter sesquiterpene lactones in chicory. *Plant Physiol.* **1998**, *117*, 1381–1392. [CrossRef]
31. Cope, A.C.; Hardy, E.M. The Introduction of Substituted Vinyl Groups. V. A Rearrangement Involving the Migration of an Allyl Group in a Three-Carbon System[1]. *J. Am. Chem. Soc.* **1940**, *62*, 441–444. [CrossRef]
32. Andersen, T.; Cozzi, F.; Simonsen, H. Optimization of Biochemical Screening Methods for Volatile and Unstable Sesquiterpenoids Using HS-SPME-GC-MS. *Chromatography* **2015**, *2*, 277–292. [CrossRef]
33. De Kraker, J.-W.; Franssen, M.C.R.; Joerink, M.; De Groot, A.; Bouwmeester, H.J. Biosynthesis of costunolide, dihydrocostunolide, and leucodin. Demonstration of cytochrome P450-catalyzed formation of the lactone ring present in sesquiterpene lactones of chicory. *Plant Physiol.* **2002**, *129*, 257–268. [CrossRef] [PubMed]
34. Kupchan, S.M.; Fessler, D.C.; Eakin, M.A.; Giacobbe, T.J. Reactions of alpha methylene lactone tumor inhibitors with model biological nucelophiles. *Science* **1970**, *168*, 376–378. [CrossRef] [PubMed]
35. Michael, A. Ueber die Addition von Natriumacetessig- und Natriummalonsaureathern zu den Aethern ungesattigter Sauren. *J. für Prakt. Chemie* **1887**, *35*, 349–356. [CrossRef]
36. Cavallito, C.J.; Haskell, T.H. The Mechanism of Action of Antibiotics. The Reaction of Unsaturated Lactones with Cysteine and Related Compounds. *J. Am. Chem. Soc.* **1945**, *67*, 1991. [CrossRef]
37. Lyss, G.; Schmidt, T.J.; Merfort, I.; Pahl, H.L. Helenalin, an anti-inflammatory sesquiterpene lactone from Arnica, selectively inhibits transcription factor NF-κB. *Biol. Chem.* **1997**, *378*, 951–962. [CrossRef]
38. Schmidt, T.J. Helenanolide-type sesquiterpene lactones-III. Rates and stereochemistry in the reaction of helenalin and related helenanolides with sulfhydryl containing biomolecules. *Bioorganic Med. Chem.* **1997**, *5*, 645–653. [CrossRef]

39. Gou, J.; Hao, F.; Kwon, M.; Chen, F.; Li, C.; Liu, C.; Ro, D.-K.; Tang, H.; Zhang, Y. Discovery of a non-stereoselective cytochrome P450 catalyzing either 8α- or 8β-hydroxylation of germacrene A acid from the Chinese medicinal plant, Inula hupehensis. *Plant J.* **2018**, *93*, 92–106. [CrossRef]
40. Pickel, B.; Drew, D.P.; Manczak, T.; Weitzel, C.; Simonsen, H.T.; Ro, D.-K. Identification and characterization of a kunzeaol synthase from Thapsia garganica: Implications for the biosynthesis of the pharmaceutical thapsigargin. *Biochem. J.* **2012**, *448*, 261–271. [CrossRef]

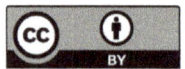 © 2020 by the author. Licensee MDPI, Basel, Switzerland. This article is an open access article distributed under the terms and conditions of the Creative Commons Attribution (CC BY) license (http://creativecommons.org/licenses/by/4.0/).

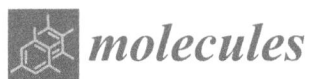

Review

Recent Achievements in Medicinal and Supramolecular Chemistry of Betulinic Acid and Its Derivatives [‡]

Uladzimir Bildziukevich [1,2,†], **Zülal Özdemir** [1,2,†] **and Zdeněk Wimmer** [1,2,*]

1. Institute of Experimental Botany of the Czech Academy of Sciences, Isotope Laboratory, Vídeňská 1083, 14220 Prague 4, Czech Republic; vmagius@gmail.com (U.B.); zulalozdemr@gmail.com (Z.Ö.)
2. Department of Chemistry of Natural Compounds, University of Chemistry and Technology in Prague, Technická 5, 16628 Prague 6, Czech Republic
* Correspondence: wimmer@biomed.cas.cz or wimmerz@vscht.cz; Tel.: +42-0241-0624-57
† These authors contributed equally.
‡ Dedicated to the memory of Professor Kenji Mori, the worldwide known natural product scientist.

Academic Editors: Pavel B. Drasar and Vladimir A. Khripach
Received: 12 September 2019; Accepted: 29 September 2019; Published: 30 September 2019

Abstract: The subject of this review article refers to the recent achievements in the investigation of pharmacological activity and supramolecular characteristics of betulinic acid and its diverse derivatives, with special focus on their cytotoxic effect, antitumor activity, and antiviral effect, and mostly covers a period 2015–2018. Literature sources published earlier are referred to in required coherences or from historical points of view. Relationships between pharmacological activity and supramolecular characteristics are included if such investigation has been done in the original literature sources. A wide practical applicability of betulinic acid and its derivatives demonstrated in the literature sources is also included in this review article. Several literature sources also focused on in silico calculation of physicochemical and ADME parameters of the developed compounds, and on a comparison between the experimental and calculated data.

Keywords: betulinic acid; structural modification; supramolecular self-assembly; cytotoxicity; antitumor activity; antiviral activity; physicochemical parameters; ADME parameters

1. Introduction

Plants represent an important challenge in searching for new plant products, of which a majority of new structures displays drug-like properties in treating serious diseases. Medicinal plants represent a diverse and rich source of bioactive plant products [1]. In this review article, attention has been focused on betulinic acid and its derivatives. Betulinic acid is a very potent plant triterpenoid compound with a broad spectrum of its own activity and a broad spectrum of pharmacologically important derivatives. The most important disadvantage of betulinic acid is its very low solubility in aqueous media, which also indicates its low bioavailability. Regardless of this disadvantage, betulinic acid displays a spectrum of biological activity that includes cytotoxicity, antitumor activity, antiviral activity, anti-diabetic activity, anti-inflammatory activity, etc. [1,2]. More details on the mode of action of **1** can be found in the original literature cited here, and it is mentioned in each paragraph dealing with different types of activity. In the natural sources, betulinic acid—like all other triterpene acids—appears in forms of more polar conjugates formed mostly with mono- and oligosaccharides or sugar esters [3]. Targeted derivation of betulinic acid may result in designing compounds displaying more favored physicochemical and ADME parameters, enhancing the potential of practical applicability of the compounds in medicinal and supramolecular chemistry.

2. Plant Sources and Discovery of Betulinic Acid

Betulinic acid, (3β)-3-hydroxy-lup-20(29)-en-28-oic acid (**1**, Figure 1), was discovered in natural plant sources long ago. It was first isolated from *Gratiola officinalis* at the beginning of the 20th century under the trivial name graciolon [4]. At the very beginning, this plant product had been subsequently isolated from different plant sources, and, therefore, described by different trivial names (e.g., platanolic acid, cornolic acid, melaleucin, etc.), however, finally identified as betulinic acid (**1**, Figure 1) [5]. It is a naturally occurring pentacyclic lupane-type triterpene, found throughout the plant kingdom (e.g., in genera *Betulla*, *Ziziphus*, *Syzygium*, *Diospiros* or *Paeonia*) [6]. However, it has also been isolated from the bark of the plane tree (*Platanus acerifolia*) [5] or from the Western Australian Christmas tree (*Nuytsia floribunda*), where it is accompanied by a small amount of betulin (**2**, Figure 1), and from the barks of six *Melaleuca* species, *M. rhaphiophylla*, *M. cuticularis*, *M. viminea*, *M. leucadendron*, *M. parvijora*, and *M. pubescens*. The first five of the *Melaleuca* species belong to the group popularly known as "paper-barks", and crystalline triterpenoid acid can be seen in places between the thin papery layers of the bark. Betulinic acid (**1**) has also been obtained from the inland form of dysentery bush (*Alyxia buxifolia*). Generally, **1** was found in different plants, both as a free aglycon and in forms of glycosylated derivatives that enhance its bioavailability [2,3]. Isolation of **1** from plant sources is not easy, because it is accompanied by a number of other terpene-based plant products. Betulin (**2**) is one of the most commonly occurring triterpene plant product often present in higher quantity than betulinic acid (**1**) itself. However, it can be converted into an aldehyde (**3**, Figure 1), followed by additional oxidation into **1** [7,8]. Purification of the target compounds can be achieved by a combination of different chromatographic methods, combined with crystallization, resulting in the white powdery compounds [5]. A new challenge may be seen in extracting the convenient plant material by supercritical carbon dioxide (SC-CO$_2$) [9], both, without or with polarity modifier, or by pressurized liquid extraction (PLE) [10].

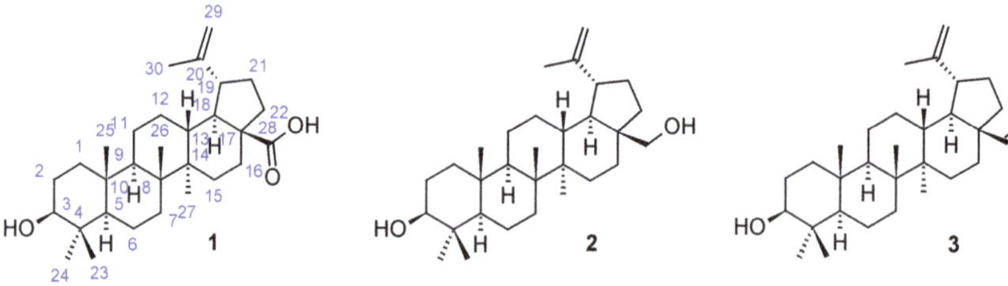

Figure 1. The structures of betulinic acid (**1**) with carbon atom numbering), betulin (**2**), and its aldehyde (**3**).

3. Pharmacological Effects of Betulinic Acid

3.1. Cytotoxicity and Antitumor Activity

Since 1970s papers appeared on the investigation of pharmacological effects of **1**. Cytotoxicity is one of the most important fields in this investigation, and it is one of the most widely investigated aspects of pharmacology of betulinic acid (**1**) [3]. At the very beginning, cytotoxicity of different plant extracts was observed, where **1** was later found in different mixtures of plant products [11,12]. Cytotoxicity of **1**, leading to apoptosis of tumor cells, was observed during the later studies [13–16]. Regardless of extensive investigation, the molecular target of **1** has not yet been identified. Speculations about the possible target(s) were based on pathway alterations like modulation of B-cell lymphoma (Bcl-2) and nuclear factor NF-κB, enhancer of activated B-cells, and antiangiogenic activity [17,18]. There is enough information about the activity of **1** and its potent derivatives, both in in vitro and in vivo models. However, it seems that in reality small changes in the chemical structure could lead to significant differences in specificity and mechanisms of action [19–21]. Nevertheless, the most recent studies indicate that the main mechanisms involved are the stimulation of apoptosis and the inhibition of kinases, both accompanied by a worthy antioxidant effect [1]. Betulinic acid (**1**) has been capable of reducing many of the toxicity indicators of the antitumor agent doxorubicin, which has been known to have strong cardiotoxic activity. These parameters, measured in human blood lymphocytes, include generation of reactive oxygen species, production of inflammatory cytokines, such as interleukin IL-12 (produced by B-lymphoblastoid cells) or tumor necrosis factor TNF-α (biosynthesized as prohormone with long and atypical signal sequence), alteration of mitochondrial membrane potential, and various morphological and histochemical changes to the apoptotic process [1].

However, it is important to stress that **1** used in these experiments consisted of a number of supramolecular aggregates formed by a process of self-assembly, which is typical for this type of triterpenoid substance in aqueous or hydroalcoholic media. These self-assembled particles were found to exert pro-apoptotic and genotoxic activity in K562 myelogenous leukemia cells, with higher efficacy than betulinic acid (**1**) itself [22].

3.2. Antiviral Activity

The absolute majority of original papers and recent reviews dealing with antiviral activity of **1** have been dealing with its anti-HIV activity [23,24]. This type of activity is a part of general antiviral activity, however, only a few reports appeared on the investigation of the general antiviral activity of **1** [5].

Human immunodeficiency virus (HIV)-caused HIV infection and acquired immunodeficiency syndrome (AIDS) were first identified over 30 years ago [25]. Global AIDS statistics estimate that 37 million people are living with HIV at present. Among them, 2 million people were newly infected with HIV, and more than 1 million died from AIDS-related illnesses [26]. Although over 30 drugs targeted at different steps of the viral life have been approved or are in experimental stages for treatment of HIV, remedy for HIV infection has not yet been found [27]. HIV therapy suffers from the rapid emergence of drug-resistant viral strains and harmful side effects caused by long-term drug treatment [27]. Therefore, a search for new and innovative anti-HIV agents has been an important research priority. Betulinic acid (**1**) represents a promising structure type for anti-HIV agents [26,28].

It acts against HIV by preventing the cleavage of the capsid-spacer peptide of the Gag protein, thereby impeding viral maturation. This causes the host cell releases virions with no infective capacity. The efficacy of **1** is influenced by various polymorphisms of this protein, especially in the residues 369–371 (QVT in wild type), with one of the best known as V370A [3]. Various structural derivatives of **1** were found to be more potent anti-HIV agents than betulinic acid (**1**) itself, however, those compounds will be discussed further in this review.

The effect of **1** against herpes viruses, especially against clinical strain HSV-1, is an example of other antiviral activity of **1** [29], the authors investigated and evaluated the in vitro experiments. They showed that after incubating the active principle with the virus, both sensitive and acyclovir-resistant strains lost their infectivity. In turn, neither pretreatment of the cell nor administrations at the time of viral propagation were effective [3,29].

Hepatitis B, which has an important health impact, represents another virus susceptible to betulinic acid (**1**). The inhibition of hepatitis B replication exerted by the triterpene is based on the downregulation of mitochondrial superoxide dismutase (SOD2) through the dephosphorylation (Ser133) of the cAMP response element-binding transcription factor at its binding site with the SOD2 promoter. Betulinic acid (**1**) has been shown to facilitate the translocation of the hepatitis B virus X protein into the mitochondria of mouse hepatocytes. The antiviral activity was strictly dependent on SOD2 because overexpression of this enzyme suppressed the effect [30].

3.3. Anti-Inflammatory Activity

The investigation of the anti-inflammatory activity of **1** was performed by focusing on the induction of inflammation by various activators of protein kinase C and other agents. Betulinic acid (**1**) inhibited the edema induced by toxic diterpene esters, mezerein, 12-deoxyphorbol-13-tetradecanoate, and 12-deoxyphorbol-13-phenylacetate, by 48, 51, and 61% (ID_{50} = 0.77 µmol/ear in this case), respectively, at a dose of 0.5 mg/ear [3]. Anti-inflammatory activity was also described in a macrolide lactone bryostatin-1-induced mouse ear edema (65% at 0.5 mg/ear), a peptide inflammatory mediator bradykinin-induced mouse paw edema (54% at 10 mg/kg), and rat skin inflammation induced by glucose oxidase (39% at 0.25 mg/site) [31,32]. In turn, no effect was observed in ear edema induced by arachidonic acid, resiniferatoxin, and xylene. Since 1 was inactive against arachidonic acid-induced inflammation, as well as in neurogenic inflammatory models, it is probable that this type of inflammation may depend on in vivo inhibition of protein kinase C [3,31,32].

3.4. Anti-Diabetic Activity

Anti-diabetic activity of betulinic acid (1) was described against type 2 of diabetes mellitus [33]. Based on different studies, both in vitro and in vivo, the mechanism of action of betulinic acid (1) was designed, reflecting glucose uptake, insulin resistance, insulin sensitivity, and glycogen biosynthesis. Those aspects were reviewed recently [3], and no substantial novel items of information have been found in the more recent literature data.

3.5. Anti-Hyperlipidemic Activity

When tested on obese mice, 1 was administered in drinking water for 15 days (50 mg·L^{-1}). It caused decreasing of total triglycerides and cholesterol levels in high fat containing diet supplied to obese mice, which resulted in decreasing of mouse body weight, abdominal fat accumulation, blood glucose increase, and content of cholesterol and triglycerides in plasma [34]. Due to the action of 1, an increase of insulin in plasma was observed [34]. Betulinic acid (1) was also able to reduce lipogenesis and lipid accumulation, which was observed during numbers of experiments in vitro and in vivo [35], in which the mechanism of action of 1 in anti-hyperlipidemic activity was studied and described.

3.6. Other Activity

The anti-parasitic and anti-infectious activity of 1 and its derivatives were also mentioned in the literature in recent time [3]. However, when searching for the details, we have found that these types of pharmacological effects were described either for various derivatives of betulinic acid (1) or for simultaneous treatments with betulinic acid (1) along with different compounds, mostly synthetic medicaments, acting in synergy. It is, therefore, no clear evidence that 1 itself is able to induce these types of activity [3]. These potential effects of 1 should be focused on more details in the future.

4. Supramolecular Characteristics of Betulinic Acid

It was already stated that 1 is the triterpene-type compound bearing a rigid pentacyclic lupane-type (6-6-6-6-5) backbone. Its molecule is 1.31 nm long [36]. Self-assembly of the molecules of 1 in aqueous media and organic solvents results in fibrous supramolecular systems. Those systems are able to present themselves as supramolecular gels. This behavior of 1 was tested with a number of organic solvents using different concentrations of 1 [36]. Since 1 is practically insoluble in water, gelling properties could not be proven in it, however, using ethanol/water mixtures (4:1 to 19:1) supramolecular gels were produced at a concentration c = 2.55% (w/v) [36]. Optical microscopy micrographs proved a formation of fibrous supramolecular systems in 1,2-dichlorobenzene [36]. More recent SEM studies of supramolecular self-assembly of 1 in mesitylene or chlorobenzene proved a formation of fibrous-like xerogels. Fibrous networks were also investigated by the AFM micrographs of 1 in *p*-xylene [37]. Self-assembly of 1 in different solvents was probably the first published example of the self-assembly of a triterpene molecule bearing no other substitution. Self-assembly characteristics of 1 in different liquids encouraged use of this type of supramolecular systems in various practical applications, namely selective damage of cancer cells without affecting the normal cells. This investigation of supramolecular behavior of 1 has been an important challenge in treating this fatally important disease [37–39].

5. Derivatives of Betulinic Acid, Their Pharmacological Effects, and Supramolecular Characteristics

5.1. Cytotoxicity and Supramolecular Characteristics

The area of monitoring cytotoxicity of different derivatives of **1** is well documented by 2015 by several review papers [1,15,39,40], as well as by a patent review [41]. Due to that fact, attention in this review article has been focused on the most recent period of several last years to cover novel betulinic acid derivatives not yet mentioned in the so-far published review papers, which have been found in the most recent literature sources. Older literature sources are cited when coherence in the text or in history requires such references.

Thus, a synthesis of novel 2,3-seco-triterpenoids and triterpenoids bearing five-membered ring A, all displaying cytotoxicity, was published (Scheme 1) [42]. The compounds were prepared on the basis of betulone (**4**) that is modified to the 2-oxime derivative of betulonic acid (**5**) by a several steps procedure [42,43]. Further structural modification of **5** (Scheme 1) resulted in a subsequent synthesis of the compounds **6–9** [42], representing the most cytotoxic structures of this series of compounds [42]. Their antiproliferative activity was tested on various human cancer cell lines. The compound **9** of this series showed adequate selectivity and cytotoxicity towards several important cancer cell lines, and, therefore, it was selected as the most active compound (IC_{50} = 3.4–10.4 µM for HEp-2, HCT116, RD TE32, and MS cancer cells). It was capable of triggering caspase-8-mediated apoptosis in HCT116 cancer cells accompanied by typical apoptotic chromatin condensation with no loss of mitochondrial membrane permeability.

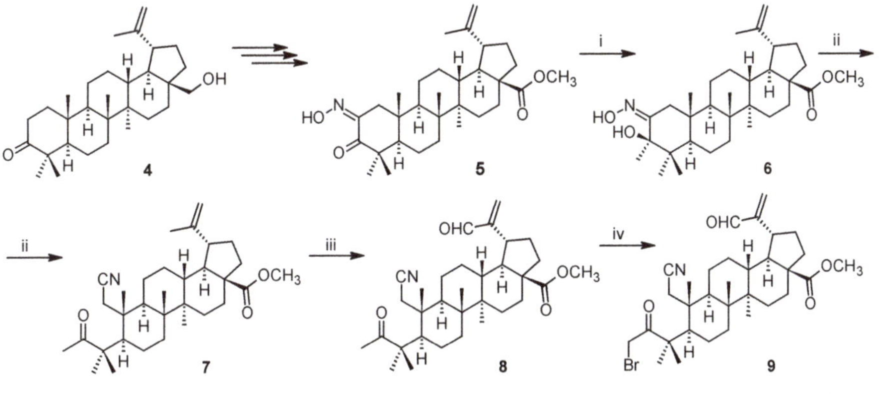

Scheme 1. Synthesis of cytotoxic derivatives based on alkylated 2,3-seco-triterpenoids. Legend: **i**: CH$_3$MgI, ether, **ii**: SOCl$_2$, DCM, **iii**: H$_2$SeO$_3$, 1,4-dioxane, **iv**: pyridinium bromide perbromide, AcOH.

To proceed with this investigation, a synthesis of a large series of novel hydrophilic esters of triterpenoid acids with cytotoxic activity was presented, and **1** was one of the natural products selected for the derivation [44]. Complex alcoholic groups (aliphatic or containing heterocycles), glycolic unit and monosaccharide groups were used as structural modifiers (Scheme 2). An easy synthetic procedure was described, in which the introduction of the above-identified substituents resulted in the preparation of the compounds with high cytotoxicity (**10a–10f**) [44]. Compound **10f** was the most selectively active compound of this series, effective against MCF7 (IC_{50} = 2.5 µM), HeLa (IC_{50} = 3.3 µM) and G-361 (IC_{50} = 3.4 µM) cancer cell lines.

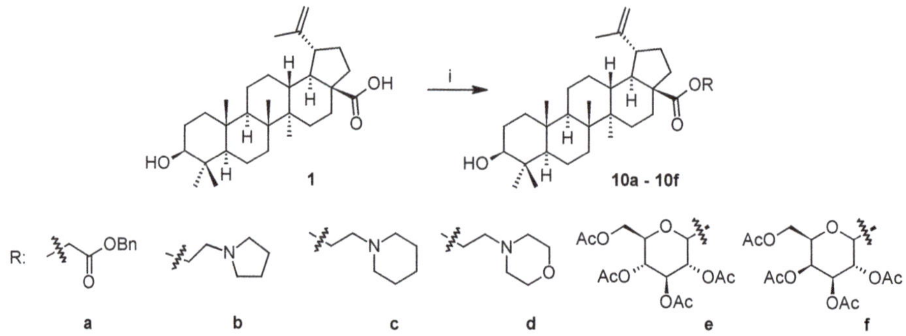

Scheme 2. Synthesis of hydrophilic esters of betulinic acid (**1**). Legend: **i**: for **a**: RBr, DBU, MeCN, DCM, 2 days, for **b–d**: Br(CH$_2$)$_2$Br, DBU, MeCN, DCM, 2 days, then piperidine (for **b**), pyrrolidine (for **c**), or morpholine (for **d**), CHCl$_3$, for **e** and **f**: 1-Br-glu(Ac)$_4$ or 1-Br-gal(Ac)$_4$, DBU, MeCN, DCM.

Diamine and polyamine derivatives of betulinic acid were also investigated for their cytotoxicity and antimicrobial activity (Scheme 3) [45]. Derivation of **1** at the C(28)-carbon center is a several steps procedure (Scheme 3), leading through the intermediates **11–14c** to the target amides **15a–15c**. Derivation of **1** at the C(3)-OH group required protection and final deprotection of the C(28)-carboxyl group. Subsequent synthesis of the intermediates **16–19c** resulted in the preparation of the target structures **20a–20c** (Scheme 3). Their cytotoxicity, antimicrobial activity, and ability to form supramolecular self-assembled systems, preferably in aqueous media, were investigated and published [45,46]. The highest cytotoxicity values of these derivatives of betulinic acid were observed with the amides formed with piperazine and spermine. When the cytotoxicity of those compounds was studied, the amides **15a–15c** were found to display micromolar or even submicromolar activity (Table 1). However, they were toxic also towards the normal fibroblasts at a comparable level, and they show no or low selectivity. In turn, amides **20a–20c** showed selectivity and no toxicity towards the normal fibroblasts. Several of those new compounds showed also antimicrobial activity [45]. The investigation of diamines and polyamines as structural modifiers was then extended to steroids with the androstene skeleton [47], and important structure-activity relations have been found, resulting in observed selectivity of several prepared compounds [45,47].

Diamine- and polyamine-based amides of betulinic acid (**1**), i.e., the compounds **15a–15c** and **20a–20c**, were subjected to the detailed studies of supramolecular self-assembly [46]. The compounds **15c** and **20c** were found to form fibrous supramolecular structures, the formation of which was proven by the UV-VIS and DOSY-NMR measurements, and, subsequently, by AFM, SEM and TEM micrographs. It seems reasonable to say that a relation exists between cytotoxicity and supramolecular characteristics because the supramolecular structures and materials have a huge potential in the area of drug delivery [37,48]. The supramolecular structures formed from triterpenoid acid derivatives can act as a pharmacologically active delivery system to the target tissues where they can directly display their pharmacological activity.

The supramolecular characteristics of those compounds were discovered when the variable temperature pulsed-field gradient diffusion ordered NMR spectroscopy (VT-DOSY-NMR) was measured, in which the dependence of diffusion coefficient on temperature showed a non-linear curve [46]. DOSY-NMR spectroscopy is generally useful in determining the species of varying size formed by the studied compounds. This non-invasive pseudo-two-dimensional (2D) NMR technique has the potential to identify and virtually separate different aggregates existing simultaneously in the samples [49]. Application of this method to the self-assembled nanostructures has been undertaken during various investigations. However, the utilization of this technique for the supramolecular gels derived from low molecular weight gelators (LMWGs) remained still less explored [49–51]. In general, when the gel is formed, the diffusion coefficient should change in a non-linear way (i.e., non-linear dependence of diffusion coefficient on temperature appeared) compared to the situation in a clear solution (linear dependence was found) because of the decreased molecular mobility and increased viscosity of the gelled system (Einstein-Stokes equation) [52]. Both investigated compounds (**15c** and **20c**) displayed a non-linear dependence of the diffusion coefficient on the temperature of the measurement indicating a formation of supramolecular networks.

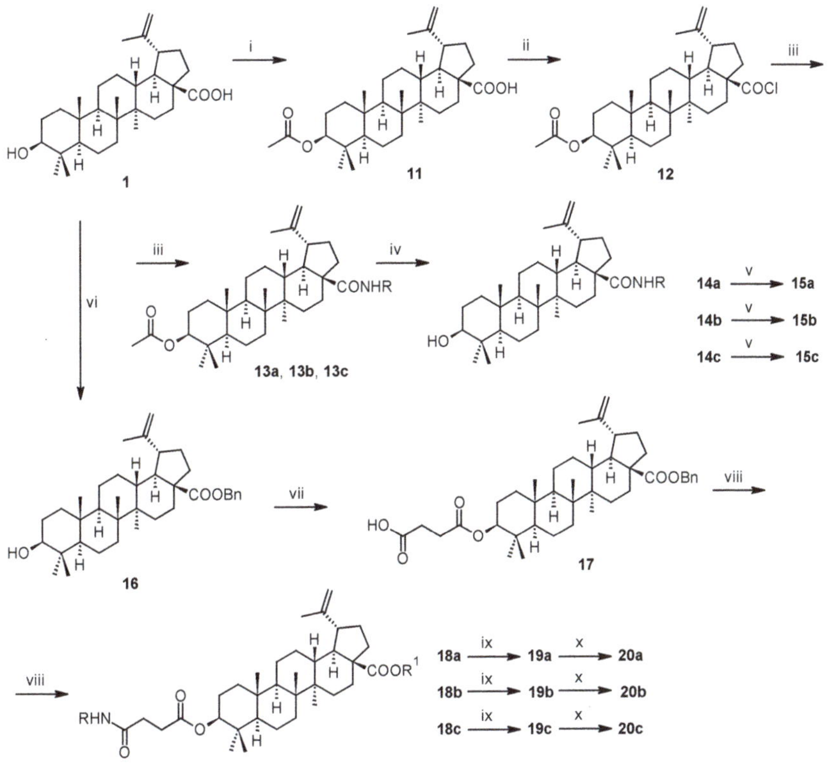

Scheme 3. Synthesis of di- and polyamine amides of betulinic acid (**1**). Legend: **i**: Ac$_2$O, EDIPA, DMAP, THF, **ii**: oxalyl chloride, DCM, **iii**: Boc-protected polyamines, EDIPA, DCM, **iv**: NaOH in water, THF/methanol (1:1), **v**: HCl (g) in diethyl ether, chloroform, **vi**: BnCl, K$_2$CO$_3$, acetone, **vii**: succinic anhydride, DMAP, pyridine, **viii**: Boc-protected polyamines, T3P, pyridine, **ix**: Pd/C, ethyl acetate/THF (1:1), 1,4-cyclohexadiene, **x**: HCl (g) in diethyl ether, CHCl$_3$.

Table 1. Experimental cytotoxicity data found for **15a–15c** and **20a–20c**.

Compound	Cytotoxicity (IC$_{50}$ [µM])			
	CEM [a]	MCF7 [b]	HeLa [c]	BJ [d]
15a	0.7 ± 0.0	2.4 ± 0.1	2.3 ± 0.0	2.6 ± 0.1
15b	0.8 ± 0.0	7.8 ± 1.1	5.7 ± 1.5	6.2 ± 2.7
15c	7.7 ± 1.6	3.3 ± 0.4	4.4 ± 1.5	3.9 ± 0.9
20a	26.8 ± 7.2	>50	>50	>50
20b	7.3 ± 0.3	35.5 ± 1.5	21.9 ± 7.0	>50
20c	5.2 ± 2.3	>50	23.8 ± 3.7	42.9 ± 3.8

[a] CEM, cells of human T-lymphoblastic leukemia, [b] MCF7, cells of human breast adenocarcinoma, [c] HeLa, cells of human cervical cancer, [d] BJ, normal human fibroblasts.

Subsequently, the compounds were subjected to a series of UV-VIS-NIR measurements, using a constant concentration of the studied compound in changing ratios of water/methanol mixtures in 10% steps, starting with pure water to pure methanol. Changes in the intensity of the peak maxima and, partly in wavelengths of those maxima also indicated a formation of supramolecular aggregates in the studied systems. The investigation was completed by visualizing the AFM, SEM, and TEM micrographs that proved a formation of fibrous supramolecular networks as well [46].

Picolyl amides of betulinic acid were investigated for their ability to cause tumor cell apoptosis (Scheme 4) [53]. The synthetic procedures described in the literature [53] in details, started at **1** and resulted in either of the target structures **22a–22c** or **24a–24c** (Scheme 4). While the picolyl amides of steryl hemiesters investigated in the past suffered from their low cytotoxicity [54], several of the picolyl amides of **1** showed high and even sub-micromolar effects [53]. The higher cytotoxicity was observed for the picolyl amine-based amides **22a–22c** in comparison with that of **24a–24c**. In the screening tests in G-361 human malignant melanoma cell line, **22b** showed therapeutic index TI = 100 (Table 2), which makes this derivative bearing the piperazine motif in the molecule to become one of the most important and most perspective compounds of this series [53].

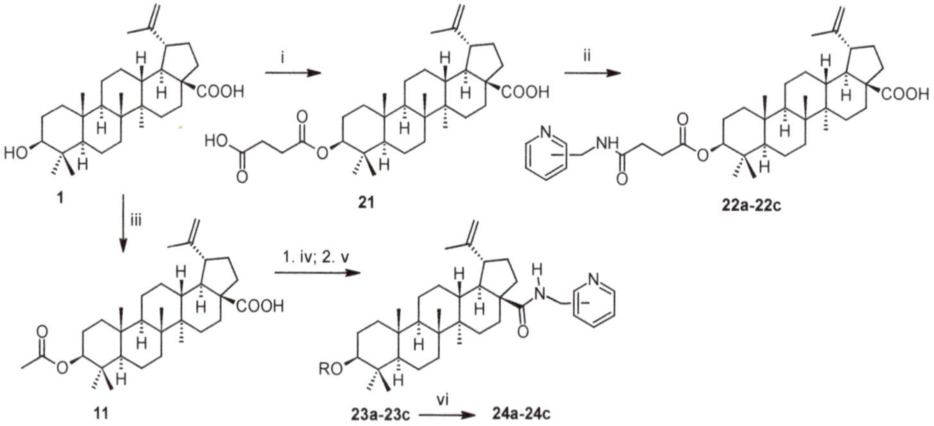

Scheme 4. Synthesis of picolyl amides of betulinic acid (**1**). Legend: **i**: succinic anhydride, DMAP, pyridine, **ii**: 2-, 3- or 4-aminomethylpyridine, T3P, dry pyridine, **iii**: Ac$_2$O, EDIPA, DMAP, THF, **iv**: oxalyl chloride, DCM, **v**: 2-, 3- or 4-aminomethylpyridine, EDIPA, DCM, **vi**: LiOH·H$_2$O, MeOH.

Table 2. Experimental cytotoxicity data found for **22a–22c** and **24a–24c** after 72 h.

Compound	Cytotoxicity (IC$_{50}$ [μM])					TI [a]
	CEM [b]	MCF7 [c]	HeLa [d]	G-361 [e]	BJ [f]	
22a	6.9 ± 0.4	2.2 ± 0.2	2.3 ± 0.5	2.4 ± 0.0	46.2 ± 2.8	19.3
22b	6.5 ± 1.5	1.4 ± 0.1	2.4 ± 0.4	0.5 ± 0.1	50.0 ± 0.0	100.0
22c	22.6 ± 5.9	>50	40.9 ± 4.7	32.1 ± 2.1	>50	ND [g]
24a	18.6 ± 1.0	27.0 ± 5.5	14.7 ± 0.2	16.4 ± 1.6	15.8 ± 1.4	1.0
24b	25.3 ± 6.9	38.7 ± 1.0	23.6 ± 2.3	18.1 ± 0.1	17.5 ± 2.7	1.0
24c	18.6 ± 3.7	21.1 ± 4.3	14.8 ± 0.2	11.6 ± 1.6	11.2 ± 1.4	1.0

[a] Therapeutic index (TI) calculated for G-361 line versus fibroblasts BJ, [b] CEM, cells of human T-lymphoblastic leukemia, [c] MCF7, cells of human breast adenocarcinoma, [d] HeLa, cells of human cervical cancer, [e] G-361, human malignant melanoma cell line [f] BJ, normal human fibroblasts, [g] ND = not determined.

Last two series of compounds derived from **1** [45,53] are the products of our team. We have also studied in silico calculations of physicochemical and ADME parameters of the target compounds **15a–15c**, **20a–20c**, **22a–22c**, and **24a–24c** (Table S1, Supplementary material). The basic details on the importance of these parameters are presented in the original papers [45,53], however, we would like to focus on the most important findings emerging from these calculated values. The recommended range for optimization of several physicochemical and ADME parameters appeared in the literature (cf. [45,53] and the literature cited therein). When comparing the recommended range for the selected parameters with their experimental data (Table S1, Supplementary material), the results can be summarized in this form: (a) molecular weight: only **15a** appears within the given range, (b) log P: all compounds appear out of the given range, (c) log S: **20b** and **24a–24c** are out of the given range, (d) the range for the number of H_{acc} and H_{don} is completed by all studied compounds, (e) all studied compounds meet the limits for log PB and log BB. The experimental results show that the range of molecular weight is less important, cytotoxicity was also found for compounds having MW > 500 (cf. Tables 1 and 2). None of the studied compounds appeared within the given range for the parameter log P, it was not the driving parameter affecting the experimental cytotoxicity values. The parameter of solubility (log S) played more important role because neither **20b** nor **24a–24c** displayed high values of cytotoxicity. Compound **22c** appeared to be surprising exception for its very low cytotoxicity. The ADME parameters did not influence these result, because all studied compounds showed their calculated values of log PB and log BB within the given range. However, these ADME parameters are connected with central nervous system (CNS) active drugs, and none of the studied compounds appeared among potentially CNS active drugs [45,53].

Chinese authors [55] designed an interesting conjugate **29** derived from **1** with diazen-1-ium-1,2-dioxolate (**28**) and found an anticancer agent releasing nitric oxide (NO) and causing cancer cell apoptosis (Scheme 5). Antiproliferative activity of **29** was tested on several cancer cell lines even with sub-micromolar concentrations. The effect of the compound **29** was compared with that of cisplatin, and it was found that the synthesized compound **29** was 20 to 2 times more active than cisplatin against different cancer cell lines, while 3 times less active on reference liver cell line [55].

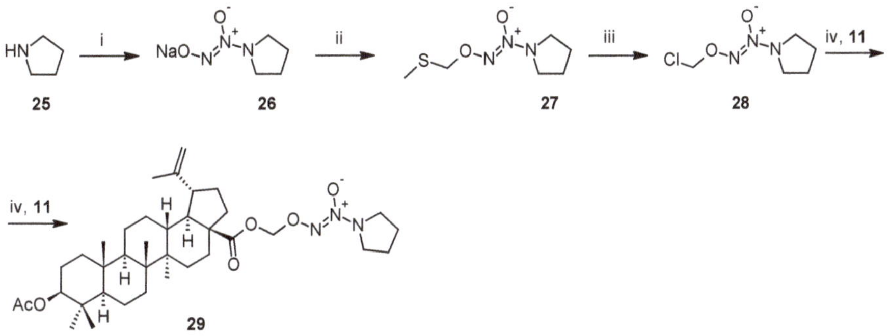

Scheme 5. Synthesis of diazen-1-ium-1,2-dioxolate nitric oxide derivative of betulinic acid (**1**). Legend: i: NO, MeONa, MeOH, nanosized TiO_2, ii: $ClCH_2SCH_3$, DMF, Na_2CO_3, iii: SO_2Cl_2, DCM, iv: **11**, Cs_2CO_3, DMF.

5.2. Antiviral Activity

5.2.1. Anti-HIV Activity

Bevirimat (**30**, Scheme 6), a derivative of **1**, is a very potent maturation inhibitor of HIV-1. It interferes with the processing of P25 (CA-SP1) to CA, leading to the accumulation of P25 and producing immature HIV-1 particles. In 2007, bevirimat (**30**) succeeded in the phases I and IIa of clinical trials [56]. However, subsequent studies resulted in observation that its effectiveness was reduced in the treatment of 40–50% of patients who carried resistant viruses associated with naturally occurring polymorphisms in the SP1 region of HIV-1 Gag [57]. This finding resulted in blocking further clinical trials with **30** to treat HIV infection.

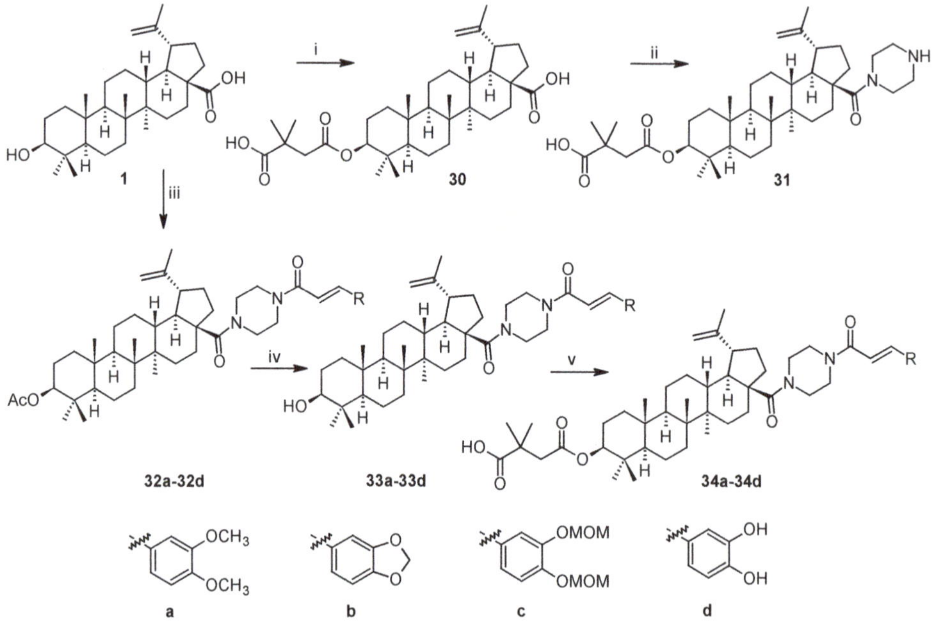

Scheme 6. Synthesis of bevirimat derivatives I. Legend: **i**: 2,2-dimethylsuccinic anhydride, DMAP, pyridine, microwave irradiation, **ii**: 1-Boc-piperazine, HOBt, EDCI, Et$_3$N, DCM, **iii**: oxalyl chloride, DCM, then a piperazine derivative, **iv**: 4 N NaOH, THF/MeOH, **v**: 2,2-dimethylsuccinic anhydride, DMAP, pyridine, microwave irradiation.

Modified bevirimat derivatives **31–34d** (Scheme 6) showed improved anti-HIV activity in comparison with **30** [58]. The procedures to synthesize **31**, **34a–34c**, and, subsequently, **34d** (Scheme 6) are described in the original literature [26]. The studied bevirimat analogs **31–34d** bear piperazine moiety in the molecule, which is quite often structural modification in drugs in general [59]. The so far made studies have resulted in a finding that piperazine can contribute to improving drug-like properties of the target compounds, namely bioavailability and metabolism [60,61]. Two nitrogen atoms located at the opposite positions in the piperazine molecule determine this compound as a convenient linker for merging desired structural motifs. Having different pharmacophores with different mechanisms of action in a single molecule may result in designing new compounds with enhanced efficacy [26]. Compound **34c** was found to be 3- to 50-times more potent than **30** against different types of the virus. A preliminary investigation of the mechanism of action indicated that **34c** is a HIV maturation inhibitor with good metabolic stability [26].

A series of C-3 phenyl- and heterocycle-substituted derivatives of the C-3 deoxybetulinic acid and C-3 deoxybetulin were also investigated for their potential as anti-HIV agents (Scheme 7) [62]. A 4-substituted benzoic acid moiety was identified as an advantageous replacement for the 3,3-dimethylsuccinate moiety present in **30**. The new analogs exhibit excellent in vitro antiviral activity against wild-type virus and a lower serum shift when compared with **30**. Compound **38** exhibits comparable cell culture potency toward wild-type virus as **30** (WT EC$_{50}$ = 16 nM for **38** compared to 10 nM for **30**). However, the potency of **38** was less affected by the presence of human serum, while the compound displayed a similar pharmacokinetic profile in rats to **30**. Thus, **38** represents a new starting point for designing the second generation of HIV maturation inhibitors.

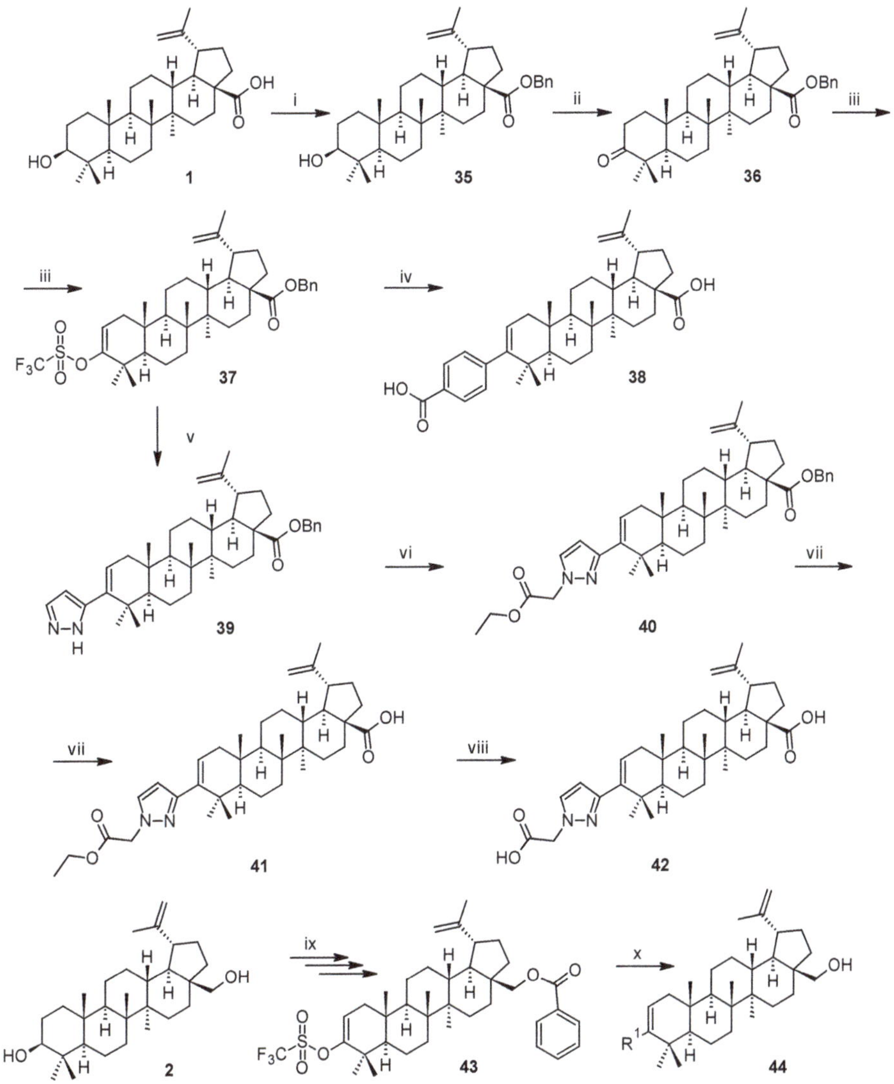

Scheme 7. Synthesis of C-3 deoxybetulinic acid derivatives I. Legend: **i**: K_2CO_3, BnBr, **ii**: PCC, CH_2Cl_2, **iii**: KHMDS, PhNTf$_2$, THF, **iv**: (a) R_1-B(OH)$_2$, Na_2CO_3, Pd(Ph$_3$P)$_4$, DME, H_2O, (b) Pd/C, H_2, EtOAc, MeOH, **v**: 1H-pyrazol-5-ylboronic acid, Pd(PPh$_3$)$_4$, $Na_2CO_3 \cdot H_2O$, dioxane, water, **vi**: BrCH$_2$COOEt, K_2CO_3, DMF, **vii**: TBDMSH, Pd(OAc)$_2$, TEA, DCE, **viii**: NaOH, 1,4-dioxane, **ix**: (a) (PhCO)$_2$O, DMAP, pyridine, (b) PCC, CH_2Cl_2, (c) KHMDS, PhNTf$_2$, THF, **x**: (a) R_1-B(OH)$_2$, Na_2CO_3, K_2CO_3 or K_3PO_4, Pd(PPh$_3$)$_4$, dioxane or DME, H_2O, (b) LiOH or NaOH, dioxane, H_2O, or (a) R_1-SnBu$_3$, LiCl, Pd(Ph$_3$P)$_4$, dioxane, (b) LiOH or NaOH, dioxane, H_2O.

The effect of a spacer between the phenyl ring and the carboxylic acid was investigated by introducing linkers with different lengths and degrees of flexibility designed to study a wide range of structural motifs [62]. As already stated above, **38** displayed sub-micromolar inhibitory activity. The effect of replacement of the phenyl ring with a series of five- and six-membered heterocycles was investigated as an additional structural modification resulted in designing another successful subseries of active compounds shown in the formula **42** and the general formula **44**. These compounds (**42** and **44**) also displayed sub-micromolar activity values accompanied by high therapeutic indices [62].

Recently, a new class of α-keto amides of **1** was developed and identified as HIV-1 maturation inhibitors [63]. The compound **53** was identified with IC_{50} values of 17 nM (HIV wild type), 23 nM (Q369H), 25 nM (V370A), and 8 nM (T371A), respectively, as a leading structure of this series of compounds (Scheme 8). When tested in a panel of 62 HIV-1 isolates covering a diversity of CA-SP1 genotypes including A, AE, B, C, and G using a PBMC-based assay, **53** was potent against a majority of isolates demonstrating an improvement over the first generation maturation inhibitor, bevirimat (**30**) [63]. The data also demonstrated that **53** shows a mechanism of action consistent with inhibition of the proteolytic cleavage of CA-SP1 [63].

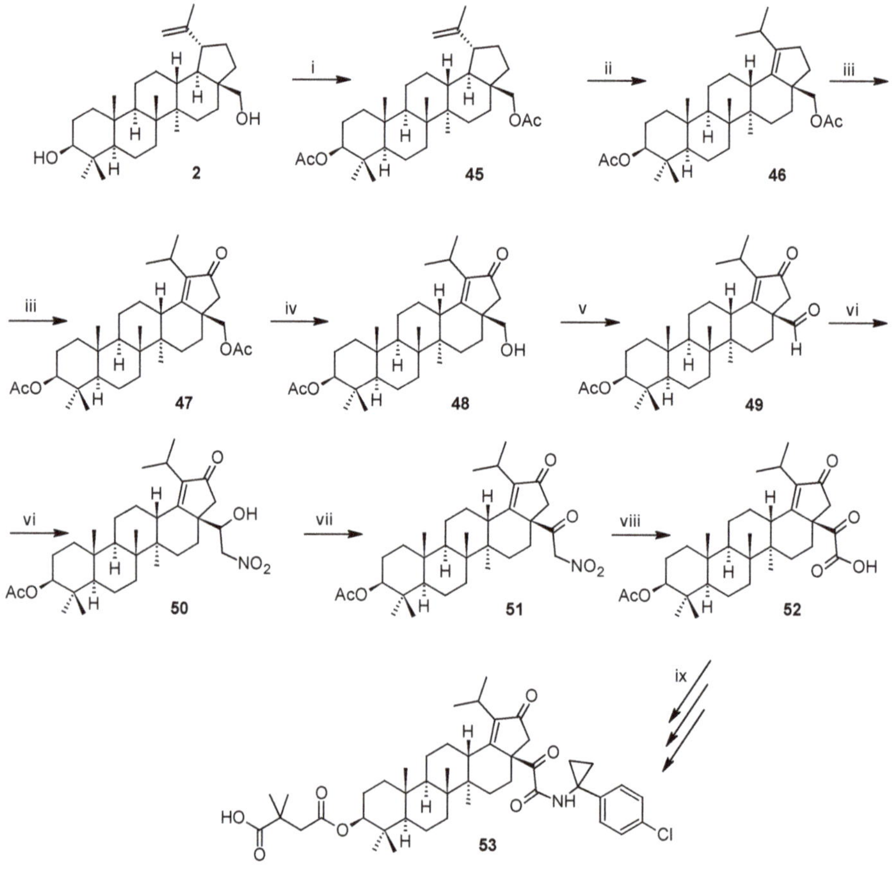

Scheme 8. Synthesis of bevirimat derivatives II. Legend: **i**: Ac$_2$O, toluene, **ii**: HBr/AcOH, AcOH, Table 2. **iii**: Na$_2$Cr$_2$O$_7$, NaOAc, toluene, AcOH, Ac$_2$O, **iv**: KOH, toluene, ethanol, **v**: PCC, silica gel, DCM, **vi**: CH$_3$NO$_2$, triethylamine, **vii**: DMP, DCM, **viii**: NaNO$_2$, AcOH, DMSO, **ix**: (**a**) oxalyl chloride, DCM, (**b**) 4-chloroaniline, TEA, DCM, (**c**) HCl (**g**) in dioxane, (**d**) 2,2-dimethylsuccinic anhydride, DMAP, pyridine.

Amides of the general formulae **54**–**57** (Figure 2), incorporating a basic side chain, provided excellent potency against both wild type and V370A viruses while maintaining a low human serum shift [64,65]. In addition, **54a** exhibited an EC_{50} = 31 nM against the ΔV370 Gag polymorphism. In turn, the structures **54** exhibited low oral exposure, attributed to a combination of poor solubility and low membrane permeability, precluding their further advancement [65]. To improve the disadvantages of the structure **54**, the structures **55** and **56** were developed. However, their antiviral activity did not increase in comparison with those of **54**. To proceed with improving the disadvantages of **54–56** again, the dibasic C-28 amine **57a** and monobasic **57b** were designed. Later on, an optimized structure **57c** showed improved antiviral profile in screening tests against three viruses [65]. However, **57c** became a subject of additional structural modification resulting finally in **57d**, which demonstrated targeted antiviral activity and improved oral exposure in rats. Installing the more basic amine closer to the lipophilic core had the effect of shielding the NH and may have a positive impact on the permeability properties of the molecule and, ultimately, on oral exposure [64,65].

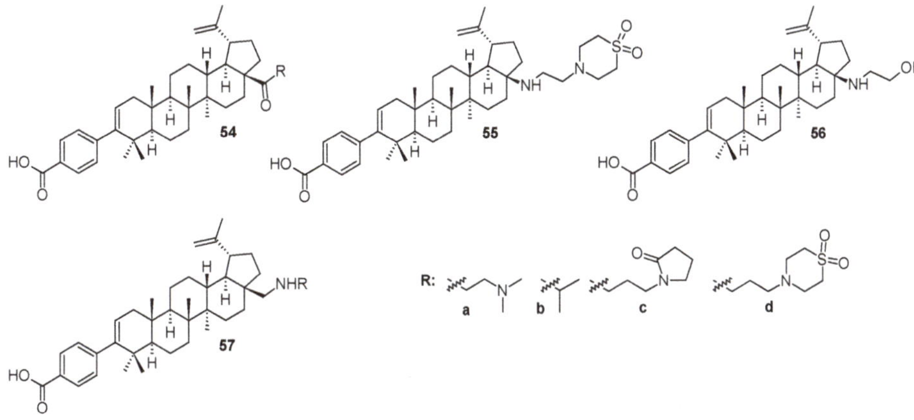

Figure 2. Structures of the HIV-1 maturation inhibitors based on betulinic acid (**1**).

A concise and scalable second-generation synthesis of HIV maturation inhibitor **64** (Scheme 9) was published in 2017 [66]. The synthesis was based on an oxidation strategy involving a CuI mediated aerobic oxidation of betulin (**2**), a highly selective PIFA mediated dehydrogenation of an oxime, and a subsequent Lossen rearrangement, which occurred through a unique reaction mechanism for the installation of the C17 amino functionality. The synthetic procedure consisted of seven steps with a 47% overall yield and it begins from the abundant and inexpensive natural product betulin (**2**) (Scheme 9) [66]. The target compound **64** became a potent HIV-1 inhibitor in cell culture that exhibited a broad spectrum of antiviral effects that encompass the V370A- and ΔV370-containing polymorphic viruses. In addition, **64** exhibited low serum binding, which resulted in the modest effect on potency in vitro, and in a preclinical suggestion of dosing once daily in humans. In the phase IIa of clinical trial, 10-days of monotherapy with two administered doses daily to the treatment-non-experienced subjects and treatment-experienced subjects, both infected with HIV-1 subtypes B or C, was generally safe and well-tolerated, and it demonstrated important reduction in viral RNA [65]. Compound **64** has currently been evaluated in the phase IIb of clinical study as a part of a treatment regimen with mechanistically different antiretroviral agents. The so far achieved values of practical importance with **64** in the HIV-1 treatment are WT EC_{50} = 1.9 nM (HIV-1 WT), and EC_{50} = 10.2 nM (HIV1 WT (HS)), which are very promising values.

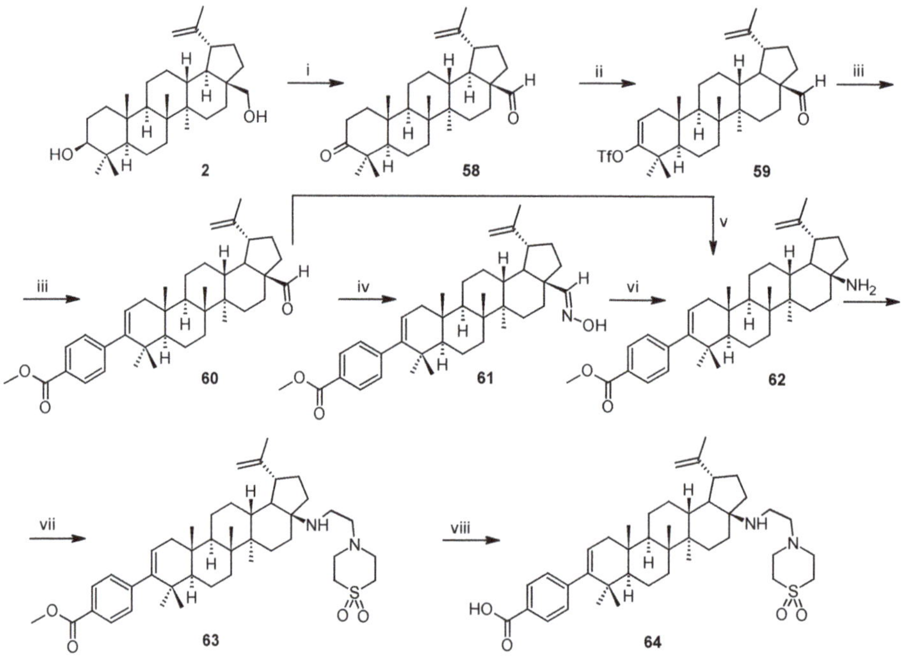

Scheme 9. Synthesis of C-3 deoxybetulinic acid derivatives II. Legend: **i**: Cu(CH$_3$CN)$_2$OTf, 4,4-dimethoxybipyridine, NMI, ABNO/TEMPO/O$_2$, **ii**: NaHDMS, PhNTf$_2$, **iii**: (**a**) Ar-B(OH)$_2$, PdCl$_2$Xantphos, **iv**: NH$_2$OH, **v**: (**a**) oxidation, (**b**) Curtius rearrangement, **vi**: (**a**) NH$_2$OH, (**b**) rearrangement, **vii**: thiomorpholine derivative, Ms$_2$O, EDIPA, reflux, **viii**: n-Bu$_4$NOH, aq. THF/CH$_3$CN.

5.2.2. Antiherpetic Activity

Herpes simplex virus types 1 and 2 (HSV-1 and HSV-2) represents other types of virus that may be treated by derivatives of betulinic acid. The developed ionic derivatives represent betulinic acid structural modification capable of improving water solubility and biological activity of the target structures **65a–66b** (Figure 3) [67]. The binding properties of these derivatives with respect to the human serum albumin (HSA) was examined and found to be similar to current anti-HIV drugs. These compounds (**65a, 65b, 66a,** and **66b**) inhibited HSV-2 replication at concentrations similar to those reported for acyclovir (IC$_{50}$ 0.1–10 µM) and with minimal cellular cytotoxicity. IC$_{50}$ values for antiviral activity against HSV-2 186 were 1.6, 0.9, 0.6, and 7.2 µM for the compounds **65a–66b**, respectively. However, these compounds did not inhibit HIV reverse transcriptase. Compound **66a** was the most active compound of this series in treating HSV-2.

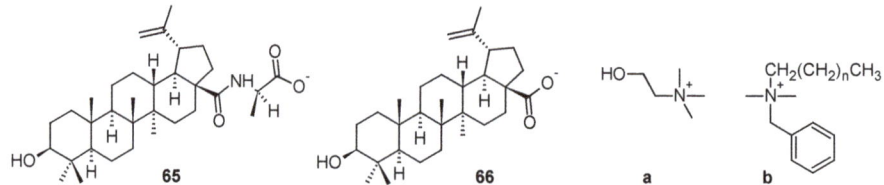

Figure 3. Ionic derivatives of betulinic acid (**1**) with antiviral activity against herpes simplex virus HSV-2.

Amide conjugates with four structural types of β-amino alcohols were synthesized from 2,3-seco-18αH-oleananoic and 2,3-seco-lupane C-3(C-28) mono- and dicarboxylic acids, in order to prepare novel agent for treating herpes simplex virus, types 1 and 2 (Scheme 10) [68]. Esters were prepared by a reaction of C(3)-hydroxy derivatives of A-seco-triterpenoids with dicarboxylic acid anhydrides. The antiviral activity of the synthesized compounds was studied against HSV-1. The most active amide (**68**) displayed antiviral effect EC_{50} = 5.7 μM). In contrast, the effect of **67** was about one order of magnitude lower than that of **68**.

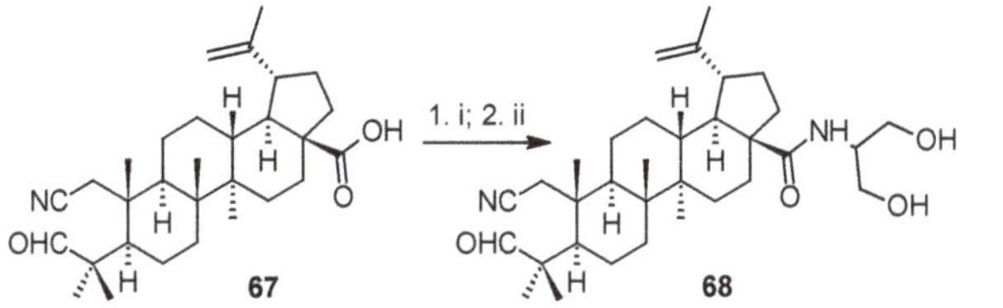

Scheme 10. Synthesis of C-3(C-28)-substituted 2,3-seco-triterpenoids. Legend: i: oxalyl chloride, DCM, ii: $(HOCH_2)_2CHNH_2$, DCM, triethyl amine.

To continue a search for agents active against herpes simplex virus, unsaturated acids, including difficultly accessible ceanothane-type ones, were prepared by the same authors, using alkaline hydrolysis of semi-synthetic triterpenoids with 1-cyano- or 3-methyl-1-cyanoalkene fragments in five-membered ring A (Scheme 11) [69]. Regioselective reduction of 1-cyano-19β,28-epoxy-2-nor-18αH-olean-1(3)-ene by DIBAL-H resulted in a synthesis of 2-aminomethyl-19β,28-epoxy-2-nor-18αH-olean-1(3)-ene. The synthesized triterpene derivatives possessed antiviral activity against HSV-1. Compound **70** (ET_{50} = 17.7 μM) was the most active compound of this small series, while **71** was less active.

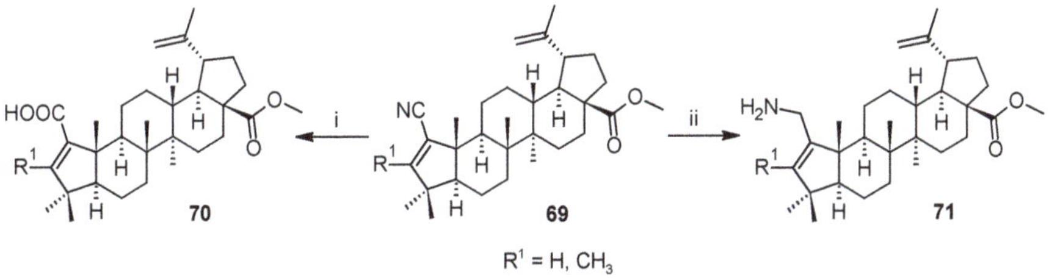

Scheme 11. Modification of the A-ring of betulinic acid. Legend: i: 15% KOH in ethanol, reflux, ii: DIBAL-H, THF, −78 °C.

5.2.3. Antihepatitic Activity

Hepatitis represents another type of virus affecting the human population. It has often been treated with oleanane derivatives (e.g., **73**, Scheme 12) [70], but betulinic acid has also been used for treating this disease [71]. Epstein-Barr virus (EBV), responsible for hepatitis and a number of other similar diseases, has widely infected more than 90% of human populations. Currently, there is no efficient way to remove the virus because the EBV carriers are usually in a latent stage that allows them to escape the immune system and common antiviral drugs. In the effort to develop an efficient strategy for the removal of the EBV virus, **1** has been shown to suppress EBV replication through SOD2 suppression slightly, with subsequent reactive oxygen species generation and DNA damage in EBV-transformed lymphoblastoid cell lines. Chidamide is a novel synthetic histone deacetylase inhibitor capable of switching EBV significantly from its latent stage to the lytic stage with increased gene expression of BZLF1 and BMRF1. However, it has a small effect on EBV replication due to the suppression effect of chidamide-mediated reactive oxygen species generation. Interestingly, a combination of **1** and chidamide synergistically inhibits EBV replication with ROS over-generation and subsequent DNA damage and apoptosis [72]. Overexpression of SOD2 diminishes this effect, while SOD2 knockdown mimics this effect. An in vivo tumor development study with the tail vein injection of EBV-transformed lymphoblastoid cell lines in nude mice proved that the combination of **1** with chidamide synergistically increased superoxide anion release in tumor tissues and suppressed EBV replication and tumor growth, prolonging significantly mouse survival. The combination of **1** with chidamide (Figure 4) could be an efficient strategy for clinical EBV removal. Unfortunately, the Chinese authors [72] did not mention clearly if they tested a mixture of **1** with chidamide that can possibly result in a formation of a pyridinium salt **74** or if they prepared the amide **75** and tested that chemical species. At the moment of finalizing this manuscript, no more details were accessible in the literature.

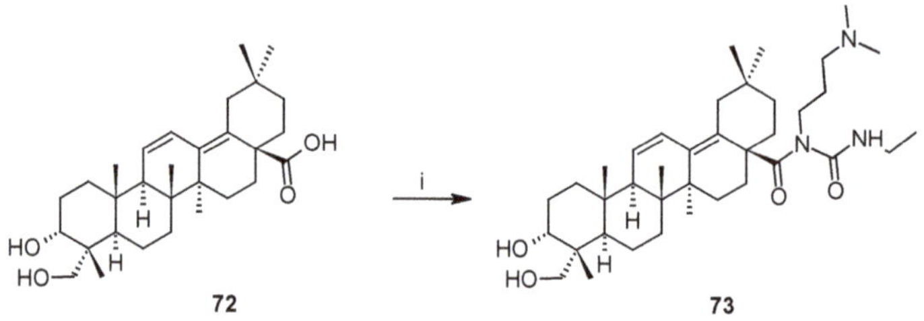

Scheme 12. Antihepatitic drug based on oleanolic acid. Legend: EDC·HCl, dichloromethane.

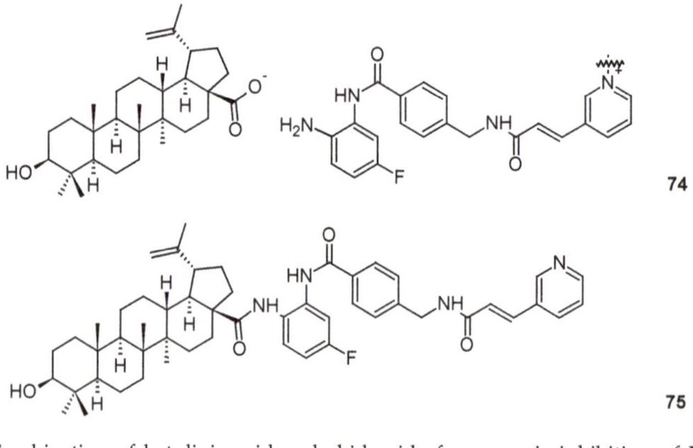

Figure 4. Combination of betulinic acid and chidamide for synergic inhibition of Epstein-Barr virus replication.

6. Conclusions

Betulinic acid (**1**) and its broad spectrum of derivatives demonstrated clearly their power in different areas of human diseases that can be successfully treated with those compounds based on a single plant product. In all areas of pharmacological applications of **1**, further development and challenge for designing novel structures are still needed. Regardless of the number of successfully active derivatives of **1**, there are still rare structures that have found their practical application in medicine. We believe that a synergic investigation of pharmacological effects and supramolecular characteristics may lead to a better understanding of the mechanism of action of those natural and semisynthetic compounds in at least several areas of treating fatal diseases mentioned in this text.

Supplementary Materials: The following are available online. Table S1: Physico-chemical and ADME parameters of the target compounds **15a–15c**, **20a–20c**, **22a–22c** and **24a–24c**.

Author Contributions: Literature search and partial draft preparation, U.B. and Z.Ö.; writing of the review article, further management and editing, Z.W.

Funding: We acknowledge funding from the MPO grants FV10599 and FV30300.

Conflicts of Interest: There are no conflicts to declare.

References

1. Ali-Seyed, M.; Jantan, I.; Vijayaraghavan, K.; Bukhari, S.N.A. Betulinic acid: Recent advances in chemical modifications, effective delivery, and molecular mechanisms of a promising anticancer therapy. *Chem. Biol. Drug Des.* **2016**, *87*, 517–536. [CrossRef] [PubMed]
2. Moghaddam, M.G.; Ahmad, J.B.H.; Samzadeh-Kermani, A. Biological activity of betulinic acid: A review. *Phamacol. Pharm.* **2012**, *3*, 119–123. [CrossRef]
3. Rios, J.L.; Manez, S. New pharmacological opportunities for betulinic acid. *Planta Med.* **2018**, *84*, 8–19. [CrossRef] [PubMed]
4. Retzlaff, F. Ueber Herba Gratiolae. *Arch. Pharm.* **1902**, *240*, 561–568. [CrossRef]
5. Šarek, J.; Kvasnica, M.; Vlk, M.; Urban, M.; Džubák, P.; Hajdúch, M. The potential of triterpenoids in the treatment of melanoma. In *Research on Melanoma—A Glimpse into Current Directions and Future Trends*; Murph, M., Ed.; InTech: Rijeka, Croatia, 2011; Chapter 7; pp. 125–158.
6. Cichewicz, R.H.; Kouzi, S.A. Chemistry, biological activity, and chemotherapeutic potential of betulinic acid for the prevention and treatment of cancer and HIV infection. *Med. Res. Rev.* **2004**, *24*, 90–114. [CrossRef]
7. Csuk, R.; Schmuck, K.; Schäfer, R. A practical synthesis of betulinic acid. *Tetrahedron Lett.* **2006**, *47*, 8769–8770. [CrossRef]
8. Krasutsky, P.A. Birch bark research and development. *Nat. Prod. Rep.* **2006**, *23*, 919–942. [CrossRef]
9. Sajfrtová, M.; Ličková, I.; Wimmerová, M.; Sovová, H.; Wimmer, Z. β-Sitosterol: Supercritical carbon dioxide extraction from sea buckthorn (*Hippophae rhamnoides* L.) seeds. *Int. J. Mol. Sci.* **2010**, *11*, 1842–1850. [CrossRef]
10. Lepojevic, I.; Lepojevic, Z.; Pavlic, B.; Ristic, M.; Zekovic, Z. Solid-liquid and high-pressure (liquid and supercritical carbondioxide) extraction of *Echinacea purpurea* L. *J. Supercrit. Fluids* **2017**, *119*, 159–168. [CrossRef]
11. Trumbull, E.R.; Bianchi, E.; Eckert, D.J.; Wiedhopf, R.M.; Cole, J.R. Tumor inhibitory agents from *Vauquelinia-Corymbosa* (Rosaceae). *J. Pharm. Sci.* **1976**, *65*, 1407–1408. [CrossRef]
12. Pisha, E.; Chai, H.; Lee, I.-S.; Chagwedera, T.E.; Farnsworth, N.R.; Cordell, G.A.; Beecher, C.W.W.; Fong, H.H.S.; Kinghorn, A.D.; Brown, D.M.; et al. Discovery of betulinic acid as a selective inhibitor of human-melanoma that functions by induction of apoptosis. *Nat. Med.* **1995**, *1*, 1046–1051. [CrossRef] [PubMed]
13. Rajendran, P.; Jaggi, M.; Singh, M.K.; Mukherjee, R.; Burman, A.C. Pharmacological evaluation of C-3 modified betulinic acid derivatives with potent anticancer activity. *Investig. New Drugs* **2008**, *26*, 25–34. [CrossRef] [PubMed]
14. Zhang, X.; Hu, J.; Chen, Y. Betulinic acid and the pharmacological effects of tumor suppression (review). *Mol. Med. Rep.* **2016**, *14*, 4489–4495. [CrossRef] [PubMed]
15. Zhang, D.M.; Xu, H.G.; Wang, L.; Li, Y.J.; Sun, P.H.; Wu, X.M.; Wang, G.J.; Chen, W.M.; Ye, W.C. Betulinic acid and its derivatives as potential antitumor agents. *Med. Res. Rev.* **2015**, *35*, 1127–1155. [CrossRef] [PubMed]
16. Gheorgheosu, D.; Duicu, O.; Dehelean, C.; Soica, C.; Muntean, D. Betulinic acid as a potent and complex antitumor phytochemical: A minireview. *Anticancer Agents Med. Chem.* **2014**, *14*, 936–945. [CrossRef] [PubMed]
17. Selzer, E.; Pimentel, E.; Wacheck, W.; Schlegel, W.; Pehamberger, H.; Jansen, B.; Kodym, R. Effects of betulinic acid alone and in combination with irradiation in human melanoma cells. *J. Investig. Dermatol.* **2000**, *114*, 935–940. [CrossRef] [PubMed]
18. Selzer, E.; Thallinger, C.; Hoeller, C.; Oberkleiner, P.; Wacheck, W.; Pehamberger, H.; Jansen, B. Betulinic acid-induced Mcl-1 expression in human melanoma-mode of action and functional significance. *Mol. Med.* **2002**, *8*, 877–884. [CrossRef] [PubMed]
19. Keller, P.W.; Adamson, C.S.; Heymann, J.B.; Freed, E.O.; Steven, A.C. HIV-1 maturation inhibitor bevirimat stabilizes the immature Gag lattice. *J. Virol.* **2011**, *85*, 1420–1428. [CrossRef]

20. Suh, N.; Wang, Y.; Honda, T.; Gribble, G.W.; Dmitrovsky, E.; Hickey, W.F.; Maue, R.A.; Place, A.E.; Porter, D.M.; Spinella, M.J.; et al. A novel synthetic oleanane triterpenoid, 2-cyano-3,12-dioxoolean-1,9-dien-28-oic acid, with potent differentiating, antiproliferative, and antiinflammatory activity. *Cancer Res.* **1999**, *59*, 336–341. [PubMed]
21. Willmann, M.; Wacheck, W.; Buckley, J.; Nagy, K.; Thalhammer, J.; Paschke, R.; Triche, T.; Jansen, B.; Selzer, E. Characterization of NVX-207, a novel betulinic acidderived anti-cancer compound. *Eur. J. Clin. Investig.* **2009**, 384–394. [CrossRef]
22. Dash, S.K.; Chattopadhyay, S.; Dash, S.S.; Tripathy, S.; Das, B.; Mahapatra, S.K.; Bag, B.G.; Karmakar, P.; Roy, S. Self-assembled nano fibers of betulinic acid: A selective inducer for ROS/TNF-alpha pathway mediated leukemic cell death. *Bioorg. Chem.* **2015**, *63*, 85–100. [CrossRef] [PubMed]
23. Yogeeswari, P.; Sriram, D. Betulinic acid and its derivatives: A review on their biological properties. *Curr. Med. Chem.* **2005**, *12*, 657–666. [CrossRef] [PubMed]
24. Aiken, C.; Chen, C.H. Betulinic acid derivatives as HIV-1 antivirals. *Trends Mol. Med.* **2005**, *11*, 31–36. [CrossRef] [PubMed]
25. Gallo, R.; Sarin, P.; Gelmann, E.; Robert-Guroff, M.; Richardson, E.; Kalyanaraman, V.; Mann, D.; Sidhu, G.; Stahl, R.; Zolla-Pazner, S.; et al. Isolation of human T-cell leukemia virus in acquired immune deficiency syndrome (AIDS). *Science* **1983**, *220*, 865–867. [CrossRef] [PubMed]
26. Zhao, Y.; Gu, Q.; Morris-Natschke, S.L.; Chen, C.-H.; Lee, K.-H. Incorporation of privileged structures into bevirimat can improve activity against wild-type and bevirimat-resistant HIV-1. *J. Med. Chem.* **2016**, *59*, 9262–9268. [CrossRef]
27. Zhan, P.; Pannecouque, C.; De Clercq, E.; Liu, X. Anti-HIV drug discovery and development: Current innovations and future trends. *J. Med. Chem.* **2015**, *59*, 2849–2878. [CrossRef]
28. Fujioka, T.; Kashiwada, Y.; Kilkuskie, R.E.; Cosentino, L.M.; Ballas, L.M.; Jiang, J.B.; Janzen, W.P.; Chen, I.-S.; Lee, K.-H. Anti-AIDS agents, 11. Betulinic acid and platanic acid as anti-HIV principles from *Syzigium claviflorum*, and the anti-HIV activity of structurally related triterpenoids. *J. Nat. Prod.* **1994**, *57*, 243–247. [CrossRef]
29. Heidary, N.M.; Laszczyk-Lauer, M.N.; Reichling, J.; Schnitzler, P. Pentacyclic triterpenes in birch bark extract inhibit early step of herpes simplex virus type 1 replication. *Phytomedicine* **2014**, *21*, 1273–1280. [CrossRef]
30. Yao, D.; Li, H.; Gou, Y.; Zhang, H.; Vlessidis, A.G.; Zhou, H.; Evmiridis, N.P.; Liu, Z. Betulinic acid-mediated inhibitory effect on hepatitis B virus by suppression of manganese superoxide dismutase expression. *FEBS J.* **2009**, *276*, 2599–2614. [CrossRef]
31. Huguet, A.; Recio, M.C.; Máñez, S.; Giner, R.; Ríos, J.L. Effect of triterpenoids on the inflammation induced by protein kinase C activators, neuronally acting irritants and other agents. *Eur. J. Pharmacol.* **2000**, *410*, 69–81. [CrossRef]
32. Gautam, R.; Jachak, S.M. Recent developments in anti-inflammatory natural products. *Med. Res. Rev.* **2009**, *29*, 767–820. [CrossRef] [PubMed]
33. Silva, F.S.; Oliveira, P.J.; Duarte, M.F. Oleanolic, ursolic, and betulinic acids as food supplements or pharmaceutical agents for type 2 diabetes: Promise or illusion? *J. Agric. Food Chem.* **2016**, *64*, 2991–3008. [CrossRef] [PubMed]
34. Thomas, C.; Gioiello, A.; Noriega, L.; Strehle, A.; Oury, J.; Rizzo, G.; Macchiarulo, A.; Yamamoto, H.; Mataki, C.; Pruzanski, M.; et al. TGR5-mediated bile acid sensing controls glucose homeostasis. *Cell Metabol.* **2009**, *10*, 167–177. [CrossRef] [PubMed]
35. Quan, H.Y.; Kim, D.Y.; Kim, S.J.; Jo, H.K.; Kim, G.W.; Chung, S.H. Betulinic acid alleviates non-alcoholic fatty liver by inhibiting SREBP1 activity via the AMPK-mTOR-SREBP signaling pathway. *Biochem. Pharmacol.* **2013**, *85*, 1330–1340. [CrossRef] [PubMed]
36. Bag, B.G.; Dash, S.S. First self-assembly study of betulinic acid, a renewable nano-sized, 6-6-6-6-5 pentacyclic monohydroxy triterpenic acid. *Nanoscale* **2011**, *3*, 4564–4566. [CrossRef] [PubMed]
37. Bag, B.G.; Majumdar, R. Self-assembly of renewable nano-sized triterpenoids. *Chem. Rec.* **2017**, *17*, 841–873. [CrossRef] [PubMed]
38. Ali, A.; Kamra, M.; Bhan, A.; Mandal, S.S.; Bhattacharya, S. New Fe(III) and Co(II) salen complexes with pendant distamycins: Selective targeting of cancer cells by DNA damage and mitochondrial pathways. *Dalton Trans.* **2016**, *45*, 9345–9353. [CrossRef]

39. Cragg, G.M.; Grothaus, P.G.; Newman, D.J. New horizons for old drugs and drug leads. *J. Nat. Prod.* **2014**, *77*, 703–723. [CrossRef]
40. Zhou, M.; Zhang, R.-H.; Wang, M.; Xu, G.-B.; Liao, S.-G. Prodrugs of triterpenoids and their derivatives. *Eur. J. Med. Chem.* **2017**, *131*, 222–236. [CrossRef]
41. Csuk, R. Betulinic acid and its derivatives: A patent review (2008–2013). *Expert Opin. Ther. Pat.* **2014**, *24*, 913–923. [CrossRef]
42. Konysheva, A.V.; Nebogatikov, V.O.; Tolmacheva, I.A.; Dmitriev, M.V.; Grishko, V.V. Synthesis of cytotoxically active derivatives based on alkylated 2,3-seco-triterpenoids. *Eur. J. Med. Chem.* **2017**, *140*, 74–83. [CrossRef] [PubMed]
43. Grishko, V.V.; Tolmacheva, I.A.; Nebogatikov, V.O.; Galaiko, N.V.; Nazarov, A.V.; Dmitriev, M.V.; Ivshina, I.B. Preparation of novel ring-A fused azole derivatives of betulin and evaluation of their cytotoxicity. *Eur. J. Med. Chem.* **2017**, *125*, 629–639. [CrossRef] [PubMed]
44. Eignerová, B.; Tichý, M.; Krasulová, J.; Kvasnica, M.; Rárová, L.; Christová, R.; Urban, M.; Bednarczyk-Cwynar, B.; Hajdúch, M. Synthesis and antiproliferative properties of new hydrophilic esters of triterpenic acids. *Eur. J. Med. Chem.* **2017**, *140*, 403–420. [CrossRef] [PubMed]
45. Bildziukevich, U.; Vida, N.; Rárová, L.; Kolář, M.; Šaman, D.; Havlíček, L.; Drašar, P.; Wimmer, Z. Polyamine derivatives of betulinic acid and β-sitosterol: A comparative investigation. *Steroids* **2015**, *100*, 27–35. [CrossRef] [PubMed]
46. Bildziukevich, U.; Kaletová, E.; Šaman, D.; Sievänan, E.; Kolehmainen, E.T.; Šlouf, M.; Wimmer, Z. Spectral and microscopic study of self-assembly of novel cationic spermine amides of betulinic acid. *Steroids* **2017**, *117*, 90–96. [CrossRef] [PubMed]
47. Özdemir, Z.; Bildziukevich, U.; Šaman, D.; Havlíček, L.; Rárová, L.; Navrátilová, L.; Wimmer, Z. Amphiphilic derivatives of (3β,17β)-3-hydroxyandrost-5-ene-17-carboxylic acid. *Steroids* **2017**, *128*, 58–67. [CrossRef] [PubMed]
48. Vashist, A.; Kaushik, A.; Vashist, A.; Bala, J.; Nikkhah-Moshaie, R.; Sagar, V.; Nair, M. Nanogels as potential drug nanocarriers for CNS drug delivery. *Drug Discov. Today* **2018**, *23*, 1436–1443. [CrossRef] [PubMed]
49. Šaman, D.; Kolehmainen, E.T. Studies on supramolecular gel formation using DOSY NMR. *Magn. Reson. Chem.* **2015**, *53*, 256–260.
50. Noponen, V.; Nonappa; Lahtinen, M.; Valkonen, A.; Salo, H.; Kolehmainen, E.; Sievänen, E. Bile acid–amino acid ester conjugates: Gelation, structural properties, and thermoreversible solid to solid phase transition. *Soft Matter* **2010**, *6*, 3789–3796. [CrossRef]
51. Svobodová, H.; Nonappa; Wimmer, Z.; Kolehmainen, E. Design, synthesis and stimuli responsive gelation of novel stigmasterol–amino acid conjugates. *J. Colloid Interface Sci.* **2011**, *361*, 587–593. [CrossRef] [PubMed]
52. Hirst, A.R.; Coates, I.A.; Boucheteau, T.R.; Miravet, J.F.; Escuder, B.; Castelletto, V.; Hamley, I.W.; Smith, D.K. Low-molecular-weight gelators: Elucidating the principles of gelation based on gelator solubility and a cooperative self-assembly model. *J. Am. Chem. Soc.* **2008**, *130*, 9113–9121. [CrossRef] [PubMed]
53. Bildziukevich, U.; Rárová, L.; Šaman, D.; Wimmer, Z. Picolyl amides of betulinic acid as antitumor agents causing tumor cell apoptosis. *Eur. J. Med. Chem.* **2018**, *145*, 41–50. [CrossRef] [PubMed]
54. Bildziukevich, U.; Rárová, L.; Šaman, D.; Havlíček, L.; Drašar, P.; Wimmer, Z. Amides derived from heteroaromatic amines and selected steryl hemiesters. *Steroids* **2013**, *78*, 1347–1352. [CrossRef] [PubMed]
55. Zhang, L.; Hou, S.; Li, B.; Pan, J.; Jiang, L.; Zhou, G.; Gu, H.; Zhao, C.; Lu, H.; Ma, F. Combination of betulinic acid with diazen-1-ium-1,2-diolate nitric oxide moiety donating a novel anticancer candidate. *OncoTargets Ther.* **2018**, *11*, 361–373. [CrossRef] [PubMed]
56. Smith, P.F.; Ogundele, A.; Forrest, A.; Wilton, J.; Salzwedel, K.; Doto, J.; Allaway, G.P.; Martin, D.E. Phase I and II study of safety, virologic effect, and pharmacokinetics/pharmacodynamics of single-dose 3-O-(3′,3′-dimethylsuccinyl) betulinic acid (bevirimat) against human immunodeficiency virus infection. *Antimicrob. Agents Chemother.* **2007**, *51*, 3574–3581. [CrossRef] [PubMed]
57. Margot, N.A.; Gibbs, C.S.; Miller, M.D. Phenotypic susceptibility to bevirimat in isolates from HIV-1-infected patients without prior exposure to bevirimat. *Antimicrob. Agents Chemother.* **2010**, *54*, 2345–2353. [CrossRef] [PubMed]
58. Qian, K.; Bori, I.D.; Chen, C.-H.; Huang, L.; Lee, K.-H. Anti-AIDS agents 90. Novel C-28 modified bevirimat analogues as potent HIV maturation inhibitors. *J. Med. Chem.* **2012**, *55*, 8128–8136. [CrossRef] [PubMed]

59. Patel, R.; Park, S.W. An evolving role of piperazine moieties in drug design and discovery. *Mini-Rev. Med. Chem.* **2013**, *13*, 1579–1601. [CrossRef]
60. Tagat, J.R.; McCombie, S.W.; Nazareno, D.; Labroli, M.A.; Xiao, Y.; Steensma, R.W.; Strizki, J.M.; Baroudy, B.M.; Cox, K.; Lachowicz, J.; et al. Piperazine-based CCR5 antagonists as HIV-1 inhibitors. IV. Discovery of 1-[(4,6-dimethyl-5-pyrimidinyl)carbonyl]-4-[4-{2-methoxy-1(R)-4-(trifluoromethyl)-phenyl}ethyl-3(S)-methyl-1-piperazinyl]-4-methylpiperidine (Sch-417690/Sch-D), a potent, highly selective, and orally bioavailable CCR5 antagonist. *J. Med. Chem.* **2004**, *47*, 2405–2408.
61. Thompson, T.N. Optimization of metabolic stability as a goal of modern drug design. *Med. Res. Rev.* **2001**, *21*, 412–449. [CrossRef]
62. Liu, Z.; Swidorski, J.J.; Nowicka-Sans, B.; Terry, B.; Protack, T.; Lin, Z.; Samanta, H.; Zhang, S.; Li, Z.; Parker, D.D.; et al. C-3 benzoic acid derivatives of C-3 deoxybetulinic acid and deoxybetulin as HIV-1 maturation inhibitors. *Bioorg. Med. Chem.* **2016**, *24*, 1757–1770. [CrossRef] [PubMed]
63. Tang, J.; Jones, S.A.; Jeffrey, J.L.; Miranda, S.R.; Galardi, C.M.; Irlbeck, D.M.; Brown, K.W.; McDanal, C.B.; Johns, B.A. Discovery of a novel and potent class of anti-HIV-1 maturation inhibitors with improved virology profile against gag polymorphisms. *Bioorg. Med. Chem. Lett.* **2017**, *27*, 2689–2694. [CrossRef] [PubMed]
64. Swidorski, J.J.; Liu, Z.; Sit, S.-Y.; Chen, J.; Chen, Y.; Sin, N.; Venables, B.L.; Parker, D.D.; Nowicka-Sans, B.; Terry, B.J.; et al. Inhibitors of HIV-1 maturation: Development of structure–activity relationship for C-28 amides based on C-3 benzoic acid-modified triterpenoids. *Bioorg. Med. Chem. Lett.* **2016**, *26*, 1925–1930. [CrossRef] [PubMed]
65. Regueiro-Ren, A.; Liu, Z.; Chen, Y.; Sin, N.; Sit, S.-Y.; Swidorski, J.J.; Chen, J.; Venables, B.L.; Zhu, J.; Nowicka-Sans, B.; et al. Discovery of BMS-955176, a second generation HIV-1 maturation inhibitor with broad spectrum antiviral activity. *ACS Med. Chem. Lett.* **2016**, *7*, 568–572. [CrossRef] [PubMed]
66. Ortiz, A.; Soumeillant, M.; Savage, S.A.; Strotman, N.A.; Haley, M.; Benkovics, T.; Nye, J.; Xu, Z.; Tan, Y.; Ayers, S.; et al. Synthesis of HIV-Maturation Inhibitor BMS-955176 from betulin by an enabling oxidation strategy. *J. Org. Chem.* **2017**, *82*, 4958–4963. [CrossRef]
67. Visalli, R.J.; Ziobrowski, H.; Badri, K.R.; He, J.J.; Zhang, X.; Arumugam, S.R.; Zhao, H. Ionic derivatives of betulinic acid exhibit antiviral activity against herpes simplex virus type-2 (HSV-2), but not HIV-1 reverse transcriptase. *Bioorg. Med. Chem. Lett.* **2015**, *25*, 3168–3171. [CrossRef] [PubMed]
68. Tolmacheva, I.A.; Igosheva, E.V.; Savinova, O.V.; Boreko, E.I.; Grishko, V.V. Synthesis and antiviral activity of C-3(C-28)-substituted 2,3-seco-triterpenoids. *Chem. Nat. Comp.* **2014**, *49*, 1050–1058. [CrossRef]
69. Konysheva, A.V.; Tolmacheva, I.A.; Savinova, O.V.; Boreko, E.I.; Grishko, V.V. Regioselective transformation of the cyano group of triterpene α,β-alkenenitriles. *Chem. Nat. Comp.* **2017**, *53*, 687–690. [CrossRef]
70. Chen, S.-Y.; Wang, C.-M.; Cheng, H.-L.; Chen, H.-J.; Hsu, Y.-M.; Lin, Y.-C.; Chou, C.-H. Biological activity of oleanane triterpene derivatives obtained by chemical derivatization. *Molecules* **2013**, *18*, 13003–13019. [CrossRef]
71. Li, N.; Zhou, Z.-S.; Shen, Y.; Xu, J.; Miao, H.-H.; Xiong, Y.; Xu, F.; Li, B.-L.; Luo, J.; Song, B.-L. Inhibition of the sterol regulatory element-binding protein pathway suppresses hepatocellular carcinoma by repressing inflammation in mice. *Hepatology* **2017**, *65*, 1936–1947. [CrossRef]
72. Yu, H.; Zhang, H.; Chu, Z.; Ruan, Q.; Chen, X.; Kong, D.; Huang, X.; Li, H.; Tang, H.; Wu, H.; et al. Combination of betulinic acid and chidamide synergistically inhibits Epstein-Barr virus replication through over-generation of reactive oxygen species. *Oncotarget* **2017**, *8*, 61646–61661. [CrossRef] [PubMed]

Sample Availability: Only samples of the compounds prepared by the authors of this review article are available from the authors.

© 2019 by the authors. Licensee MDPI, Basel, Switzerland. This article is an open access article distributed under the terms and conditions of the Creative Commons Attribution (CC BY) license (http://creativecommons.org/licenses/by/4.0/).

MDPI
St. Alban-Anlage 66
4052 Basel
Switzerland
Tel. +41 61 683 77 34
Fax +41 61 302 89 18
www.mdpi.com

Molecules Editorial Office
E-mail: molecules@mdpi.com
www.mdpi.com/journal/molecules

www.ingramcontent.com/pod-product-compliance
Lightning Source LLC
LaVergne TN
LVHW070429100526
838202LV00014B/1554